ADVANCES IN THE BIOSCIENCES

Volume 79

CONTROL OF BREATHING AND DYSPNEA

ADVANCES IN THE BIOSCIENCES

Latest volumes in the series:

CONTROL OF BREATHING AND DYSPNEA

An International Symposium held in Sendai, Japan,
27 & 28 October 1989

Editors:

T. TAKISHIMA

Tohoku University, Sendai, Japan

N.S. CHERNIACK

Case Western Reserve University, Ohio, USA

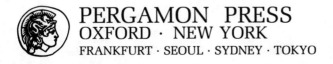

PERGAMON PRESS
OXFORD · NEW YORK
FRANKFURT · SEOUL · SYDNEY · TOKYO

U.K.	Pergamon Press plc, Headington Hill Hall, Oxford OX3 0BW, England
U.S.A	Pergamon Press Inc., Maxwell House, Fairview Park, Elmsford, New York 10523, U.S.A.
GERMANY	Pergamon Press GmbH, Hammerweg 6, D-6242 Kronberg, Germany
KOREA	Pergamon Press Korea, KPO Box 315, Seoul 110-603, Korea
AUSTRALIA	Pergamon Press Australia Pty Ltd, P.O. Box 544, Potts Point, N.S.W. 2011, Australia
JAPAN	Pergamon Press, 5th Floor, Matsuoka Central Building, 1-7-1 Nishishinjuku, Shinjuku-ku, Tokyo 160, Japan

Copyright © 1991 Pergamon Press plc

First edition 1991

ISBN: 0–08–040786–2

ISSN: 0065–3446

In order to make this volume available as economically as possible the author's typescripts have been reproduced in their original forms. This method unfortunately has its typographical limitations but it is hoped that they in no way distract the reader.

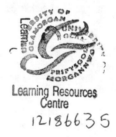
Printed in Great Britain by BPCC Wheatons Ltd, Exeter

Contents

Abnormality of Respiratory Control

Respiratory Muscles and Dyspnea

Contributors

Abe, T., Department of Medicine, School of Medicine, Kitasato University, Sagamihara, Kanagawa 228, Japan

Adachi, M., Medical Institute of Bioregulation, Kyushu University, Beppu 874, Japan

Akiyama, Y., First Department of Medicine, School of Medicine, Hokkaido University, Sapporo 060, Japan

Altose, M.D., Department of Medicine, Case Western Reserve University, Cleveland, OH 44106, USA

Aoki, M., Department of Physiology, Sapporo Medical College, Sapporo 060, Japan

Arata, A., Department of Physiology, Showa University School of Medicine, Tokyo 142, Japan

Arita, H., Institute of Basic Medical Sciences, University of Tsukuba, Tsukuba 305, Japan

Asakura, K., Department of Otolaryngology, Sapporo Medical College, Sapporo 060, Japan

Bruce, E.N., Departments of Medicine and Biomedical Engineering, Case Western Reserve University, Cleveland, OH 44106, USA

Cerretelli, P., Department of Physiology, Faculty of Medicine, University of Geneve, Geneve, Switzerland

Cherniack, N.S., Department of Medicine, Case Western Reserve University, Cleveland, OH 44106, USA

Chin, K., Department of Clinical Pulmonary Physiology, Chest Disease Research Institute, Kyoto University, Kyoto 606, Japan

Chonan, T., First Department of Internal Medicine, Tohoku University School of Medicine, Sendai 980, Japan

Chou, W., Division of Pulmonary and Critical Care Medicine, Department of Medicine, and Department of Pharmacology, University of Medicine and Dentistry of New Jersey-Robert Wood Johnson Medical School, New Brunswick, NJ, USA

Dick, T.E., Department of Medicine, Case Western Reserve University, Cleveland, OH 44106, USA

Edelman, N.H., Division of Pulmonary and Critical Care Medicine, Department of Medicine, and Department of Pharmacology, University of Medicine and Dentistry of New Jersey-Robert Wood Johnson Medical School, New Brunswick, NJ, USA

Eguchi, K., Department of Nervous and Sensory Functions, Research Institute of Environmental Medicine, Nagoya University, Nagoya 464-01, Japan

Euler, C. von, Nobel Institute for Neurophysiology, Karolinska Institutet, Stockholm, Sweden

Fujieda, K., Department of Respiratory Diseases, Tokyo Teishin Hospital, Tokyo 102, Japan

Fujimoto, S., First Department of Internal Medicine, Osaka City University Medical School, Osaka 545, Japan

Fujimura, S., Department of Surgery, Research Institute for Chest Disease and Cancer, Tohoku University, Sendai 980, Japan

Fukuba, Y., Dept. Biometrics, Res. Inst. Nuclear Med. Biol., Hiroshima University, Hiroshima 730, Japan

Fukuda, Y., Department of Physiology II, School of Medicine, Chiba University, Chiba 280, Japan

Fukunaga, T., Division of Respiratory Diseases, Department of Internal Medicine, Kanazawa Medical University, Ishikawa 920-02, Japan

Gandevia, S.C., Department of Clinical Neurophysiology, Institute of Neurological Sciences, The Prince Henry and Prince of Wales Hospitals and School of Medicine, University of New South Wales, Sydney, N.S.W. 2036, Australia

Geller, H.M., Division of Pulmonary and Critical Care Medicine, Department of Medicine, and Department of Pharmacology, University of Medicine and Dentistry of New Jersey-Robert Wood Johnson Medical School, New Brunswick, NJ, USA

Gleeson, K., Division of Pulmonary/Critical Care Medicine, Pennsylvania State University College of Medicine, Hershey, PA, USA

xiii

Gonsalves, S., Division of Pulmonary and Critical Care Medicine, Department of Medicine, and Department of Pharmacology, University of Medicine and Dentistry of New Jersey-Robert Wood Johnson Medical School, New Brunswick, NJ, USA

Haga, T., Tokyo National Chest Hospital, Tokyo 204, Japan

Haji, A., Department of Pharmacology, Faculty of Medicine, Toyama Medical and Pharmaceutical University, Toyama 930-01, Japan

Harasawa, M., Department of Respiratory Diseases, Tokyo Teishin Hospital, Tokyo 102, Japan

Hazama, H., Department of Neuropsychiatry, Tottori University School of Medicine, Yonago 683, Japan

Hida, W., First Department of Internal Medicine, Tohoku University School of Medicine, Sendai 980, Japan

Hiraga, T., First Department of Medicine, School of Medicine, Hokkaido University, Sapporo 060, Japan

Hirano, T., Department of Nervous and Sensory Functions, Research Institute of Environmental Medicine, Nagoya University, Nagoya 464-01, Japan

Hirayama, H., Department of Cardiovascular Medicine, Hokkaido University School of Medicine, Sapporo 060, Japan

Homma, I., Department of Physiology, Showa University School of Medicine, Tokyo 142, Japan

Honda, K., Department of Neuropsychiatry, Fukushima Medical College, Fukushima 960, Japan

Honda, Y., Department of Physiology, School of Medicine, Chiba University, Chiba 280, Japan

Horikoshi, R., Department of Neuropsychiatry, Fukushima Medical College, Fukushima 960, Japan

Hua, S., Department of Medicine, School of Medicine, Kitasato University, Sagamihara, Kanagawa 228, Japan

Huang, J., Division of Respiratory Diseases, Department of Internal Medicine, Kanazawa Medical University School of Medicine, Ishikawa 920-02, Japan

Hukuhara,T., Jr., Department of Pharmacology II, The Jikei University School of Medicine, Tokyo 105, Japan

Ichimaru, Y., Medical Institute of Bioregulation, Kyushu University, Beppu 874, Japan

Ide, T., Department of Anesthesiology, Chiba University School of Medicine and the Department of Anesthesiology, National Cancer Center Hospital, Chiba 280, Japan

Inoue, Y., Department of Neuropsychiatry, Tottori University School of Medicine, Yonago 683, Japan

Ishida, K., Research Center of Health, Physical Fitness and Sports Nagoya University, Nagoya 464-01, Japan

Ishii, T., First Department of Internal Medicine, Yokohama City University School of Medicine, Yokohama 232, Japan

Isono, S., Department of Anesthesiology, Chiba University School of Medicine and the Department of Anesthesiology, National Cancer Center Hospital, Chiba 280, Japan

Itasaka, Y., Department of Otolaryngology, Akita University Hospital, Akita 010, Japan

Iwanaga, K., Saga Res. Inst., Otsuka Pharmaceutical Ltd., Japan

Iwase, N., First Department of Internal Medicine, Tohoku University School of Medicine, Sendai 980, Japan

Izumiyama, T., First Department of Internal Medicine, Tohoku University School of Medicine, Sendai 980, Japan

Kagawa, S., Department of Anesthesiology, The Jikei University School of Medicine, Tokyo 105, Japan

Kamide, M., Department of Anesthesiology, The Jikei University School of Medicine, Tokyo 105, Japan

Kaminuma, O., Department of Animal Environmental Physiology, Faculty of Agriculture, University of Tokyo, Tokyo 113, Japan

Kanamaru, A., Department of Physiology, Showa University School of Medicine, Tokyo 142, Japan

Kaneko, M., Department of Neuropsychiatry, Fukushima Medical College, Fukushima 960, Japan

Kaneko, Y., Department of Neuropsychiatry, Fukushima Medical College, Fukushima 960, Japan

Kanno, T., Department of Physiology, Fukushima Medical College, Fukushima 960-12, Japan

Kataura, A., Department of Otolaryngology, Sapporo Medical College, Sapporo 060, Japan

Kato, F., Department of Pharmacology II, The Jikei University School of Medicine, Tokyo 105, Japan

Kawabe, Y., Tokyo National Chest Hospital, Tokyo 204, Japan

Kawahara, K., Department of Information, Faculty of Engineering, Yamagata University, Yonezawa 992, Japan

Kawakami, Y., First Department of Medicine, School of Medicine, Hokkaido University, Sapporo 060, Japan

Kikuchi, Y., First Department of Internal Medicine, Tohoku University School of Medicine, Sendai 980, Japan

Kimura, N., Department of Pharmacology II, The Jikei University School of Medicine, Tokyo 105, Japan

Kishi, F., First Department of Medicine, Hokkaido University School of Medicine, Sapporo 060, Japan

Kitagawa, S., Division of Respiratory Diseases, Department of Internal Medicine, Kanazawa Medical Univeristy, Ishikawa 920-02, Japan

Koba, T., Saga Res. Inst., Otsuka Pharmaceutical Ltd., Japan

Kobayashi, I., Department of Medicine, School of Medicine, Tokai University, Isehara, Kanagawa 259-11, Japan

Kobayashi, K., Department of Anesthesiology, The Jikei University School of Medicine, Tokyo 105, Japan

Kobayashi, S., First Department of Medicine, School of Medicine, Hokkaido University, Sapporo 060, Japan

Kobayashi, T., Department of Cardiovascular Medicine, Hokkaido University School of Medicine, Sapporo 060, Japan

Kochi, T., Department of Anesthesiology, Chiba University School of Medicine and the Department of Anesthesiology, National Cancer Center Hospital, Chiba 280, Japan

Koga, S., Dept. Physical Education Ergonomics, Kobe Design University, Kobe, Japan

Koh, S.O., Department of Anesthesia, University of California, San Francisco, CA 94143-0542, USA

Koike, K., Department of Surgery, Research Institute for Chest Disease and Cancer, Tohoku University, Sendai 980, Japan

Kondo, T., Department of Medicine, School of Medicine, Tokai University, Isehara, Kanagawa 259-11, Japan

Konno, K., First Department of Internal Medicine, Tokyo Women's Medical College, Tokyo 162, Japan

Kozaki, Y., Department of Nervous and Sensory Functions, Research Institute of Environmental Medicine, Nagoya University, Nagoya 464-01, Japan

Kumashiro, H., Department of Neuropsychiatry, Fukushima Medical College, Fukushima 960, Japan

Kumazawa, T., Department of Nervous and Sensory Functions, Research Institute of Environmental Medicine, Nagoya University, Nagoya 464-01, Japan

Kuno, K., Department of Clinical Pulmonary Physiology, Chest Disease Research Institute, Kyoto University, Kyoto 606, Japan

Kurihara, N., First Department of Internal Medicine, Osaka City University Medical School, Osaka 545, Japan

Kuriyama, T., Department of Chest Medicine, School of Medicine, Chiba University, Chiba 280, Japan

Kusuhara, N., Department of Chest Medicine, School of Medicine, Kitasato University, Sagamihara, Kanagawa 228, Japan

Ma, J., 1st Affiliated Hospital, Suzhou Medical College, Suzhou, China

Machida, K., Tokyo National Chest Hospital, Tokyo 204, Japan

Maruyama, R., Department of Physiology, School of Medicine, Chiba University, Chiba 280, Japan

Matsumoto, S., Department of Physiology, Fukushima Medical College, Fukushima 960-12, Japan

Matsushita, H., First Department of Internal Medicine, Osaka City University Medical School, Osaka 545, Japan

Mead, J., Harvard School of Public Health, Boston, MA, USA

Mier, A., Department of Medicine, Charing Cross Hospital, Fulham Palace Road, London W6 8RF, UK

Mikami, T., Division of Biomedical Systems Engineering, Faculty of Engineering, Hokkaido University, Sapporo 060, Japan

Miki, H., First Department of Internal Medicine, Tohoku University School of Medicine, Sendai 980, Japan

Miura, C., First Department of Internal Medicine, Tohoku University School of Medicine, Sendai 980, Japan

Miyamoto, Y., Department of Information, Faculty of Engineering, Yamagata University, Yonezawa 992, Japan

Miyamura, M., Research Center of Health, Physical Fitness and Sports Nagoya University, Nagoya 464-01, Japan

Miyazaki, S., Department of Otolaryngology, Akita University Hospital, Akita 010, Japan

Mizuguchi, A., Department of Physiology, Sapporo Medical College, Sapporo 060, Japan

Mizuguchi, T., Department of Anesthesiology, Chiba University School of Medicine and the Department of Anesthesiology, National Cancer Center Hospital, Chiba 280, Japan

Morinari, H., Department of Respiratory Diseases, Tokyo Teishin Hospital, Tokyo 102, Japan

Mukai, C., Kaseikai Mukai Clinic, Mukai Research Institute of Microbiology, Yamato, Kanagawa 242, Japan

Mukai, S., Kaseikai Mukai Clinic, Mukai Research Institute of Microbiology, Yamato, Kanagawa 242, Japan

Munaka, M., Dept. of Biometrics, Res. Inst. Nuclear Med. Biol., Hiroshima University, Hiroshima 730, Japan

Nagasaka, Y., Division of Respiratory Diseases, Department of Internal Medicine, Kanazawa Medical University School of Medicine, Ishikawa 920-02, Japan

Nagayama, N., Tokyo National Chest Hospital, Tokyo 204, Japan

Nagayama, T., Department of Physiology, Fukushima Medical College, Fukushima 960-12, Japan

Nakada, T., Department of Surgery, Research Institute for Chest Disease and Cancer, Tohoku University, Sendai 980, Japan

Nakano, Y., Department of Otolaryngology, Sapporo Medical College, Sapporo 060, Japan

Nakazono, Y., Department of Information, Faculty of Engineering, Yamagata University, Yonezawa 992, Japan

Neubauer, J.A., Division of Pulmonary and Critical Care Medicine, Department of Medicine, and Department of Pharmacology, University of Medicine and Dentistry of New Jersey-Robert Wood Johnson Medical School, New Brunswick, NJ, USA

Nishimura, M., First Department of Medicine, School of Medicine, Hokkaido University, Sapporo 060, Japan

Nishino, T., Department of Anesthesiology, National Cancer Center Hospital, Chiba 280, Japan

Ohi, M., Department of Clinical Pulmonary Physiology, Chest Disease Research Institute, Kyoto University, Kyoto 606, Japan

Ohta, Y., Department of Medicine, School of Medicine, Tokai University, Isehara, Kanagawa 259-11, Japan

Ohya, N., Division of Respiratory Diseases, Department of Internal Medicine, Kanazawa Medical University School of Medicine, Ishikawa 920-02, Japan

Okabe, S., First Department of Internal Medicine, Tohoku University School of Medicine, Sendai 980, Japan

Okawa, M., Department of Neuropsychiatry, Akita University Hospital, Akita 010, Japan

Oku, Y., Departments of Medicine and Biomedical Engineering, Case Western Reserve University, Cleveland, OH 44106, USA

Okubo, S., Department of Respiratory Diseases, Tokyo Teishin Hospital, Tokyo 102, Japan

Okubo, T., First Department of Internal Medicine, Yokohama City University School of Medicine, Yokohama 232, Japan

Onimaru, H., Department of Physiology, Showa University School of Medicine, Tokyo 142, Japan

Orem, J.M., Department of Physiology, Texas Tech University Health Sciences Center, Lubbock, TX 79430, USA

Otsuka, Y., Tokyo National Chest Hospital, Tokyo 204, Japan

Remmers, J.E., Department of Medicine, University of Calgary, Calgary, Alberta, Canada

Sagara, Y., Department of Surgery, Research Institute for Chest Disease and Cancer, Tohoku University, Sendai 980, Japan

Saidel, G.M., Department of Biomedical Engineering, Case Western Reserve University, Cleveland, OH 44106, USA

Saito, I., Sapporo Meiwa Hospital, Sapporo 062, Japan

Saito, Y., Sapporo National Hospital, Sapporo 003, Japan

Sakai, Y., Department of Pharmacology, Saitama Medical School, Saitama 350-04, Japan

Sakurai, M., First Department of Internal Medicine, Tohoku University School of Medicine, Sendai 980, Japan

Sakurai, S., Division of Respiratory Diseases, Department of Internal Medicine, Kanazawa Medical University School of Medicine, Ishikawa 920-02, Japan

Sato, H., Department of Medicine, School of Medicine, Kitasato University, Sagamihara, Kanagawa 228, Japan

Sato, M., Department of Anesthesiology, The Jikei University School of Medicine, Tokyo 105, Japan

Sato, Y., Medical Institute of Bioregulation, Kyushu University, Beppu 874, Japan

Satoh, M., First Department of Internal Medicine, Tohoku University School of Medicine, Sendai 980, Japan

Schaefer, T., Department of Applied Physiology, Ruhr-University Bochum, Bochum 1, Germany

Schena, F., Department of Physiology, Faculty of Medicine, University of Geneve, Geneve, Switzerland

Schlaefke, M.E., Department of Applied Physiology, Ruhr-University Bochum, Bochum 1, Germany

Severinghaus, J.W., Cardiovascular Research Institute, University of California, San Francisco, CA 94143-0542, USA

Shen, H., Division of Respiratory Diseases, Department of Internal Medicine, Kanazawa Medical University, Ishikawa 920-02, Japan

Shimizu, T., Department of Physiology, Fukushima Medical College, Fukushima 960-12, Japan

Shindoh, C., First Department of Internal Medicine, Tohoku University School of Medicine, Sendai 980, Japan

Shintani, T., Department of Otolaryngology, Sapporo Medical College, Sapporo 060, Japan

Sibuya, M., Department of Physiology, Showa University School of Medicine, Tokyo 142, Japan

Sibuya, M.B., Department of Physiology, Showa University School of Medicine, Tokyo 142, Japan

Simbulan, D.G., Jr., Department of Nervous and Sensory Functions, Research Institute of Environmental Medicine, Nagoya University, Nagoya 464-01, Japan

Sterbenz, G., Division of Pulmonary and Critical Care Medicine, Department of Medicine, and Department of Pharmacology, University of Medicine and Dentistry of New Jersey-Robert Wood Johnson Medical School, New Brunswick, NJ, USA

Suzuki, A., First Department of Medicine, School of Medicine, Hokkaido University, Sapporo 060, Japan

Suzuki, H., Department of Medicine, School of Medicine, Tokai University, Isehara, Kanagawa 259-11, Japan

Suzuki, J., First Department of Internal Medicine, Yokohama City University School of Medicine, Yokohama 232, Japan

Suzuki, S., First Department of Internal Medicine, Yokohama City University School of Medicine, Yokohama 232, Japan

Tada, H., Department of Otolaryngology, Akita University Hospital, Akita 101, Japan

Tadaki, E., Dept. of Nervous and Sensory Functions, Research Inst. of Environmental Medicine, Nagoya Univ., Nagoya 464-01, Japan

Taguchi, O., First Department of Internal Medicine, Tohoku University School of Medicine, Sendai 980, Japan

Takahashi, E., Division of Biomedical Systems Engineering, Faculty of Engineering, Hokkaido University, Sapporo 060, Japan

Takano, K., Department of Pharmacology II, The Jikei University School of Medicine, Tokyo 105, Japan

Takano, N., Physiology Laboratory, Department of School Health, Faculty of Education, Kanazawa University, Kanazawa 920, Japan

Takaoka, K., Japan Steel Memorial Hospital, Sapporo, Japan

Takeda, R., Department of Pharmacology, Faculty of Medicine, Toyama Medical and Pharmaceutical Univ., Toyama 930-01, Japan

Takeda, T., First Department of Internal Medicine, Osaka City University Medical School, Osaka 545, Japan

Takishima, T., First Department of Internal Medicine, Tohoku University School of Medicine, Sendai 980, Japan

Tamura, T., Department of Neuropsychiatry, Tottori University School of Medicine, Yonago 683, Japan

Tanaka, M., Department of Medicine, School of Medicine, Kitasato University, Sagamihara, Kanagawa 228, Japan

Tanifuji, Y., Department of Anesthesiology, The Jikei University School of Medicine, Tokyo 105, Japan

Tateishi, I., Division of Biomedical Systems Engineering, Faculty of Engineering, Hokkaido University, Sapporo 060, Japan

Toga, H., Division of Respiratory Diseases, Department of Internal Medicine, Kanazawa Medical University School of Medicine, Ishikawa 920-02, Japan

Togawa, K., Department of Otolaryngology, Akita University Hospital, Akita 020, Japan

Tojima, H., Department of Chest Medicine, School of Medicine, Chiba University, Chiba 280, Japan

Tomita, T., Department of Medicine, School of Medicine, Kitasato University, Sagamihara, Kanagawa 228, Japan

Tsubone, H., Department of Animal Environmental Physiology, Faculty of Agriculture, University of Tokyo, Tokyo 113, Japan

Tsuji, T., Lab. Biol. Engineering, Faculty of Engineering, Hiroshima University, Hiroshima 730, Japan

Tsukamoto, Y., Department of Pharmacology II, The Jikei University School of Medicine, Tokyo 105, Japan

Ueda, K., Department of Neuropsychiatry, Tottori University School of Medicine, Yonago 683, Japan

Usui, S., Lab. Exercise Physiol. Biomechanics, Faculty of Integrated Arts and Sciences, Hiroshima University, Hiroshima 730, Japan

Wiegand, L., Division of Pulmonary/Critical Care Medicine, Pennsylvania State University College of Medicine, Hershey, PA, USA

Xi, L., Department of Physiology, Faculty of Medicine, University of Geneve, Geneve, Switzerland

Yaginuma, M., Department of Neuropsychiatry, Fukushima Medical College, Fukushima 960, Japan

Yamabayashi, H., Department of Medicine, Tokai University, Isehara, Kanagawa 259-11, Japan

Contributors   xix

Yamakawa, K., Department of Otolaryngology, Akita University Hospital, Akita 010, Japan

Yamamoto, M., First Department of Medicine, Hokkaido University School of Medicine, Sapporo 060, Japan

Yamanouchi, K., Division of Respiratory Diseases, Department of Internal Medicine, Kanazawa Medical University, Ishikawa 920-02, Japan

Yamasaki, M., Department of Physiology, Fukushima Medical College, Fukushima 960-12, Japan

Yamauchi, Y., Department of Information Engineering, Yamagata University, Yonezawa 992, Japan

Yanaga, T., Medical Institute of Bioregulation, Kyushu University, Beppu 874, Japan

Yasuda, H., Department of Cardiovascular Medicine, Hokkaido University School of Medicine, Sapporo 060, Japan

Yoshino, K., First Department of Internal Medicine, Tokyo Women's Medical College, Tokyo 162, Japan

Yoshioka, A., First Department of Medicine, Hokkaido University School of Medicine, Sapporo 060, Japan

Yuan, W.-J., Department of Pharmacology II, The Jikei University School of Medicine, Tokyo 105, Japan

Zwillich, C.W., Division of Pulmonary/Critical Care Medicine, Pennsynvania State University College of Medicine, Hershey, PA, USA

Preface

Dyspnea is one of the major symptoms in many respiratory and cardiovascular diseases, and it interferes greatly with the patient's quality of life; however its causal mechanism has still not been sufficiently clarified. Moreover, in recent years, not only dysfunction of the respiratory centers in respiratory disease, but also ventilatory dysfunction accompanying respiratory control abnormalities such as sleep apnea syndrome as well as impairments of gas exchange have been gaining attention. Patients with diseases involving dyspnea or respiratory control abnormalities may present themselves to physicians in a number of medical disciplines, including internal medicine, psychoneurology, gerontology, pediatrics, otorhinolaryngology, etc., and in this regard, both basic and clinical research is making steady progress. With this background in mind, an 'International Symposium on Control of Breathing and Dyspnea' was held on 27 and 28 October 1989, in Sendai, Japan.

The Symposium consisted of four sessions:
    I. Respiratory rhythm generation
    II. Abnormality of respiratory control
    III. Respiratory muscle and dyspnea
    IV. Behavioral control of breathing and dyspnea

About two hundred scientists from seven countries were able to participate in this symposium, which was a great success.

The proceedings contain the papers presented at this symposium. Research on respiratory control and dyspnea is becoming more and more intensive, covering a large number of fields from molecular biology to integrated brain function. We sincerely hope that this volume will contribute to the development of such research.

Finally, we would like to express our deep gratitude to all contributors to this book, the individuals and organizations who supported this symposium, and to Drs. Wataru Hida, Yoshihiro Kikuchi, and Tatsuya Chonan for their invaluable help in making this publication possible.

Tamotsu Takishima
Neil S. Cherniack

Section 1
RESPIRATORY RHYTHM

Neural Organization and Rhythm Generation

Curt von Euler

Nobel Institute for Neurophysiology,
Karolinska Institutet, Box 60400, S-104 01 Stockholm, Sweden

ABSTRACT

Breathing is a complex behavior, the control of which engages large and widespread parts of the central nervous system from cerebral cortex down to the lumbar segments. Even purely automatic breathing for metabolic purposes is a complex motor act. The breathing patterns depends on a host of feedback circuits, reflexes and higher central control mechanisms for optimization of the ventilatory performance and for adaptation to prevailing and anticipated metabolic needs. The most basic mechanisms for respiratory rhythm generation seems to be located in the medulla oblongata. Recent advances concerning the physiological and morphological properties of the respiration-related neurons in the brain stem, on the one hand, and the 'systems behavior' on the other, has provided the basis for current concepts on the construct of the central pattern generator and its different part-mechanisms for inspiratory on-switch, inspiratory 'ramp' generation, inspiratory off-switch, post-inspiration inspiratory activity and control of expiratory motor activity in the 2nd part of expiration.

KEYWORDS

Neural organization of respiratory control; Respiratory rhythm generation; Breathing behavior; Adaptive control; Pattern generation; Pattern formation.

INTRODUCTION - CONTROL OF BREATHING BEHAVIOR

Superficially breathing may appear as a fairly simple, unsophisticated motor act. At a closer look, however, it becomes apparent that breathing is a complex behavior which can exhibit a variety of different patterns dependent on the prevailing situation. The generation and adaptive control of the breathing pattern are governed by a multitude of intricate neural mechanisms hierarchically organized to adjust the magnitude of ventilation and the pattern of the respiratory movements so as to match optimally the ever changing energy requirements and the many non-metabolic demands on the breathing apparatus.

For optimal performance during all conditions the respiratory controllers need continuous re-calibrations and re-adjustments by a host of feedback and feedforward circuits, integrating mechanisms and inputs from higher brain structures and spinal levels. Among these important mechanisms seem to adapt the systems also according to anticipated changes in metabolic rate,

Advances in the Biosciences Vol. 79
© 1991 Pergamon Press plc.
Printed in Great Britain.

4   C. von Euler

e.g. at the initiation of exercise (e.g. DiMarco et al., 1983). These mechanisms, largely under the supervision of different forebrain structures, are prerequisites for the great adaptability characteristic of the human respiratory control system.

In addition to the bulbar respiratory mechanisms for the basic rhythm generation these respiratory control functions involve many parts of the central nervous system such as different cortical, amygdalar, hypothalamic and other limbic areas, mesencephalic, pontine and cerebellar structures. The precise co-ordination of the different respiratory muscles and their adjustments to trunk movements and postural activities require intricate neural spinal and supraspinal mechanisms capable of immediate automatic compensations for any changes in muscle length, direction of muscle forces and other factors of chest wall mechanics. A detailed knowledge of the mechanics of this system is an absolutely prerequisite for a full understanding of its neural control. There is still a long way to go, however, before that level of knowledge is reached.

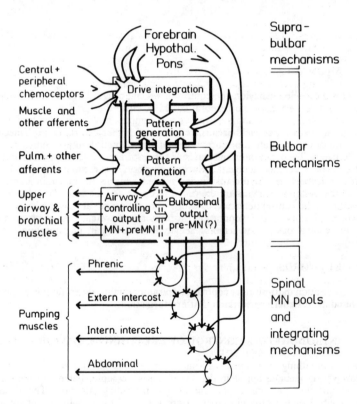

Fig. 1. The main features of the functional organization of the neural control of breathing discussed in the text. Emphases are put on the mechanisms for drive integration, pattern generation, pattern formations, and their influences on the two main output systems for the airway-controlling and pumping muscles. The scheme further emphasizes the great influences originating from forebrain and other suprabulbar structures, and the importance of the internuncial networks of the bulbar, airway-controlling, and spinal pump-muscle-controlling motoneuron (MN) pools. Hypothal.: Hypothalamus; Pulm.: pulmonary; extern.intercost.: external intercostal; intern.intercost.: internal intercostal. (From Euler, 1988).

Thus, it seems both conceptually justified and practicle to discuss the control of breathing behavior in terms of 1) mechanisms for the basic pattern generation, and 2) mechanisms for the adaptive control of breathing and optimal pattern formation. A third set of mechanisms, hitherto fairly neglected, are those concerned with the ventilatory drive integration (e.g. Budzinska et al., 1985b). Certainly there is a great deal of overlap and interaction between these three sets of mechanisms diagrammatically depicted in Fig. 1. This paper will deal mainly with the first mentioned of these mechanisms, i.e. for the basic pattern or rhythm generation.

GENERAL PROPERTIES OF RHYTHM GENERATING MECHANISMS

One of the most challenging problems of the neurosciences of today concerns the question of how networks of neurons are designed and operate to generate behavior. To reach such an understanding about the construct and function behind even a relatively simple behavior such as an alternating motor activity in breathing or locomotion, and how it may fail, due to disease or injury, it is necessary to acquire knowledge both on the overriding principles of neuronal functions, and how these principles are implemented by the individual building blocks of neurons and synapses in the particular network. Knowledge of anatomical connectivity is essential but not enough; functional connectivity and functional network operation depends critically upon the synaptic and cellular properties. Also the flow of activity within the circuit must be defined e.g. by assessing the temporal sequence of activity of the circuit elements using such criteria as changes in membrane potential, membrane conductance, firing frequency and the onset and termination of firing (Getting, 1989).

The functional connectivity, and thus the operation of the network, can be altered in many ways e.g. by modulation of the intrinsic properties of neurons and of synaptic efficiency (facilitation, depression, potentiation, and 'reflex reversal') e.g. by neuromodulators. Acting on surface receptors these can change the kinetics of certain ion channels, either by direct actions or by way of second messenger induction. These effects can be strong enough to provide a neuron with properties not present in the absence of the modulator. Thus, the functional connectivity is under dynamic control and dependent on the prevailing tasks but, of course, within the constraints of its anatomical organization. This provides possibilities not only for adaptive control of the output activity of the network but also for it to generate different behaviors during different conditions (Getting, 1989). This implies that a separate neural network is not necessary for each behavior or for each behavioral modification, such as breathing for gas exchange, breathing for the purpose of speech and singing or breathing for thermoregulatory panting. Certain inputs to a network may be both instructive and permissive in that they may both re-organize the functional interactions within the network to fit the task at hand, activate the network to perform the task.

CURRENT CONCEPTS ON THE DESIGN OF THE RESPIRATORY RHYTHM GENERATING NETWORKS

The Anatomical Organization of Respiration-Related Neuronal Populations in the Medulla Oblongata

The central pattern generator, CPG, for automatic breathing and its main output system of premotor neurons is located in the lower brainstem, probably within the medulla oblongata. This location in close approximation to the motoneuron pools for the upper airway and bronchial muscles is, however, at a considerable distance from the spinal motoneuron pools for the volume driving muscles. This organization, which appears to contrast with the spinal localization of the CPGs for locomotion, reflects the phylogenetic origin of large parts of the respiratory apparatus from the brancheal structures. It forms the basis for a close co-ordination of the airway-controlling and the volume driving muscles which is of fundamental importance both in breathing and in the different non-respiratory reflexes and functions especially these involving vocalization (cf. Euler, 1986).

It would seem likely, although still uncertain, that the neurons constituting the building blocks of the basic pattern generator for breathing and its different part mechanisms can be found among the respiration-related, RR, neurons in medulla (Cohen, 1979, Euler, 1986, 1991). At the present state of our knowledge, however, the location of the CPG for breathing cannot be defined in terms of any circumscribed region of the main populations, or aggregates, of respiration-related neurons, i.e. the Dorsal and the Ventral Respiratory Groups, DRG and VRG (including the Bötzinger Complex) or any other anatomically specified bulbar structure. Rather, the CPG seems to be organized in a wide spread manner and with a great deal of redundancy. This view is based on the findings that it is difficult to abolish rhythmic activity by circumscribed lesions or focal cold blocks within the VRG or DRG (e.g. Speck & Feldman, 1982, Budzinska et al., 1985a).

During the last decade a great deal of knowledge has been obtained from intracellular studies of the different types of known RR neurons with respect to membrane potential, membrane conductance and firing patterns (e.g. Ballantyne & Richter, 1984, 1986, Bianchi et al., 1988, Richter, 1982). These have revealed characteristic phase-related patterns of excitatory and inhibitory post-synaptic modulations with a preponderance of inhibitory interactions. This has led to hypotheses that the respiratory pattern generating networks might be composed of groups of neurons interacting with each other largely through inhibitory synaptic connections in parallel with excitatory, mainly drive-dependent inputs.

For several reasons, however, the classical concepts that the breathing rhythm depends on reciprocal inhibition between two symmetrical populations of inspiratory and expiratory premotor neurons forming an inspiratory and an expiratory "half-center" has been found untenable in the proposed form.

Instead Richter and his co-workers (1986) have argued that the respiratory cycle should be regarded as consisting of three phases: 1) the inspiration, 2) the post-inspiratory, or the first expiratory phase (E-phase I) characterized by the re-appearance of some declining inspiratory activity, the post-inspiration inspiratory activity, PIIA, and 3) the second expiratory phase (E-phase II) during which expiratory motor activity may be recruited in conditions of increased drive for ventilation. These three phases are considered to be delimited by four sequentially activated sub-mechanisms causally involved in the phase transitions. These sub-mechanisms are those responsible for 1) the sudden onset and progressive augmentation of the inspiratory ramp, i.e. the central inspiratory activity (CIA), 2) the termination of the inspiratory activity, i.e. the inspiratory "off-switch" mechanisms, 3) the events occurring during the early part of E-phase I, such as the PIIA and the laryngeal adductor activation, and 4) the control of E-phase II and the expiratory motor output (Euler, 1986, 1991). For this operation the following six types of neurons (see Fig. 2) have been proposed to serve as the main neuronal building elements. These are: 1) "Early inspiratory", or "early burst", interneurons, 2) "Inspiratory ramp interneurons", 3) "Late-onset inspiratory interneurons", 4) "Early expiratory", or "post-inspiration (PI)-related interneurons", 5) "Early peak whole expiratory interneurons", 6) "Expiratory ramp interneurons".

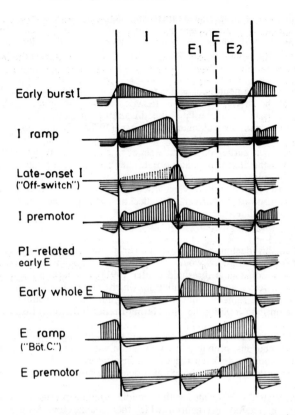

Fig. 2. Excitatory and inhibitory activity patterns of main types of inspiration- and expiration-related neurons in medulla during inspiratory (I) and expiratory (E) phases (E_1 and E_2 denote subdivisions of this phase). PI: post-inspiration; Böt.C., Bötzinger Complex. See text for further explanation. Vertical hatching represents excitatory synaptic activity and discharge rate; horizontal hatching denotes synaptic inhibition. During main part of inspiratory phase late-onset neurons receive an augmenting excitation but are kept silent by an inhibition which may emanate from early burst neurons. (From Euler, 1991).

The Sub-Mechanisms of the Pattern Generator - Possible Neural Correlates

The Ramp Generation. Following a fairly synchronous onset the augmentation rate of inspiratory activity is proportional to the respiratory drive. At conditions with stable drive put, the inspiratory trajectory is usually fairly linear, with but small breath-to-breath variations. The underlying progressively augmenting pattern of excitatory postsynaptic potentials, EPSPs, is damped somewhat by a simultaneous weaker barrage of inhibitory postsynaptic potentials, IPSPs (Richter, 1982, Ballantyne and Richter, 1984) probably derived from the early inspiratory neurons.

The Inspiratory "Off-Switch" Mechanisms. Inspiratory activity is terminated either when it has produced a sufficient tidal volume, or when it has proceeded for a predetermined duration of time as "deamed adequate" for the prevailing condition by the respiratory controller. These settings seem to be expressed in terms of a centrally controlled threshold, the off-switch threshold, attained by some progressively increasing activities. The level of this threshold is subject to adaptive control. Its adjustment according to the prevailing conditions is one of the important means by which depth and rate of breathing is regulated (Euler, 1986, 1991). The fact that the off-switch excitability is continuously and progressively increasing during the course of the inspiratory phase precludes a timing device acting through trigger signals.

With respect to the possible neural correlates to the inspiratory off-switch mechanisms it has been postulated that the reversible Stage 1 off-switch events (Remmers et al., 1979) correspond closely to the discharge of the late-onset inspiratory neurons, also referred to as the "putative off-switch" neurons by Feldman and Cohen (1978). Their onset and time-activity profile is strongly influenced by pulmonary stretch receptor inputs: lung inflation causes facilitation resulting in an earlier onset and steeper rate of rise of firing, while withholding lung inflation causes disfacilitation and later onset. They receive a ramp-like increase of EPSPs during the whole of inspiration but this excitatory input is counteracted by an initially strong but decrementing postsynaptic inhibitory activity which starts off and reaches its peak at the very beginning of the inspiratory phase and then declines. The time course of this IPSP activity seems to correspond to that of the discharge rate of the early inspiratory ("early burst") interneurons (Ballantyne and Richter, 1984; see Fig. 2).

It would seem that this declining inhibitory power provides the progressively increasing excitability of the "off-switch". This would imply that the firing threshold of the late-onset neurons constitutes the off-switch threshold (Euler 1991). The facilitation of the late-onset inspiratory neurons in response to lung inflation, which mimics the inhibition of the early inspiratory neurons to the same stimulus, is providing the off-switch function with its well-known dependence on lung inflation i.e. the Hering-Breuer inflation reflex.

The final, irreversible Stage 2 off-switch (Remmers et al., 1979) might be executed by the early expiratory PI-related neurons, probably in combination with early whole expiratory neurons which may have the capacity to keep the central inspiratory inhibition, CII, (Knox, 1979), during the whole expiratory phase, although at a declining power.

The inspiratory "off-switch" is associated with a rapidly rising deep wave of hyperpolarization of the inspiratory-ramp, I-ramp, interneurons which then declines towards the end of E-phase I. Possibly, this hyperpolarization is mediated by the late-onset inspiratory neurons followed by the action of the PI-related neurons and the early whole expiratory neurons (Ballantyne and Richter, 1986).

The E-Phase I is characterized by the post-inspiration inspiratory activity, PIIA, and the initially strong but declining activity of the underlying early expiratory PI-related interneurons. The declining activity during E phase I might be caused by an augmenting inhibitory input from ramp expiratory interneurons (see Fig. 2). During E-phase II these neurons receive a progressively increasing postsynaptic inhibition. During inspiration they receive an initially strong but declining postsynaptic inhibition.

The time - activity profile of the PI-related expiratory interneurons is modulated by pulmonary stretch receptor input: Lung inflation brakes the rate of decline of their discharge and causes prolongation of this phase. Conversely, procedures preventing an inflation of the lung to occur during inspiration, e.g. tracheal occlusion, causes a more rapid decline of the firing rate of these cells and a shortening of this phase (Feldman and Cohen, 1978).

The E-Phase II. The inhibitory activity that depresses the various inspiration-promoting influences and reflexes during the expiratory phase acts during the whole expiratory phase, although with a declining power. This inhibitory activity which has been referred to as the central inspiratory inhibition, CII (Knox, 1979), seems to control the whole expiratory duration.

The rate of decay of this inhibition is strongly modulated by pulmonary reflexes. It is slowed down by lung inflations, causing prolongation of the expiratory duration, while inspiration-facilitating reflexes, e.g. those mediated by rapidly adapting pulmonary receptors, accelerates the decay rate and shortens the expiratory phase (Knox, 1979).

The studies of the decay rate of the inhibitory power of CII and its reflex pertubations have shown that it is more closely related to the time course of the early-peak whole expiratory neurons than to that of the PI-related ones. The pattern of postsynaptic inhibition observed in some of these expiration-related, ER, neurons seems to correspond to the discharge pattern of I ramp interneurons, while in other ER neurons the pattern of IPSPs was similar to the firing pattern of early-onset inspiratory neurons. Furthermore it has been reported that inspiration-related, IR, neurons of the VRG and DRG send inhibitory projections to ER neuron populations. Similarly early-onset inspiratory neurons appear to project to the contralateral ER neurons of the caudal part of the VRG (Long and Duffin, 1986).

IN SUMMARY

On this hypothesis, then, the early and the late-onset inspiratory neurons together with the early expiratory PI-related neurons can be regarded as key elements in the rhythm generating network. The decremental post-synaptic inhibition of the ER neurons, except the PI-related ones, during inspiration is caused by the early inspiratory ("early burst") neurons which also would seem likely candidates for the cause of the decremental inhibition of the late-onset inspiratory neurons and their modulation by lung inflations. It is further suggested that the postsynaptic inhibition during E-phase I of the various IR neurons, and of the expiratory premotor neurons is caused by the early expiratory PI-related neurons. The PI-related interneurons have been postulated to have important roles in the rhythm generating network also by suppressing, or "gating", the inputs to the system from the drive-integrating mechanisms in the ventral rostrolateral structures of medulla (Richter et al., 1986).

The above hypotheses have been subjected to model simulations by Botros and Bruce (1990). The results of these quantitative studies have demonstrated the feasibility of most of the qualitative concepts discussed above. However, so far it has not been firmly established that any of these neurons really are functionally involved in the pattern generating networks nor that they are connected as proposed. More investigations are required in order to discern which neurons are involved in the basic pattern generator and their anatomical connectivity as well as their functional connectivity and interactions within this network under different conditions. It should be kept in mind also that new hitherto unknown types of respiration-related neurons may still be discovered and found to be of importance in the rhythm generating mechanisms. Moreover, it seems quite possible that the pattern generator consists of many parallel, self-sustaining oscillating networks organized as a set of coupled but not necessarily identical oscillators.

So far there is no conclusive evidence that pacemaker cells are involved. However, participation of such elements cannot be excluded at the present state of knowledge, and it does not seem unlikely that unstable or bistable membrane properties, electrical coupling, and local circuit mechanisms influencing only parts of neurons may be found to be involved. Recent results (e.g. by Onimaru and Homma, 1987) obtained on in vitro preparations of neonatal rat brainstem have shown that in a Cl⁻-free medium or a medium containing antagonists to the inhibitory neurotransmitters GABA or glycine rhythmic activity can still be recorded which thus seems to be independent of Cl⁻-dependent post-synaptic inhibition. This suggest the possibility that neurons with pace-maker properties might be involved in the rhythm generating networks. However so far there are no confirmative evidence to prove this hypothesis from intracellular recordings from such elements.

REFERENCES

Ballantyne, D. and D.W. Richter (1984). Post-synaptic inhibition of bulbar inspiratory neurones in the cat. J. Physiol. (London), 348, 67-88.

Ballantyne, D. and D.W. Richter (1986). The non-uniform character of expiratory synaptic activity in expiratory bulbospinal neurones of the cat. J. Physiol. (London), 370, 433-456.

Bianchi, A.L., L. Grélot, S. Iscoe and J.E. Remmers (1988). Electrophysiological properties of rostral medullary respiratory neurones in the cat: an intracellular study. J. Physiol. (London), 407, 293-310.

Botros, S.M. and E.N. Bruce (1990). Neural network implementation of a three-phase model of respiratory rhythm generation. (Submitted).

Budzinska, K., C. von Euler, F.F. Kao, T. Pantaleo and Y. Yamamoto (1985a). Effects of graded focal cold block in the solitary and para-ambigual regions of the medulla in the cat. Acta Physiol. Scand., 124, 317-328.

Budzinska, K., C. von Euler, F.F. Kao, T. Pantaleo and Y. Yamamoto (1985b). Effects of graded focal cold block in rostral areas of the medulla. Acta Physiol. Scand., 124, 329-430.

Cohen, M.I. (1979). Neurogenesis of respiratory rhythm in the mammal. Physiol. Rev., 59, 1105-1173.

DiMarco, A.F., J.R. Romaniuk, C. von Euler and Y. Yamamoto (1983). Immediate changes in ventilation and respiratory pattern associated with onset and cessation of locomotion in the cat. J. Physiol. (London), 343, 1-16.

Euler, C. von (1986). Brainstem mechanisms for generation and control of breathing pattern. In: Handbook of Physiology. The Respiratory System (Cherniack, N.S. and Widdicombe, J.G., eds). vol. 2 Control of Breathing, pp 1-67. American Physiological Society, Bethesda.

Euler, C. von (1988). Introduction: forebrain control of breathing behaviour. In: Respiratory Psychophysiology (Euler, C. von and Katz-Salamon, M., eds). Wenner-Gren International Symposium Series, vol. 50, pp 1-14. Macmillan Press, London.

Euler, C. von (1991). Neural organization and rhythm generation. In: The Lung: Scientific Foundations (Crystal, R.G., West, J.B. et al., eds). Raven Press, New York (In press).

Feldman, J.L. and Cohen, M.I. (1978). Relation between expiratory duration and rostral medullary expiratory neuronal discharge. Brain Res., 141, 172-178.

Getting, P.A. (1989). Emerging principles governing the operation of neural networks. Ann. Rev. Neurosci., 12, 185-204.

Knox, C.K. (1979). Reflex and central mechanisms controlling expiratory duration. In: Central Nervous Control Mechanisms in Breathing (Euler, C. von and Lagercrantz, H., eds.), Wenner-Gren International Symposium Series, vol. 32, pp 203-216. Pergamon Press, Oxford.

Long, S. and Duffin, J. (1986). The neuronal determinants of respiratory rhythm. Progr. Neurobiol., 27, 101-182.

Onimaru, H. and Homma, I. (1987). Respiratory rhythm generator neurons in medulla of brainstem - spinal cord preparation from newborn rat. Brain Res., 403, 380-384.

Remmers, J.E., Baker Jr, J.P. and Younes, M.K. (1979). Graded inspiratory inhibition: the first stage of inspiratory "off-switching". In: Central Nervous Control Mechanisms in Breathing (Euler, C. von and Lagercrantz, H., eds.), Wenner-Gren International Symposium Series, vol. 32, pp 195-201. Pergamon Press, Oxford, UK.

Richter, D.W. (1982). Generation and maintenance of the respiratory rhythm. J. Expt. Biol., 100, 93-107.

Richter, D.W., Ballantyne, D. and Remmers, J.E. (1986). How is the respiratory rhythm generated? NIPS, 1, 109-112.

Speck, D.F. and Feldman, J.L. (1982). The effect of microstimulation and microlesions in the dorsal and ventral respiratory groups in medulla of cat. J. Neurosci., 2, 744-757.

Organization of the Neural Mechanisms for Generation of Respiratory Rhythm in the Brain Stem

T. Hukuhara, Jr.

Department of Pharmacology II, Jikei University School
of Medicine, Minato-ku, Tokyo 105, Japan

ABSTRACT

The present neurophysiological aspects and the essential experimental results on the anatomical localization, functional and neuronal organization of the central respiratory mechanisms in the brain stem were discussed. The brain stem neural mechanism for central regulation of breathing is regarded as a complex neuronal mechanism consisting of several functional subsystems subserving different functions. One of these functions is the generation of the respiratory rhythm. The subsystem for respiratory rhythm generation is located in the lateral region of the medullary reticular formation outside the areas in which DRG and VRG are located. DRG and VRG are thought to be premotor neuron pools. Rhythmic activity originating in this subsystem is dominant in terms of the spontaneity over other rhythmic activities in the pontine and spinal cord mechanisms. Evidences for functional heterogeneity of brain stem respiratory neurons are demonstrated. Neuronal mechanisms involving respiratory neurons identified as members of primary respiratory neuron populations or primary respiratory neuron networks located in the lateral region of the medullary reticular formation may play essential roles in the generation of respiratory rhythms. These views contribute to providing important prerequisites for further studies on the mechanisms for the respiratory rhythm generation within the neuronal network of the central respiratory mechanisms.

KEYWORDS

Respiratory rhythmogenesis; respiratory neurons; respiratory center; phrenic nerve; cranial nerves; autocorrelation function; Fourier analysis; brain stem; respiratory system; medullary reticular formation.

INTRODUCTION

Respiratory movements are continuously adjusted in response to physiological demands of the organism by neural and chemical respiratory control mechanisms. These dynamic regulatory processes are maintained involving the entire neuroaxis, although the central respiratory mechanisms in the brain stem play a main role in the regulation of breathing (Cohen, 1979; Euler, 1986; Wyss, 1964). Rhythmic control of the act of breathing is performed by a rhythmic nervous activity which originates in the medulla oblongata, preferentially, in the lateral region of the bulbar reticular formation taking priority in respect to the spontaneity of the respiratory rhythmicity (Hukuhara <u>et al.</u>, 1954; Hukuhara Jr., 1973, 1976, 1988; Hukuhara Jr. <u>et al.</u>, 1981).

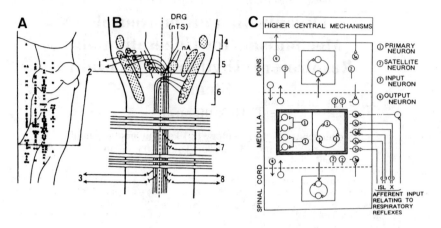

Fig. 1. Localization of respiratory neurons in the brain stem of the cat. A: location of respiratory neurons in the right half of the dorsal projection of the brain stem of cats. A total of 149 sites, where single respiratory unit activity was recorded, was found by systematic exploration experiments by 244 dorsoventral microelectrode tracks from the dorsal surface of the brain stem over the pontine and bulbar reticular formation as well as the neighboring structures in 15 cats, lightly anesthetized, paralyzed, vagotomized, and ventilated artificially. Each of the following symbols indicates respectively the site where different types of single respiratory unit activity were recorded. Symbols: filled circle, inspiratory; cross, expiratory; filled triangle, inspiratory-expiratory and expiratory-inspiratory phase-spanning unit activity (Hukuhara Jr., 1973). B: schematic diagram of the two main aggregates (stippled areas) of respiration-related neurons: the longitudinal zone in the lateral part of the diagram constituting the ventral respiratory group (VRG) with its subdivisions [4, 5, 6, and nA (the nucleus ambiguus)], and the dorsal respiratory group (DRG) in the medial part to the vicinity of the obex. The diagram further shows the locations of the main group by symbols: open circles, expiratory; open triangle, inspiratory with their decussating, descending axons projecting to the spinal motoneurons (filled small circles and triangles). In nA, laryngeal motoneurons are indicated. For simplicity, the presence of neurons and axons are represented on only one side. 1, 10th cranial nerve; 2, horizontal level of the obex in A and B for comparison; 3, internal intercostal nerve; 4, Boetzinger complex (rostral VRG); 5, nucleus paraambigualis (intermediate VRG); 6, nucleus retroambigualis (caudal VRG); 7, phrenic nerve; 8, external intercostal nerve; nTs, nucleus tractus solitarius (Euler, J. Auton. Nerv. Syst., Suppl., 1986, p. 55). C: functional organization of respiratory neurons in the central respiratory mechanisms in the brain stem. ISL, internal branch of the superior laryngeal nerve; X, vagus

nerve; 3a-3g, subtypes of the input respiratory neuron population. The block circumscribed by the shaded belt zone in the medulla suggests two possibilities of the neuronal organization of primary respiratory neurons for the respiratory rhythm generation. Left half, network model for respiratory rhythm production generated by primary respiratory neurons as pacemaker neurons in the neuronal network of the medulla oblongata; right half, oscillator circuitry model triggered by extrinsic tonic excitatory inputs. For further explanation see text.

NEUROPHYSIOLOGICAL ASPECTS AND THE ESSENTIAL EXPERIMENTAL EVIDENCES

Multiplicity of the Function of the Central Respiratory Mechanisms

In viewing the present status of our knowledge concerning the functional organization of the central respiratory mechanisms, it seems reasonable to understand that generation of an autonomous rhythmic nervous activity in the lower brain stem is one of the functions of the central respiratory mechanisms. Thereupon we would like to propose a view that the neuronal network of the central respiratory mechanisms might be regarded as a complex neural organization consisting of several functional subsystems (Fig. 1, C; Hukuhara Jr., 1973, 1988; Hukuhara Jr. et al., 1981). These subsystems are functional in nature and engage mainly the following functions operating in dynamic interactions with other subsystems to a greater or lesser degree. These subsystems are virtually different from the classical subcenters such as pneumotaxic, apneustic, inspiratory, expiratory, gasping centers which have been hypothesized as the subcenters of the classical respiratory centers in terms of the neural organization for the respiratory rhythm generation (Cohen, 1979; Wyss, 1964). Multiple functions of 6 of the central respiratory mechanisms are as follows (Hukuhara Jr., 1988):

Generation of the respiratory rhythm. The production of the rhythmic nervous activity is autonomous and intrinsic within the neuroaxis, most probably in the lower brain stem. This rhythmic activity may serve a prototype of the respiratory rhythms and be modified to respiratory rhythms of a normal character by interactions with other subsystems of the central respiratory mechanisms and the related compartment of the respiratory regulatory systems.

Production of respiratory pattern. Respiratory rhythmic activity produced and modified within the central respiratory mechanisms is transmitted to premotor neuron pools such as the dorsal and ventral respiratory groups in the brain stem resulting in production of respiratory patterns.

Coordinated control of motoneuronal pools innervating respiratory muscles and respiration-related muscles.

Integration of centripetal influences converging to the central respiratory mechanisms.

Interactions between the central control mechanisms for the functions regulated by the autonomic nervous systems.

Possible involvement of the central respiratory mechanisms to unspecific ascending control for neural mechanisms in the forebrain.

Spatial Distribution of Respiratory Neurons in the Central Nervous System

The majority of respiratory neurons have been found mainly in the neural structures of the pons, medulla and spinal cord (Cohen, 1979; Euler, 1986; Hukuhara Jr., 1973; Hukuhara et al., 1954). However it should be noted that respiratory neuronal discharges have been recorded from various regions in the forebrain: neocortex, hippocampus, midbrain, hypothalamus and thalamus (Cohen, 1979; Hukuhara Jr., 1973, 1988).

Respiratory Neuron Groups in the Relatively Higher Density Regions in the Brain Stem. When the whole pontine and medullary regions were systematically explored for spontaneously active respiratory unitary discharges, respiratory neurons are located almost in the entire area of the pontine and medullary structures displaying considerable different densities (Fig. 1 A, B; Cohen, 1979; Euler, 1986; Hukuhara Jr., 1973; Wyss, 1964).

Respiratory Neurons in the Reticular Formation of the Brain Stem. It has been reported that reticular neurons displaying respiratory rhythmic activities were located in the bulbar, pontine and mesencephalic reticular formations in cats, rabbits, rats, dogs and monkeys (Cohen, 1979; Euler, 1986; Hukuhara Jr., 1973, 1988; Wyss, 1964).

According to recent findings in cats, rabbits and rats, respiratory reticular neurons were scattered and intermingled throughout most regions of the mesencephalic, pontine and bulbar reticular formation. In contrast to the findings described in previous reports, no circumscribed regions where respiratory units were grouped according to discharge type were found, although inspiratory and expiratory units were found predominantly in the bulbar reticular formation (A of Fig. 1; Hukuhara Jr., 1973). However, neurons were found more frequently in the lateral as compared with in the medial region of the bulbar reticular formation in the pontine and mesencephalic reticular formation.

Respiratory Neuron Groups in the Relatively High-Density Regions in the Lower Brain Stem (B of Fig. 1). In the pons and medulla of cats respiration neurons are concentrated in, but not restricted to, several clusters. Within the explored area respiratory neurons distributed with a relatively higher density in the following structures: nucleus parabrachialis and Koelliker-Fuse nucleus; ventrolateral part of the nucleus of solitary tract [Fig. 1, B, DRG (nTS)]; nuclei ambiguus (Fig. 1, B, nA), paraambigus, and retroamgigualis; motoneuronal pools of the cranial nerves. Based on assumptions that some neurons in the DRG (dorsal respiratory group), VRG (ventral respiratory group), and PRG (pontine respiratory group) the respiratory neurons population might relate specifically to the central respiratory control.

Changes of Bulbar Respiratory Neuronal Discharge, Hypoglossal and Phrenic Nerve Activity before and after Transection at the Bulbo-Spinal Junction (Hukuhara Jr., 1976)

In a series of experiments the spontaneous periodic discharge of bulbar inspiratory or expiratory neurons, the hypoglossal nerve activity and the phrenic nerve discharge were recorded after brain stem transection at the level of the ponto-bulbar junction and then changes of these discharges were investigated in mid-course of simultaneous recording by transection at the bulbo-spinal junction or rostral medulla caudal to the lowermost border of the Boetzinger complex (Fig. 1, B, 4) in some cases. The bulbar inspiratory neuron (1 in Fig. 2A and B) had continued to discharge in synchronization with the hypoglossal (Fig. 2A, 2) and phrenic nerve discharge (Fig. 2A, 3) even after the brain stem transection . After bulbo-spinal transection the phrenic burst discharge was abolished (3 in B of Fig. 2), while the bulbar inspiratory unitary activity (1 in B of Fig.2) and the hypoglossal nerve activity (2 in B of Fig. 2) were maintained with their spontaneous discharges. No alteration of spontaneous discharges of the phrenic nerve activity was observed after 4.10% CO_2 inhalation.

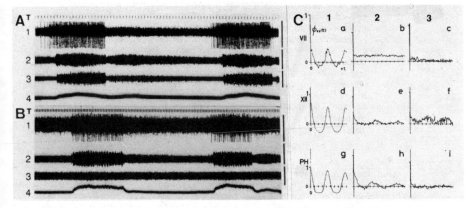

Fig. 2. Changes of a bulbar inspiratory discharge and discharge
pattern of the phrenic, hypoglossal nerve activity caused
by brain stem transection in the rostral medulla at a level
caudal to the lowermost border of the Boetzinger complex
and additional transection of the neuroaxis at the bulbospinal junction in mid-course of simultaneous recording in
an anesthetized, paralyzed, and artificially ventilated cat.
T, each division represents 0.1 s; 1, a bulbar inspiratory
unitary discharge recorded from an inspiratory neurons located in the lateral part of the bulbar reticular formation
in the right side; 2. right hypoglossal nerve efferent
activity; 3, right efferent phrenic nerve activity; 4, integrated neurogram of right hypoglossal nerve efferent activity. A: after transection of the brain stem at the
pontobulbar junction in a cat whose vagosympathetic nerve
trunks and the carotid sinus nerves were cut bilaterally. B:
after additional transection of the neuraxis at the bulbo-
spinal junction and 9 min after 4.10% CO_2 inhalation for
15 min. Calibration, vertical bars in the right-hand side of
the tracings 1,2 and 3 indicate 100 uV. Values of various
factors related to experimental conditions in A: end-tidal
O_2 level=15.8%, end-tidal CO_2 level=2.79%; Pao_2=96% of
the control value (100%) before transections; medullary
tissue Po_2 as measured by a polarographic technique=79%
of the control (100%); arterial blood pressure=65 mmHg;
2.79%, 65 mmHg; in B: 18.5%, 4.50%, 53%, 51%, 72
mmHg, respectively. Note the persistence of spontaneous
rhythmic discharges of the bulbar inspiratory neuron and
the hypoglossal nerve similar to that of control and of a
normal character, not a gasping type activity in A and B,
and the disappearance of the phrenic rhythmic discharge in
the same time in B. For further explanations, see text. C:
autocorrelation analysis of spontaneous activities recorded
simultaneously from the facial (VII), hypoglossal (XII), and
phrenic (PH) nerves in a anesthetized, paralyzed and artificially ventilated cat in the course of transections of
the neuroaxis. The autocorrelograms in 1 (a, d, g) were
obtained after cutting the vagosympathetic trunks and the
carotid sinus nerves bilaterally. Those in 2 (b, e, h) represent results obtained during 6.50% CO_2 in O_2 inhalation
after transection of the brain stem in the rostral medulla
at a level caudal to the lowermost border of the Boet-

zinger complex. Note the persistent rhythm which seems to be synchronized periodic fluctuations in both the hypoglossal (e) and phrenic nerve activities (h). 3 (c, f, i) represents results obtained during 4.10% CO_2 in O_2 inhalation after the additional neuroaxis transection at the bulbo-spinal junction. Note that the periodic fluctuation of the value of autocorrelation function which means the existence of rhythmic activity in the nerve discharges is solely maintained in the hypoglossal nerve activity (f) in 3 of C. The ordinates indicate the autocorrelation function in relative units and one division on the time axis of the abscissae represents 900 ms (Hukuhara Jr., 1976).

Conditions for Occurrence of Patterns of Apneusis, Apneustic Breathing and Gasping in the Isolated Medulla. In some cases after a lapse of time after brain stem transection the phrenic and hypoglossal nerve discharges had altered spontaneously to an apneustic breathing pattern, but not the facial nerve activity. Then the phrenic and hypoglossal nerve activity changed into a gasping pattern following by cessation of the discharge as the arterial and bulbar tissue Po_2 lowered below ca. 50% of the value before transection. On the basis of these evidences it is very likely that each of the apneusis, apneustic breathing pattern and the gasping pattern (Cohen, 1979; Euler, 1986; Wyss, 1964) is not a definite breathing pattern being produced on the basis of the activity of the classical subcenters such as the apneustic and the gasping center, but rather they are a transient activity patterns representing each step of graded changes of the level of the overall activity of the respiratory neuronal network in correspondence to the particular functional state of the central respiratory mechanisms (Hukuhara et al., 1951; Hukuhara Jr., 1973, 1976, 1988).

Changes of Cranial Nerve Activity before and after Neuroaxis Transection at Pontobulbar and Bulbo-spinal Junction (Hukuhara Jr., 1976)

Changes of these spontaneous respiratory activities of the cranial-facial and hypoglossal nerves and the phrenic nerve activity with simultaneous recording were investigated before and after brain stem transection at the level of the pontobulbar Fig. 2C, 2) and additional bulbospinal (Fig. 2C, 3) junction. As shown in Fig. 2C, the rhythmic burst in the facial nerve activity was abolished after the pontobulbar junction transection (b in Fig. 2C), whereas the respiratory discharges in the phrenic and hypoglossal nerve activity were maintained (d, e in Fig. 2C). Subsequent transection at bulbo-spinal junction abolished phrenic rhythmic discharges, while hypoglossal rhythmic activity continued (f in Fig. 2C). This evidences support the fact that there exists a dominant nature with respect to the spontaneity of the respiratory rhythm originating in the bulbar mechanisms within the bulbar compartment of the respiratory neuronal network over other rhythms which are displayed in the presumed oscillatory circuitry in the pons (Cohen, 1979) and in the ponto-bulbar respiratory complex (Euler, 1986). Based on this evidence it would be proposed that there exists an hierarchical functional organization between the respiratory neurons in the bulbar, pontine and spinal cord compartment of the respiratory neuronal network as far as the primary.

Correlation between Correlation Coefficient of Autocorrelation (CC) and Coefficient of Variation (CV) (Fig. 3a). The relation between the CC of autocorrelation and CV for the period of the volley for a total of 172 respiratory units (bulbar 159, pontine 13). There was a significant correlation (r=-0.48, P<0.001, Y= -0.03X+0.70) between the two variables. The coefficient of variation for the period of the phrenic burst discharges in 85 rabbits ranged from 0.9 to 9.1% and the mean with standard deviation of CV was 3.0±1.6% with the 99% confidence interval from 2.5% to 3.5%. The correlation coefficients of autocorrelation of the phrenic nerve activity in these 85 experiments ranged from 0.51 to 0.96 giving the mean and the standard deviation of 0.80±0.09 with the 99% confidence interval from 0.78 to 0.82. Four bulbar inspiratory and five bulbar expiratory neurons were spontaneously discharging stably with a CV for the period in a range from 1.3% to 2.1% smaller than the lower limit of the 99% confidence interval of the phrenic CV for the volley period of 2.5% indicated by the vertical broken line in Fig. A, while their CCs of autocorrelation ranging from 0.83 to 0.94 were larger than the upper limit of the 99% confidence interval of the phrenic CC of 0.82 indicated by the horizontal broken line in Fig. A. These inspiratory and expiratory neurons discharging stably were located in the nucleus reticularis parvocellularis or subnucleus reticularis ventralis medullae oblongatae (Hukuhara Jr. et al., 1981; Hukuhara Jr., 1988).

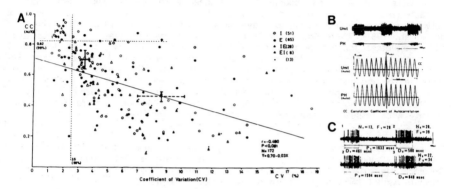

Fig. 3. Correlation diagram (A) and identification of respiratory unitary discharge in terms of its temporal stability (B and C). A: correlation diagram between correlation coefficient of autocorrelation of pulse-density (CC) of respiratory unitary discharges (ordinate) and coefficient of variation (CV=100·SD/Mean) for the volley period of respiratory unit activity in the course of 7-10 consecutive respiratory cycles (abscissa) in the bulbar and pontine reticular formations in anesthetized, vagotomized, paralyzed and artificially ventilated rabbits. Each symbol represents a respiratory unit displaying periodic burst discharges: open circle, inspiratory; Filled circle, expiratory; open triangle, inspiratory-expiratory phase-spanning; filled triangle, expiratory-inspiratory phase-spanning; asterisk, pontine unit. Note that nine respiratory units (1-9 in A in the upper, left part) among 172 units are discharging constantly with a small coefficient of variation (CV) and a large autocorrelation coefficient (CC). B: identification of a inspiratory unit activity by means of quantitative measurement of its temporal stability. Unit, a bulbar inspiratory unit activity; PH, phrenic nerve discharge; unit (Auto), autocorrelogram of unit; PH (Auto), autocorrelogram of PH. The ordinate of autocorrelograms indicates the autocorrelation function and the abscissa is time axis. C: variability of a bulbar expiratory unit activity in the course of two respiratory cycles. The first and last spike in volley numbered from 1 to 3 are each indicated by a short vertical line. Ni, number of spikes in volley; Fi, mean frequency in volley; Pi, period of volley; Di, duration of volley. Note the remarkable fluctuation in the four variables (Hukuhara Jr. et al., 1981).

18   T. Hukuhara, Jr.

Localization and Discharge Type of Respiratory Neurons Discharging with High
Stability

Stably discharging inspiratory and expiratory neurons having a small CV for the volley period and a large CC of autocorrelation were found in the bulbar reticular
formation, but not in corresponding areas in the medulla described as the high density regions in cats and in pontine structures. This fact is not contradictory to and
in accordance with the results of previous experiments obtained by brain stem transection techniques (Fig. 2).

The neuronal network for the central respiratory mechanisms may involve the
primary respiratory neuron population as a neuronal functional subsystem which is
characterized in its specified relations to the rhythmogenesis within the neuronal
network of the central respiratory mechanisms (Hukuhara Jr., 1973, 1988; Hukuhara
Jr. et al., 1981). These stably discharging inspiratory neurons may be the most possible candidates for the primary neurons. Thus, the respiratory neurons, inspiratory
and expiratory, which are discharging stably with a large correlation coefficient of
autocorrelation and a small coefficient of variation for the volley period, and are
found in the medullary reticular formation, may play an essential role as the members of primary respiratory neuron population in generating the respiratory rhythm
in the lateral region of the medullary reticular formation preferentially taking
priority with respect to spontaneity of respiratory periodicity.

Reviewed research from this department was partly supported by the Ministry of
Education, Science and Culture, Japan, Grant-in-Aid for Developmental Scientific
Research No. 01870012 and by the Science Research Promotion Foundation, Japan,
Grant-in-Aid of the Science Research Promotion Fund 1988.

The valuable help given by Miss Takako Sato in the preparation of the manuscript
is gratefully acknowledged.

        REFERENCES

Cohen, M. I. (1979). Neurogenesis of respiratory rhythm in the mammal. Physiol.
   Rev., 59, 1105-1173.
Euler, C. von (1986). Brain stem mechanisms for generation and control of breath-
   ing pattern. In: Hdb. Physiol. (A.P. Fishman et al., eds.), Sect. 3, Vol.II, Part I,
   Amer. Physiol. Soc., pp. 1-67. Bethesda.
Hukuhara, T., Jr. (1973). Neuronal organization of the central respiratory
   mechanisms in the brain stem of the cat. Acta Neurobiol. Exp., 33, 19-244. War-
   saw.
Hukuhara, T., Jr. (1976). Functional organization of brain stem respiratory neurons
   and its modulation induced by afferences. In: Coll Inst Nat'l Sante Rech Med. (E.
   Duron, ed.), Vol. 59, pp. 49-53. INSERM, Paris.
Hukuhara, T., Jr. (1988). Organization of the brain stem neural mechanisms for
   generation of respiratory rhythm - Current problems.Jpn. J. Physiol., 38, 753-776.
Hukuhara, T., T. Sumi and H. Okada (1954). Action potentials in the normal
   respiratory centers and its centrifugal pathway in the medulla oblongata and spinal
   cord. Jpn. J. Physiol., 4, 145-153.
Hukuhara, T., S. Nakayama, S. Baba and T. Odanaka (1951). On the localization of
   the respiratory center. Jpn. J. Physiol., 2, 44-49.
Hukuhara, T., Jr., K. Goto, K. Takano and Y. Hattanmaru (1981). Localization and
   functional organization of bulbar and pontine respiratory neurons in the rabbit. In:
   Advances in Physiol. Sci., 10, 579-586.
Wyss, O. A. M. (1964). Die nervoese Steuerung der Atmung. Ergeb. Physiol., 54, 1-
   398.

Chemosensitivity of Medullary Neurons in Tissue Cultures

J.A. Neubauer, W. Chou, S. Gonsalves,
G. Sterbenz, H.M. Geller and N.H. Edelman

Division of Pulmonary and Critical Care Medicine,
Department of Medicine, and Department of
Pharmacology, University of Medicine and Dentistry of
New Jersey-Robert Wood Johnson Medical School, New
Brunswick, New Jersey, USA

ABSTRACT

Although it is generally accepted that structures near the surface of the ventral medulla function as respiratory chemoreceptors, the nature of the stimulus
(fixed acid versus CO_2), the site of chemosensitivity (extracellular versus
intracellular), and whether chemosensitivity is a function of a few unique cells
remains unelucidated. In order to examine these questions, we have prepared two
reduced medullary neuronal preparations (tissue explants and dissociated cell
cultures) and have determined that chemosensitivity is retained in culture.
Further, we have found that ventral medullary neurons in culture respond only
to CO_2 and not fixed acid and that neurons cultured from the dorsal medulla
also respond to changes in CO_2. In addition, since a previous study had
demonstrated that carbonic anhydrase may be dynamically involved in CO_2
transduction (Mishra et al., 1985) and that carbonic anhydrase is present in
sensory neurons of peripheral ganglia (Riley et al., 1984; Wang et al., 1983),
we tested whether the neurons from the chemosensitive areas contain carbonic
anhydrase using immunocytochemistry in dissociated cell cultures of ventral
medulla. To determine whether the presence of carbonic anhydrase is unique
to the ventral medulla, we examined other brain regions (dorsal medulla, cortex and hypothalamus) for the presence of neuronal carbonic anhydrase. Immunocytochemical studies in dissociated cultures indicated that a small population
of neurons cultured from the chemosensitive regions of the ventral medulla
contain carbonic anhydrase. However, carbonic anhydrase was found in neurons
cultured from all regions with the largest percentage in the anterior hypothalamus. The presence of carbonic anhydrase in about 25% of the ventral
medullary neurons suggests that only a subpopulation of the cultured neurons
are responsible for the central respiratory activity. The presence of carbonic
anhydrase in subpopulations of neurons in other CNS regions suggests that CO_2
chemosensitivity may be a more distributed neuronal function within the CNS,
which may or may not be important in respiratory responses.

KEYWORDS

Chemosensitivity; in vitro; extracellular recordings; carbonic anhydrase II,
neurons; immunocytochemistry.

The majority of central nervous system neurons respond to extracellular acidosis
with membrane hyperpolarization and a reduction in excitability. However, classical respiratory physiology has shown that there exists a unique subset of
neurons which are excited by hypercapnia and which participate in exciting the
central respiratory neurons. These neurons have been shown experimentally to
reside in the ventral medulla but can not be ascribed to a discrete nucleus.
In addition, in vivo studies (Eldridge et al., 1985; Shams, 1985; Teppema et
al., 1983) and in vitro tissue slice studies (Fukuda, 1983) have demonstrated
a differential sensitivity to equal extracellular pH changes induced by CO_2
versus fixed acid with a greater response to CO_2 induced pH changes. The
mechanism of signal transduction for acid sensitivity has remained elusive
in terms of the particular stimulus sensed (CO_2, HCO_3^-, or H^+), the site
of sensitivity (extracellular versus intracellular), and in regards to whether
it is an intrinsic function of a few unique cells or requires a synaptically
intact network.

Some of the earliest work of chemosensitive cells in vitro was done by Fukuda
(1983) using a tissue slice preparation of the medulla. He found evidence of
cells which responded to CO_2 and not HCO_3^- as well as cells which
responded to HCO_3^- and not CO_2. We sought to examine the mechanisms of
chemosensitivity in even more reduced preparations and thus we have adapted
tissue culture and cell culture preparations which have been used successfully
to characterize the electrophysiology and pharmacology of warm and cold temperature sensitive neurons in the hypothalamus (Baldino and Geller, 1982).
The first of these was to utilize the technique of tissue culture by preparing
primary tissue cultures of medullary explants and determining whether these
explants contain spontaneously active neurons which alter their firing frequency
with reductions in extracellular pH and whether these cells exhibit differential
sensitivity to CO_2 and fixed acid. To determine whether "chemosensitivity" in
culture is specific to the ventral medulla, we characterized the pH responses of
both the ventral and dorsal medullary neurons in explant cultures.

Tissue explant cultures of the ventral and dorsal medulla were prepared from
the medullas of one-day old neonatal rats from regions dissected from either
the ventrolateral surface or from the dorsal medulla corresponding as closely
as possible to the region of the nucleus tractus solitarius. The tissue sections were minced and placed on collagen-coated plastic coverslips. These
coverslips were placed in culture tubes with supplemented culture medium and
incubated at 37°C with 5% CO_2. After allowing 24 hours for adhesion, the
cultures were rotated for 2 to 3 weeks.

Neurons in these roller-tube cultures survive for up to several months and
exhibit a pattern of thinning, from several cell layers to just a few cells
deep, as the cells migrate away from the original explant site. After the
cultures thinned out sufficiently for individual neurons to be observed under
phase contrast optics, the cultures were placed in a recording chamber, superfused with mock CSF and temperature maintained at a constant 37°C. The pH in
the chamber and the spontaneous action potentials, recorded extracellularly,
were continuously monitored. To characterize the neuronal response to changes
in extracellular pH, the pH of the superfusate was varied either by changing
PCO_2 at constant HCO_3^- or by changing HCO_3^- at constant PCO_2.

A representative response of a spontaneously active ventral medullary neuron
which was excited by a decrease in extracellular pH by varying the PCO_2 is
shown in Fig. 1. This cell increased its spontaneous spike activity from an
average of 3 Hz to 6 Hz when pH was lowered 0.4 pH units. The response to CO_2
was determined in 27 spontaneously active ventral medullary neurons. Of these,
10 demonstrated an increase in firing frequency. In contrast, 15 of the ventral
medullary neurons decreased their spontaneous firing frequency when the pH was
lowered with CO_2 and two neurons had firing frequencies which were unaffected
by CO_2.

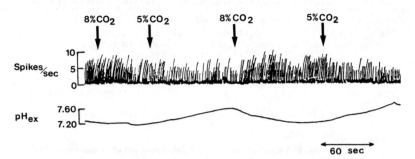

Fig. 1. CO_2 response of integrated spike activity in a spontaneously active ventral medullary neuron in explant culture.

Neurons cultured from the dorsal medulla also responded to pH changes induced
with CO_2, with either excitation or depression of their spontaneous firing
frequency. Figure 2 illustrates the CO_2 response of two dorsal medullary
cells. In Fig. 2A, increasing CO_2 of the perfusate resulted in an increase in
the firing frequency and was associated with a nearly continuous firing pattern.
In contrast, the cell shown in Fig. 2B was depressed at higher CO_2 levels and
stimulated when the pH was reduced by lowering CO_2. In addition, note that
the pattern of activity of this cell was also CO_2 dependent, firing with a
bursting pattern with the decrease in CO_2. This bursting pattern of activity
was a very typical pattern of activity in dorsal medullary neurons being
demonstrable in 12 out of 23 spontaneously active neurons cultured from the
dorsal medulla. These cells had a wide range of burst durations and cycling
times with the mean duration of the burst activity about 0.8+0.1 min and the
mean cycle time of 1.7+0.4 min. In addition, in some of these neurons, there
was a persistence of the bursting activity after synaptic transmission was
blocked with a low Ca++-high Mg++ perfusate suggesting that the spontaneous
activity was an intrinsic function of some of these cells.

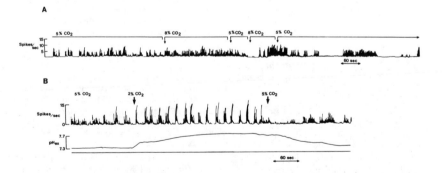

Fig. 2. CO_2 responses of integrated spike activity in spontaneously active dorsal medullary neurons in explant cultures. (A) illustrates a neuron which increased its
spike activity with increased CO_2; (B) demonstrates a
neuron which was depressed by increased CO_2.

Figure 3 illustrates the effect of altering the extracellular HCO3$^-$ on the
spontaneous activity of a ventral medullary neuron in 3A, and two dorsal
medullary neurons, in 3B a non-bursting neuron and in 3C a bursting dorsal
medullary neuron. Although spontaneously active neurons from both ventral and
dorsal medulla tissue cultures responded to changes in extracellular pH induced
with CO_2, changing the HCO3$^-$ of the perfusate had no consistent effect on
the amount of spontaneous neuronal activity in either the ventral or dorsal
medulla.

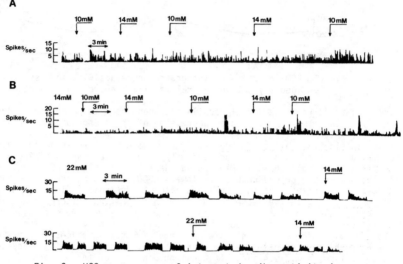

Fig. 3.   HCO3$^-$ responses of integrated spike activity in
          spontaneously active medullary neurons cultured
          from ventral medulla (A) and dorsal medulla (B&C).

Thus, the extracellular recordings in these organotypic cultures revealed that
chemosensitive neurons are present in both ventral and dorsal medulla and that
these cells only responded to changes in pH induced with CO_2 with about 30% of
neurons exhibiting excitation. The observation that chemosensitive neurons were
found in both ventral and dorsal medulla cultures suggests that chemosensitivity
may be a distributed function within the medulla.

We have begun some studies to determine whether isolated neurons in dissociated
cell cultures also retain the function of chemosensitivity with the eventual aim
to characterize the cellular mechanisms responsible for acid sensitivity. Cultures were prepared from 1-2 day old neonatal rats. The minced tissue was subjected to gentle enzymatic treatment by incubation with trypsin and collagenase
for 20 minutes at 37°C. Cells were then dispersed mechanically by trituration.
Cells were plated on either polylysine or astrocyte coated coverslips and incubated at 37°C and 5% CO_2 in a supplemented DMEM culture medium. After 1-3
weeks in culture spontaneous neuronal activity was measured using the loose-cell
patch recording technique (Hamill et al., 1981). This technique yields a very
high-resolution extracellular recording. Preliminary studies on spontaneously
active neurons have shown that neurons dissociated in this manner retain the
sensory property of chemosensitivity. Figure 4 illustrates the response of
ventral medullary neurons cultured from the chemosensitive regions to CO_2
induced changes in the extracellular pH of the superfusate. The firing rate of
the neuron in (A) was inversely proportional to extracellular pH, being greatest
(1.7+0.2 Hz) when pH was lowest (7.4) and least (0.5+0.1 Hz) when pH was highest
(7.67). In contrast, the firing rate of the neuron in (B) was proportional to

extracellular pH with a firing rate of 0.4+0.04 Hz at low pH and increasing to
1.2+0.2 Hz when pH was higher. Thus, analogous to spontaneous active neurons
in tissue explant cultures, neurons in dissociated cell cultures exhibit the
characteristics of both acid excitation and acid depression. Currently we have
examined the CO_2 response of 8 spontaneously active neurons and found that 2
of these increase and 4 decrease their firing rates with a decrease in the
extracellular pH.

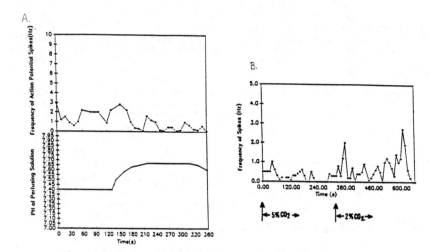

Fig. 4. CO_2 responses of spontaneously active neurons in
          dissociated ventral medullary cultures. The neuron
          in (A) increased its mean frequency of action poten-
          tials when pH was decreased (CO_2 excited) while the
          neuron in (B) increased its mean frequency of firing
          when pH was increased (CO_2 depressed).

We thought that we could explore the suggestion of a distributed CO_2 sensitivity if we could further characterize chemosensitive neurons by identifying
specific markers. Based on our previous work which suggested that carbonic
anhydrase was dynamically involved in the respiratory response to CO_2, carbonic anhydrase was one possible marker for chemosensitive neurons. Although
it was generally thought that carbonic anhydrase is not present in CNS neurons,
subsequent work from several groups including those of Riley et al. (1984) and
Wong et al. (1983) have shown that while carbonic anhydrase is not present in
peripheral motor neurons, it is present in the sensory neurons of peripheral
ganglia. Thus, we hypothesized that sensory neurons involved in chemosensitivity contain carbonic anhydrase. Since previous histochemical techniques in tissue slices had failed to identify carbonic anhydrase in CNS neurons primarily
because of the very high background level of carbonic anhydrase in oligodendro-
cytes, we used the dissociated cell culture technique to enhance the sensitivity
of the immunocytochemical methods since culturing in this manner results in the
growth of isolated neurons on a principally astrocytic substratum. In addition,
we were again interested in whether the presence of carbonic anhydrase in
neurons would be specific to the ventral medulla or whether it is present in
the dorsal medulla or other brain regions.

Dissociated cell cultures of the ventral and dorsal medulla, the premotor cortex, the hypothalamus, optic nerve and the dorsal root ganglia were prepared
from one-day old rat pups as described above. Cultures of optic nerve and
dorsal root ganglia were prepared to serve as positive controls for CNS oligo-
dendrocytes from optic nerves and peripheral sensory neurons from dorsal root
ganglia. After 1-3 weeks in culture, the coverslips were stained for the
presence of carbonic anhydrase. In addition, neurons were identified by
staining for the presence of phosphorylated neurofilament using the specific
polyclonal antibody RT97.

Staining was accomplished using an immunocytochemical peroxidase anti-peroxidase
technique. Cultures were fixed and permeabilized. Cultures were then incubated
with a blocking buffer of 5% normal goat serum. The primary antibody of carbonic anhydrase II or RT97 was applied for 12-18 hours. After incubation with
a biotinylated secondary antibody, the conjugate, avidin-horseradish peroxidase,
was applied and the peroxidase reaction product was visualized by using DAB and
hydrogen peroxide.

Immunocytochemical staining for carbonic anhydrase in dissociated cell cultures
of the ventral medulla revealed the presence of neurons in this region which
stained intensely for carbonic anhydrase. Although only 25% of the ventral
medullary neurons stained for carbonic anhydrase, if these neurons are the
chemosensitive cells, this observation would be consistent with the percentage
of chemosensitive neurons reported by Pokorski (1976). In addition to the
positive staining in the ventral medulla, neurons in the dorsal medulla also
stained for carbonic anhydrase. However, again most of the dorsal medullary
neurons did not stain positive for carbonic anhydrase with only 18% of the
dorsal medullary neurons staining positive. A slightly greater percentage of
cortical neurons (35%) stained positive for carbonic anhydrase; however, this
staining tended to be less intense than the staining in the medulla. The
greatest amount of neuronal staining that we observed was in the hypothalamus
with 60% of the hypothalamic neurons staining positive for carbonic anhydrase.
This large degree of carbonic anhydrase positive neurons may be consistent with
both its sensory functions and its apparent activation with changes in CO_2
which has been shown by Tamaki and his co-workers (1986).

In summary, we feel that in using these two reduced models to study "chemosensitivity" that we have shown evidence suggesting that chemosensitivity is probably
not unique to the ventral medulla and the respiratory system and may very well
be a distributed CNS function, that extracellular acidosis induced by fixed acid
may not be a chemosensitive stimulus, and that with this very first demonstration of carbonic anhydrase in CNS neurons that this enzyme may play a role in
setting up or maintaining pH gradients in CO_2 sensitive neurons distributed
throughout the CNS.

REFERENCES

Baldino, F. Jr. and H.M. Geller (1982). Electrophysiological analysis of
   neuronal thermosensitivity in rat preoptic and hypothalamic tissue cultures.
   J. Physiol. (London), 327, 173-184.
Eldridge, F.L., J.P. Kiley and D.E. Millhorn (1985). Respiratory responses to
   medullary hydrogen ion in cats: different effects of respiratory and metabolic
   acidosis. J. Physiol. (London), 358, 258-297.
Fukuda, Y. (1983). Difference between actions of high PCO_2 and low HCO_3 on
   neurons in the rat medullary chemosensitive areas in vitro. Plugers Arch.,
   398, 324-330.
Hamill, O.P., A. Marty, E. Neher, B. Sakmann and F.J. Sigworth (1981). Improved
   patch-clamp techniques for high-resolution current recordings from cells and
   cell-free membrane patches. Pflugers Arch., 391, 85-100.

Mishra, J., J.A. Neubauer, J.K-J. Li and N.H. Edelman (1985). Relationship of the dynamic characteristics of ventral medullary (Vm) pH and respiratory center output during CO_2 forcing. Fed. Proc., 44, 1583.
Pokorski, M. (1976). Neurophysiological studies on central chemosensor in medullary ventrolateral areas. Am. J. Physiol., 230, 1288-1295.
Riley, D.A., S. Ellis and J.L.W. Bain (1984). Ultrastructural cytochemical localization of carbonic anhydrase activity in rat peripheral sensory and motor nerves, dorsal root ganglia and dorsal column nuclei. Neuroscience, 13, 189-206.
Shams, H. (1985). Differential effects of CO_2 and H+ as central stimuli of respiration in the cat. J. Appl. Physiol., 58, 357-364.
Tamaki, Y., T. Nakayama and K. Matsumura (1986). Effects of carbon dioxide inhalation on preoptic thermosensitive neurons. Pflugers Arch., 407, 8-13.
Teppema, L.J., P.W.J.A. Barts, H.Th. Folgering and J.A.M. Evers (1983). Effects of respiratory and (isocapnic) metabolic arterial acid-base disturbances on medullary extracellular fluid pH and ventilation in cats. Respir. Physiol., 53, 379-395.
Wong, V., C.P. Barrett, E.J. Donati, L.F. Eng and L. Guth (1983). Carbonic anhydrase activity in first-order sensory neurons of the rat. J. Histochem. Cytochem., 31, 293-300.

Central Chemosensitivity

M.E. Schlaefke

Department of Applied Physiology, Ruhr-University
Bochum, D-4630 Bochum 1, Germany

ABSTRACT

The mechanism: The central pH sensitive mechanism as an important respiratory drive is responsible for the precision of central acid base homeostasis. The mechanism is of cholinergic nature, and according to our present
knowledge not the specialization of one neuronal element but a complex
system making use of various appropriate morphological, physico-chemical,
neurophysiological and neurochemical specificities within the ventral region of the medulla oblongata. Tonically firing neurons within the surface
layer respond to changes of pH in blood and extracellular fluid, others
respond to chemical as well as to different unspecific stimuli. Pathophysiology: With the loss of the central chemosensitive drive the rhythm
generator is dependent upon peripheral chemoreceptors, the function of
which involves the ascending reticular activating system. In Ondine's
Curse Syndrome the rise of the peripheral chemoreceptor threshold during
sleep causes excessive increases of pCO_2 with highest values during
NREM-sleep, aggravating the hypoxemia and resulting in life threatening
events. This pathomechanism also seems to play a role in certain forms of
sudden infant death. A therapeutic approach: Taking into consideration the
danger of hypoxic damage, continuous measurement of oxygen saturation was
used for a feed back to support the critically reduced peripheral chemoreceptor function during sleep. In case the saturation fell below a
threshold value, paired stimulation in combination with oxygen supply was
triggered. A reset of the peripheral chemoreceptor threshold was observed.
Whether the central chemosensitive mechanism may recover by training or
whether the central processing of chemoreceptor input may become optimized
during sleep by the described manoeuver is still an open question.

KEYWORDS

central chemosensitivity; Ondine's Curse Syndrome; Sudden Infant Death
Syndrome; plasticity; chemoreceptor threshold; conditioning.

INTRODUCTION

The central chemosensitive mechanism challenges respiratory physiologists throughout our century. The concept developed by Winterstein and continued by Loeschcke was established by physico-chemical, respiratory, neurophysiological, and morphological data as well as by a mathematical model. At present this concept is useful to interprete clinical observations in patients with central respiratory disorders and Ondine's Curse Syndrome, it suggests experimental therapeutic approaches, and provides us with a model for the Sudden Infant Death Syndrome.

THE MECHANISM

Winterstein (1911) assumed that pO_2 and pCO_2 act by a single mechanism, and assumed the common denominator to be the hydrogen ion, either dissociated from carbonic acid or from acids formed during oxygen deficiency. After the discovery of the carotid and aortic glomera, Winterstein reformulated his reaction theory accepting that peripheral and central chemoreceptors had to be considered separately. The central chemoreceptor is not sensitive to hypoxia. The question now is restricted to the alternatives that hydrogen ion or molecular CO_2 is the adequate stimulus. Experimental and theoretical approaches took into consideration a unique pH sensitive receptor which would be able to signalize both the respiratory and the metabolic acidosis (Loeschcke, 1982).

Today pH can be measured directly, either within the tissue of the brain or on the surface, e.g. within the H^+ sensitive areas. The noninvasive technique is based on the observation that there is free access to the glass electrode from the intercellular compartment (Dermietzel, 1976). The time course of ventilation and of brain extracellular pH using the surface technique followed step-changes of inspired CO_2 (Ahmad and Loeschcke, 1982). The tidal volume especially after denervation of the peripheral chemoreceptors followed closely the pH. Tidal volume and pH measured on the cortical surface, however, were unrelated. Loeschcke's theory claims the 'receptor' in the brain tissue responding to H^+-ions (Loeschcke, 1982). The local extracellular pH is only partly under the influence of the CSF because the tissue is perfused by the blood. Loeschcke assumes that the local pCO_2 is determined by local metabolism, CO_2 binding capacity of the blood, blood flow and the distance to the capillaries. The average tissue pCO_2 in the brain under steady state conditions has been proposed as the algebraic means of venous and arterial pCO_2 of cerebral blood plus 1 Torr (Ponten and Siesjö, 1966). Bicarbonate in response to acid-base changes in CSF varies by only 40 % as much as in blood plasma (Fencl, 1971; Pappenheimer et al., 1965). The HCO_3^- exchange between blood and brain is a fast process occurring simultaneously with an exchange of Cl^- in the opposite direction. (Ahmad and Loeschcke, 1982). The exchange possibly uses a protein carrier through an anion exchange channel of the endothelium of the brain capillaries (Wieth et al., 1980). When CO_2 is inhaled the increase of bicarbonate concentration in ECF is greater than in blood plasma, even if the plasma bicarbonate is kept constant. Ahmad and Loeschcke (1982) demonstrated, that HCO_3^- in this case is exchanged for Cl^- in a one to one fashion between ECF and cells. Extracellular pH depends on the two types of anion exchange between plasma and endothelium and through endothelium to the extracellular fluid and between cells and extracellular fluid. In the ECF five compartments, namely red cells, plasma, endothelium, extracellular fluid, and glia cells must be considered for the pH kinetics. This is true for metabolic as well as respiratory acidosis.

A mathematical model made use of the bicarbonate relation between plasma and CSF (Middendorf and Loeschcke, 1976). Hereby was shown that the ventilatory response to respiratory acidosis is much higher than that to metabolic acidosis. The increase of ventilation, however, is more effective in

regulating blood pH in metabolic than in respiratory acidosis (Middendorf and Loeschcke, 1978).
The responsible chemosensitive site for the respiratory system has been localized within the superficial tissue layer of the ventral medullary surface (reviewed by Schlaefke, 1981). Tonically firing neurones within the ventral medullary areas (rostral, intermediate (S) and caudal) change their frequency in correspondence to the pH measured on the ventral medullary surface, whether pH is varied by local superfusion of artificial cerebrospinal fluid (fig. 1), by inhalation of CO_2 or by injection of fixed acid (reviewed by Schlaefke, 1981).

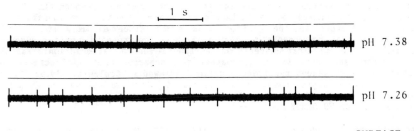

SURFACE pH

Fig. 1: Extracellular recording of a neuron within the superficial tissue of area S during variation of surface pH by local superfusion of artificial CSF. pH is measured on the surface.

Blood flow of the ventrolateral surface is CO_2- sensitive as well, and this more than the blood flow in the adjacent white matter (Feustel et al., 1984).

In vitro and in vivo experiments with cholinergic drugs on the ventral surface and on H^+ sensitive neurons within the superficial layer resulted in the following conclusion: The chemosensitive mechanism uses cholinergic synapses on which H^+ ions act like acetylcholine (ACh) and can be replaced by it. Blockade is possible by mecamylamine, atropine and partly also by hexamethonium, which suggests the presence of both muscarinic and nicotinic receptors (Fukuda and Loeschcke, 1979; Dev and Loeschcke, 1979). The topical distribution of ACh showed two peaks of maximal effect coinciding with the reactions to hydrogen ions. Also nicotine was found to mimic the effect of ACh and physostigmine enhanced its action. The presence of atropine inhibits the ventilatory effect of CSF acidosis and local application of atropine counteracts the stimulating effect of progesterone (Burton et al., 1989; Tok and Loeschcke, 1981). Yamada et al. (1982) localized GABA receptors with respiratory and cardiovascular functions within the intermediate area. GABA acts on ventral medullary structures especially in relation to inhibitory functions of the sympathetic activity (Mc Gall and Humphrey, 1985; Keeler et al., 1984; Ruggiero et al., 1985). Cholinoceptive and nicotinoceptive neurons have been mapped systematically (Willenberg et al., 1985). Further neuropeptides and ß-endorphine positive cells were localized within the chemosensitive fields. There were also detected vasoactive intestinal peptide, substance P and somatostatin (Leibstein et al., 1985).

Errington and Dashwood (1979) traced interconnections between the ventral medullary surface and the NTS as well as with the dorsal nucleus of the vagus using horseradish peroxidase. Latencies of 5 – 15 ms were recorded from neurons within the NTS when the caudal area was stimulated (Davies and Loeschcke, 1977). Procaine on the ventral surface was followed by a decrease of the neuronal activity of inspiratory, expiratory and reticular neurons, some nonrespiratory neurons were activated (Schwanghart et al., 1974). Peskow and Piatin (1976) recorded complete cessation of inspiratory activity, brought about by cold block of the intermediate area. The strongest inhibition was observed in the discharge of early and late inspiratory neurons. Expiratory neurons either became silent or continued to exhibit tonic firing with reduced impulse frequency. Functional interconnections between the Bötzinger complex regarding the influence on the respiratory rate and the respiratory motor output and the central chemosensitive mechanism seem to exist (Budzinska et al., 1985). Tonically firing neurons within the paragigantocellular nucleus respond to H^+ as well as to peripheral nerve stimulation and to chemical stimulation of polymodal receptors in the gastrocnemius muscle (See et al., 1982). Cold block within the intermediate area abolishes the respiratory response to CO_2 and the respiratory effect of peripheral nerve stimulation. Further effects are an increase of sympathetic discharge, and an increase of hyperthermically induced respiratory drive (reviewed by Schlaefke, 1981).

PATHOPHYSIOLOGY

Complete loss of central chemosensitivity is the main symptom of patients suffering from the Ondine's Curse Syndrome. Reduced CO_2 responses have been observed in infants with an apparent life threatening event during the first month of life. Transiently reduced CO_2 responses were recorded in infants during the first year of life, which were evaluated as risk for the sudden infant death syndrome (Schlaefke et al., 1990). Symptomes like periodic breathing, insensitivity to CO_2, apneas, and irreversible respiratory and circulatory arrest by mild hypoxia were induced by superficial lesion of the intermediate area in chronic nonanaesthetized cats or by local application of glycine in acute experiments (Schlaefke, 1989). The peripheral chemoreceptors in the animal model guarantee the continuation of breathing (Schlaefke, 1981). These findings coincide with the observation that the ventral medullary superficial layer in victims of SIDS and Ondine's Curse Syndrome was impoverished of nerve cells compared with controls (Kille and Schlaefke, 1986).

In 14 infants, aged between 5 weeks and 12 years, we found complete insensitivity to CO_2 measured during NREM-sleep or during sleep onset. The peripheral chemoreceptors were intact in these patients. The degree of respiratory acidosis varies with sleep phases and is severe in NREM- and less severe in REM-sleep. With sleep onset and in light NREM-sleep the peripheral chemoreflex initiated sighs down to a tcpO₂ of 19 mmHg improving the blood gas situation for a moment. This may occur several times. Deeper sleep phases with further increases of pCO₂ and hypoxia impede the performance of the peripheral chemoreceptor reflex and arousals. These dangerous phases in infants often remain undiscovered on behalf of 'normal' skin colour, absence of prolonged apneas and brady- or tachycardia, and may precede artificial ventilation during sleep and so contribute to the development of pulmonary hypertension in these patients.

A THERAPEUTIC APPROACH

In patients with Ondine's Curse Syndrome and in cats after elimination of the area S we trained the respiratory system during sleep combining unspecific and chemical respiratory stimuli in analogy to the classical conditioning. As trigger for the application of paired stimuli we used transcutaneous pulse oximetry. When the oxygen saturation fell under a

threshold of e.g. 91 % a computer started the paired stimuli: an unspecific stimulus of 1 s, e.g. sound, light, an air jet versus the mouth-nose
region, or electrical stimulation of the femoral nerve (2V, 20 Hz, 1 ms),
respectively. The first stimulus caused a 'respiratory arousal'. The
second stimulus was a 'specific' 1.5 s lasting chemical stimulus, O_2 or
1,5 % CO_2 in O_2 following the unspecific stimulus after a pause of 0.5 s.
The stimulation was interrupted as long as SaO_2 exceeded the trigger
threshold. To avoid a questioned respiratory muscle fatigue we generally
run periods of 20 minutes for training during sleep (Burghardt and
Schlaefke, 1986; Schlaefke et al., 1987; 1990).

Two 24-month-old boys with an Ondine's Curse Syndrome had normal blood gas
values when awake, they were able to breathe spontaneously during sleep
but developed severe hypercapnia (100 mmHg) and hypoxemia (15 mmHg). They
did not respond to CO_2 but showed initial inhibition to hyperoxia. We used
a trigger threshold of SaO_2 of 91 %, an air jet and oxygen as paired
stimuli. In both infants already after a few minutes of training sighs as
a peripheral chemoreceptor response were observed shortly before the SaO_2
fell down and could trigger the next stimulation. Less stimuli were
necessary with time of training (fig. 2).

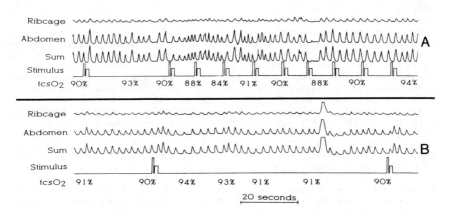

Fig. 2. Paired stimuli (air jet of 0.5 s to mouth-nose
        region followed by an increase of FIO_2 2 l/min
        for 1.5s) triggered by pulse oximetry (SaO_2 91%)
        during sleep of an Ondine's Curse patient 12
        months of age and the effect on ventilation
        (induction plethysmography). Start (A) and
        40 min after start of training (B).

The sequence of a general and a chemical respiratory stimulus seems to
improve the processing of the central respiratory apparatus during sleep
when the central acid base homeostate is lost. Whether this is obtained by
an optimization of peripheral chemoreceptor contribution, working as long
as the controller is not out of range, or by a convalescence of the central chemosensitive mechanism is still an open question. Spontaneous recovery of central chemosensitivity, however, we did never observe, either in
control studies with cats, nor in infants, in whom the respiratory
response to CO_2 was missing after birth as well as eight years later.

ACKNOWLEDGEMENTS

Supported   by   Ministerium   für   Wissenschaft   und   Forschung   NRW: IV
A6-40102187. In cooperation with Hellige GmbH, D-7800 Freiburg, FRG.

REFERENCES

Ahmad, H.R. and H.H. Loeschcke (1982). Transient and steady state response
of pulmonary ventilation to the medullary extracellular pH. *Pfluegers
Arch.*, *395*, 285-292.
Burghardt, F. and M.E. Schlaefke (1986). Loss of central chemosensitivity:
an animal model to overcome respiratory insufficiency. *J. Autonom. Nerv.
Syst. Suppl.*, 105-109.
Budzinska, K., C. von Euler, F.F. Kao, T. Pantaleo and Y. Yamamoto (1985).
Effects of graded focal cold block in rostral areas of the medulla. *Acta
Physiol. Scand.*, *124*, 329-340.
Davies, R.O. and H.H. Loeschcke (1977). Neural activity evoked by electri-
cal stimulation on the chemosensitive areas on the ventral medullary
surface. *Proc. IUPS*, *13*, 164.
Dermietzel, R. (1976). Central   chemosensitivity,   morphological   studies.
In: *Acid-base homeostasis of the brain extracellular fluid and the
respiratory control system.* (H.H. Loeschcke, ed.), pp. 52-66. Thieme,
Stuttgart.
Dev, N.B. and H.H. Loeschcke (1979). A cholinergic mechanism involved in
the respiratory chemosensitivity. *Pfluegers Arch.*, *379*, 29-36.
Fencl, V. (1971). Distribution of H^+ and HCO_3^- in cerebral fluids. In: *Ion
homeostasis of the brain.* (O.K. Siesjoe and S.C. Sorensen, eds), pp.
175-195. Munksgaard, Kopenhagen.
Feustel,   P.J.,   M.J.   Stafford,   J.S.   Allen   and   J.W.   Severinghaus   (1984).
Ventrolateral   medullary   surface   blood   flow   determined   by   hydrogen
clearance. *J. Appl. Physiol.*, *56*, 150-154.
Fukuda, Y. and H.H. Loeschcke (1979). A cholinergic mechanism involved in
the   neuronal   excitation   by H^+ in   the   respiratory   chemosensitive
structures of the ventral medulla oblongata of rats in vitro. *Pfluegers
Arch.*, *379*, 125-135.
Errington, M.L. and M.R. Dashwood (1979). Projections to the ventral
surface of the cat brain stem demonstrated by horseradish peroxidase.
Neurosci. Lett., *12*, 153-158.
Keeler, J.R., C.W. Shults, T.N. Chase and C.J. Helke (1984). The ventral
surface of the medulla in the rat: Pharmacologic and autoradiographic
localization of GABA induced cardiovascular effects. *Brain Res.*, *297*,
217-224.
Kille, J.F. and M.E. Schlaefke (1986). Do ventral medullary neurones
control the cardiorespiratory system in man? *Pfluegers Arch.*, *406*, R25.
Leibstein, A.G., I.M. Willenberg and R. Dermietzel (1981). Morphology of
the medullary chemosensitive fields. I. Mapping of the neuronal matrix
by a horseradish peroxidase technique. *Pfluegers Arch.*, *391*, 226-230.
Loeschcke, H.H. (1982). Central chemosensitivity and the reaction theory.
J. Physiol., *332*, 1-24.
Mc Gall, R.B. and S.J. Humphrey (1985). Evidence for GABA mediation of
sympathetic   inhibition   evoked   from   midline   medullary - depressor   sites.
Brain Res., *339*, 356-360.
Middendorf, T. and H.H. Loeschcke (1976). Mathematische Simulation des
Respirationssystems. *J. Math. Biol.*, *3*, 149-177.
Middendorf, T. and H.H. Loeschcke (1978). Cooperation of the peripheral
and central chemosensitive mechanisms in the control of the extracellu-
lar pH in brain in non-respiratory acidosis. *Pfluegers Arch.*, *375*,
257-260.

Pappenheimer, J.R., V. Fencl, S.R. Hasey and D. Held (1965). Role of cerebral fluids in the control of respiration as studied in unanaesthetized goats. *Am. J. Physiol., 208*, 436-450.

Peskow, B.J. and W.F. Piatin (1976). Reactions of neurons of the respiratory center to local cooling of the ventral surface of the medulla oblongata. *Sechenov Physiol. J., UDSSR, 62/7*.

Ponten, U. and B.K. Siesjö (1966). Gradients of CO_2 tension in the brain. *Acta Physiol. Scand., 67*, 129-140.

Ruggiero, D.A., M.P. Meeley, M. Anwar and D.J. Reis (1985). Newly identified GABAergic neurons in regions of the ventrolateral medulla which regulate blood pressure. *Brain Res., 339*, 171-177.

Schlaefke, M.E. (1981). Central chemosensitivity: A respiratory drive. *Rev. Physiol. Biochem. Pharmacol., 90*, 172-244.

Schlaefke, M.E. (1989). Plötzlicher Kindstod: Klinische Physiologie und Modelle. In: *Der plötzliche Kindstod* (W. Andler, M.E. Schlaefke and E. Trowitzsch, eds.), pp. 135-147. Acron, Berlin/New York.

Schlaefke, M.E. and F. Burghardt (1981). Training of central chemosensitivity in infants with sleep apnea. In: *Central neurone environment* (M.E. Schlaefke, H.P. Koepchen and W.R. See, eds.), pp. 74-81. Springer, Berlin Heidelberg.

Schlaefke, M.E., T. Schaefer, H. Kronberg, G.J. Ullrich and J. Hopmeier (1987). Transcutaneous monitoring as trigger for therapy of hypoxemia during sleep. *Adv. Exp. Med. Biol., 220*, 95-100.

Schlaefke, M.E., T. Schaefer, B. Nebel, D. Schaefer and C. Schaefer (1990). Development, disturbances, and training of respiratory regulation in infants. In: *Sleep and health risk* (J.H. Peter, T. Penzel and P. von Wichert, eds.). Springer, Berlin.

Schwanghart, F., R. Schroeter, D. Klüssendorf and H.P. Koepchen (1974). The influence of novocaine block of superficial brain stem structures on discharge pattern of specific respiratory and unspecific reticular neurons. In: *Central rhythmic and regulation* (W. Umbach and H.P. Koepchen, eds.), pp. 104-110. Hippokrates, Stuttgart.

See, W.R., T. Kumazawa and M.E. Schlaefke (1982). Modulation of neural activity in the central chemosensitive structures by peripheral nerve afferents. *Neurosci. Lett., 10*, S441.

Tok, T. and H.H. Loeschcke (1981). Untersuchung über die zentrale Wirkung von Progesteron auf die Atmung und Vasomotorik bei Katzen. *Z. Atemwegs- und Lungenkrankheiten, 7*, 148-153.

Wieth, J.O., J. Brahm and J. Funder (1980). Transport and interactions of anions and protons in the red blood cell membrane. *Ann. N.Y. Acad. Sci., 341*, 394-418.

Willenberg, I.M., R. Dermietzel, A.G. Leibstein and M. Effenberger (1985). Mapping of cholinoceptive (nicotinoceptive) neurones in the lower brain stem: with special reference to the ventral surface of the medulla. *J. Autonom. Nerv. Syst., 14*, 299-313.

Winterstein, H. (1911). Die Regulierung der Atmung durch das Blut. *Pfluegers Arch., 138*, 167-184.

Yamada, K.A., W.P. Norman, P. Hamosh and R.A. Gillis (1982). Medullary ventral surface GABA receptors affect respiratory and cardiovascular function. *Brain Res., 248*, 71-78.

Locations of Central Chemoreceptors

H. Arita and H. Yamabayashi

Institute of Basic Medical Sciences, University of
Tsukuba, Tsukuba, Ibaraki 305, and Department of
Medicine, Tokai University, Isehara, Kanagawa,
259-11 Japan

ABSTRACT

Locations of the central chemoreceptors have been evaluated in anesthetized or decerebrated, spontaneously breathing cats using three distinct experimental techniques: 1) extracellular recording of medullary reticular neurons with non-phasic discharges excited exclusively by stimulation of central chemoreceptors, 2) systematic search for medullary micro regions showing acidic shift of ECF pH during intravertebral arterial injection of CO_2-saturated saline, and 3) identification of H^+-sensitive cells by direct application of acidified mock CSF using micro pressure-ejection method; these cells are also found to be excited by transcapillary stimulation of the central chemoreceptors. All these results have indicated a possibility that pH-dependent central chemoreceptors, if any, would be located in two separate areas, i.e., in the ventrolateral medulla and in the dorsal medulla.

KEYWORDS

Central chemoreceptors; ventrolateral medulla; brain ECF pH; pH-sensitive microelectrode; H^+-sensitive cell; micro pressure-ejection method; control of breathing.

INTRODUCTION

It is generally known that the brain is supplied by two pairs of arterial trunks, the carotid arteries and the vertebral arteries. Heymans et al. (1930) have discovered the carotid bodies as respiratory chemoreceptors near the bifurcations of the common carotid arteries. On the other hand, Loeschcke's group (1958) has later identified other chemoceptive areas located on the ventral surface of the medulla, which are the regions perfused by the vertebral arteries. These data imply that Po_2, Pco_2 and/or pH of internal environment would be mainly checked at those two (ventral and dorsal) sites where arterial blood enters the brain. As for the medullary chemoceptive areas, i.e., so-called central chemoreceptors, the precise locations still remain unknown, although many physiological and histological investigations have been made. However, there are accumulating data concerning that the central chemoreceptors play an essential role in regulation of respiration during hypercapnia. Under these circumstances we have recently done three distinct experiments which are focused upon the question about location of the central chemoreceptors. First, we have made extracellular recording of tonically active medullary neurons which are excited by stimulation of the central chemoreceptors. Second, using liquid membrane pH-sensitive microelectrodes, we have studied ECF pH dynamics within the medulla during CO_2 loading. Third, we have tried to identify H^+-sensitive cells in vivo by direct application of acidified mock CSF with

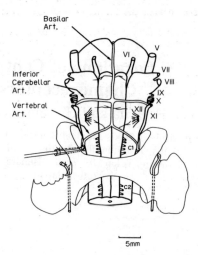

Fig. 1. Schematic drawing of medulla with ventral view showing site where
an injection catheter was placed. Note that a lateral part of right
transverse process of atlas was removed to expose vertebral artery.

micro-ejection technique. In all these experiments described herein we have used a
technique of transcapillary stimulation of the central chemoreceptors, namely an
intravertebral arterial injection of saline saturated with CO_2. This technique is
characterized by the fact that the CO_2 source injected into the vertebral artery can
alter transiently acid-base homeostasis of the perfusion area including the whole
medulla. Note that the area is not restricted to the superficial ventral areas of the
medulla. As a result, we have found two distinct intramedullary regions which are
involved in function of the central chemoreceptors.

MATERIALS AND METHODS

Experiments were performed on anesthetized (dial-urethane i.p.) and/or midcollicular
decerebrated cats. The animals were tracheotomized and allowed to breathe air
spontaneously. Respiratory flow was measured using a hot-wire flowmeter attached to the
tracheal cannula. The C_5 branch of right phrenic nerves (PN) was isolated; the PN
activity was amplified and integrated using an RC circuit (a time constant 200 ms).

To stimulate the central chemoreceptors, the right vertebral artery was isolated and
cannulated at the C1 level (Fig. 1). We determined a minimal volume (0.2-0.6 ml) of CO_2
-saturated saline for each animal, which produced a clear (rapid and transient)
excitation of respiration (Arita et al., 1988a). As the control, the same amount of
saline saturated with 3-4% CO_2 in O_2 buffered by HCO_3^- (pH=7.38-7.45) was used, and it
was confirmed that the control injections did not evoke any changes in respiration.
Another fine catheter was inserted into the common carotid artery through the thyroid
artery. The peripheral chemoreceptors were stimulated by injecting warm saline
saturated with CO_2.

The animals were suspended prone in a stereotaxic frame. To expose the dorsal surface
of the medulla, occipital craniotomy was performed and the dura overlying the brainstem
was opened. Single units with non-phasic discharges were systematically searched in the
area between 6.5 mm rostral and 3.0 mm caudal to the obex, and between 2.0 and 5.5 mm
lateral to the midline from the dorsal surface to the ventral bottom using glass
microelectrodes. Once a spontaneous non-phasic firing was detected, we gave an
injection of CO_2-saturated saline into the vertebral artery to stimulate the central
chemoreceptors. After a 2-3 min recovery period, another injection was given into the

carotid artery to stimulate the peripheral chemoreceptors. The effects on neuronal activity were assessed with the firing rate changes (the 1st experiment).

In another experiments studying medullary ECF pH dynamics (the 2nd experiment), we made double-barreled pH-sensitive microelectrodes (Arita et al., 1989), i.e., a liquid membrane pH-electrode using neutral carrier. H^+-sensitive ligand was injected into one barrel for pH electrode and the other barrel for reference electrode was filled with 3M KCl. Each electrode was calibrated in vitro with phosphate buffer (pH 6.2-7.8). The electrodes used in this study gave a mean slope of 59.8±6.0mV/pH, and the 90% response time was about 5s. Before and after measurements of ECF pH deep in the medulla, the electrode was kept in the pool of mock CSF on the dorsal surface, whose pH was simultaneously determined by Corning pH/blood gas analyzer: this was a basis for determination of an absolute value of ECF pH. The electrode was inserted dorsoventrally down to the ventral bottom using a micromanipulator, and it was held at various depths along the track. We first obtained a baseline value of ECF pH at each depth, and then we evaluated ECF pH responses to injections of CO_2-saturated saline into the vertebral artery. Once we found the regions where ECF pH change (acidity) coincided with respiratory increase during the CO_2 loading, we made intensive examinations of ECF pH responses near the region.

In the other experiments using micro pressure-ejection technique (the 3rd experiment), four-barreled micropipettes were made. One barrel for recording was filled with 0.5 M sodium acetate, and other barrels for ejections were filled with the following three kinds of mock CSF: control mock CSF (pH=7.45±0.16), acidified mock CSF (pH=6.98±0.07), and glutamate-dissolved mock CSF. The barrels containing these solutions were attached to polyethylene tubes for pressure ejection. Compressed nitrogen gas was applied via the tubes by means of a pneumatic pump which regulated the ejection pressure and the duration of pressure pulse. Ejection volume from each barrel was determined after successful recordings; 70-100 picoliter/sec per kg/cm². Single units with non-phasic discharges were systematically searched in the forementioned area. When a spontaneous non-phasic firing was detected, we first of all applied glutamate to prove that the recording was made from cell body rather than fiber. If the response was positive, then acidified mock CSF and, in turn, control mock CSF were applied in the vicinity of the cell. Thereafter, we evaluated responses to injections of CO_2-saturated saline into the vertebral artery and the carotid artery. The effects were assessed with the firing rate changes.

RESULTS AND DISCUSSION

The activity of 146 units with non-phasic discharges was recorded extracellularly in the 1st experiment (Arita et al., 1988b). Thirty-nine of the 146 units were excited by

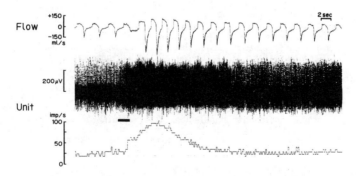

Fig. 2. Effect of intravertebral arterial injection of CO_2-saturated saline on a spontaneously active unit with non-phasic discharges. Traces are from the top downwards: respiratory flow with inspiration up; unit activity; its pulse-counter output. Bar below unit activity trace indicates the period of intravertebral arterial injection.

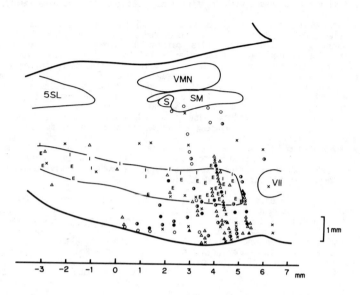

Fig. 3. Anatomical maps of sites at which various types of unit were
recorded: open circles, the units which responded exclusively to
central chemoreceptor stimulation; half filled circles, the units
with integrations of central and peripheral chemoreceptor inputs;
triangle, the units with nociceptive action. For simplicity the
recoding sites are projected onto the standard sagittal plane of
the medulla 3 mm lateral to the midline.

the intravertebral arterial injecions of CO_2-saturated saline in the same time course
as ventilatory augmentation (Fig. 2). Eighteen of the 39 units did not react to
peripheral chemoreceptor stimulation, i.e., they responded exclusively to central
chemoreceptor stimulation. These 18 units were distributed in the caudal chemoceptive
area of the ventral surface, in the vicinity of ventral respiratory group (VRG)
neurons, and in the dorsal area ventral to the solitary tract (Fig. 3). Twenty-one of
the 39 units were excited by peripheral chemoreceptor stimulation, i.e., neurons with
integrations of central and peripheral chemoreceptor inputs. They were densely packed
in the nucleus paragigantocellularis lateralis, although also found in and around the
rostral VRG neurons (Fig. 3). Fifty-one of the 146 non-phasic units were excited (44
units) or inhibited (7 units) immediately after the intravertebral arterial injections,
and their discharges returned to pre-injection levels prior to or during the early
period of ventilatory augmentation (Arita et al., 1988b). They also reacted to skin
pinching, i.e., neurons with nociceptive action, and were found scattered variously in
the ventral half of the medulla. Fourteen of the 146 units reacted to both
chemoreceptor and nociceptor stimulation. The remaining 42 units were non-responsive.
In summary, the distributions of the tonically active neurons excited exclusively by
the central chemoreceptors were located in the ventrolateral medulla and in the dorsal
medulla.

In the 2nd experiment we evaluated ECF pH dynamics within the medulla during the
intravertebral arterial injections of CO_2-saturated saline (Arita et al, 1989). Most of
the tested regions elicited no or only small changes in ECF pH, whereas ventilation
exhibited a clear excitation (lower panel in Fig. 4). However, we were able to find
responsive micro regions where ECF pH shifted to the acid side in the time course
analogous to respiratory excitation during the CO_2 loadings (upper panel in Fig. 4):

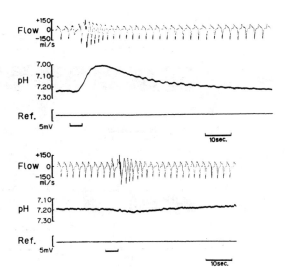

Fig. 4. Representative patterns of ECF pH changes in response to intravertebral arterial injections of CO_2-saturated saline. Each bar indicates the injection period. Flow, respiratory flow with inspiration upwards; pH, medullary ECF pH; Ref, voltage from reference microelectrode.

the acidic shift occurred just before the respiratory excitation. The correlation between the acidic changes in ECF pH and the ventilatory augmentation implies that the responsive regions (47 regions) would be specific local environments fitting the central chemoreceptors. Forty (85%) out of the 47 responsive regions were found to be scattered in the ventrolateral medulla, i.e., a long narrow zone extending from the ventrolateral surface to the VRG areas. The responsive regions were not necessarily restricted to the superficial ventral layers. We were also able to find the responsive regions in the dorsal area ventral to the nucleus tractus solitarii (NTS), though they were fewer in number (7/47). The distributions corresponded roughly to the areas where we had identified the tonically firing neurons excited exclusively by stimulation of the central chemoreceptors, as described above.

In the 3rd experiment using micro pressure-ejection technique, we examined responses of medullary neurons with non-phasic discharges (164 units) to direct application of acidified mock CSF (pH 6.85-7.05). We found only sixteen H^+-sensitive cells (16/164). The typical example is shown in Fig. 5. This cell was excited promptly on application ($\sim$500 picoliter) of acidified mock CSF, whereas it was unaffected by micro-ejection of the control mock CSF. This means that the effect can be attributed to an increase in hydrogen ion or low pH. Ten out of the 16 H^+-sensitive cells were further excited by transcapillary stimulation of the central chemoreceptors using a method of intravertebral arterial injection of CO_2-saturated saline. The discharges increased in a similar time course to that of respiratory augmentation (Fig. 5C). The present results indicate that the 10 cells are H^+-sensitive neurons whose activity is linked with respiratory change.

Distributions of these ten specific H^+-sensitive cells were found deep in the ventrolateral medulla and in the vicinity of the NTS, as illustrated in Fig. 6.

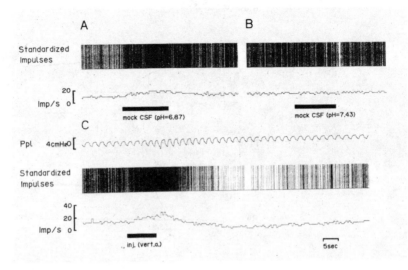

Fig. 5 A typical example of medullary H^+-sensitive neuron. which was
recorded extracellularly through one barrel of a four-barreled
micropipette in decerebrated, spontaneously breathing cat. The
neuronal activity is expressed by standardized impulses (top trace)
and the pulse-counter output (second trace). A, application (580
picoliter) of acidified mock CSF (pH 6.87) increased the firing rate
promptly. Bars below the traces indicate the duration of ejection.
B, application of control mock CSF (pH 7.43) did not evoke any
significant changes in the discharge. C, intravertebral arterial
injection of CO_2-saturated saline increased the firing rate
correlatively with ventilatory augmentation which is represented by
change in intrapleural pressure (Ppl).

Regarding the H^+-sensitive neurons situated in the ventrolateral medulla, the present
results seem compatible with the previos report by Marino and Lamb (1975). That is, two
H^+-sensitive neurons identified by them are situated approximately 3 mm from the
ventral surface of the medulla, while five H^+-sensitive neurons identified herein were
also located deep in the ventrolateral medulla. As for the other five H^+-sensitive
neurons situated in the dorsal medulla, we are interested in the previous in vitro
studies (Fukuda et al., 1975; Miles, 1983; Dean et al., 1989) demonstrating that there
exist CO_2/H^+-sensitive cells in and around the NTS. The dorsal distributions of H^+
-sensitive neurons identified in this in vivo study were also found near the NTS. The
similarity in the locations implies that both chemoceptive cells might belong to the
same neuronal population. We would like to emphasize that the H^+-sensitive   neurons
identified in the present study were shown to be excited by transcapillary stimulation
of the central chemoreceptors.

In summary, all these data obtained in the different experiments suggest a possibility t
hat the pH-dependent central chemoreceptors, if any, might be situated in the ventrolate
ral medulla and in the dorsal medulla.

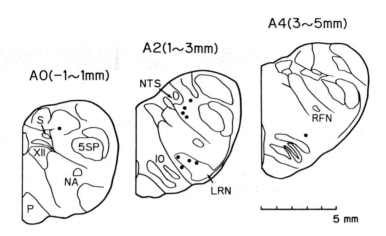

Fig. 6. Transverse sections of the medulla showing locations of ten H^+
-sensitive neurons. The recording sites are projected onto the
three standard frontal planes. A0; a section between 1 mm caudal
and 1 mm rostral to the obex. A2; a section between 1-3 mm rostral
to the obex. A4; a section between 3-5 mm rostral to the obex.

REFERENCES

Arita, H., N. Kogo and K. Ichikawa (1988a). Rapid and transient excitation of
respiration mediated by central chemoreceptor. J. Appl. Physiol., 64, 1369-1375.
Arita, H., N. Kogo and K. Ichikawa (1988b). Locations of medullary neurons with
nonphasic discharges excited by stimulation of central and/or peripheral chemoreceptor
and by activation of nociceptors in cat. Brain Res., 442, 1-10.
Arita, H., K. Ichikawa, S. Kuwana and N. Kogo (1989). Possible locations of
pH-dependent central chemoreceptors: intramedullary regions with acidic shift of ECF pH
during hypercapnia. Brain Res., 485, 285-293.
Dean, J. B., W. L. Lawing and D. E. Millhorn (1989). CO_2 decreases membrane conductance
and depolarizes neurons in the nucleus tractus solitarii. Exp. Brain Res., 76, 656-661
Fukuda, Y., Y. Honda, M. E. Schläfka and H. Loeschcke (1978). Effect of H^+ on the
membrane potential of silent cells in the ventral and dorsal surface layers of the rat
medulla in vitro. Pflügers Arch., 376, 229-235.
Heymans, C., J. J. Bouckaert and L. Dautrebande (1930). Sinus carotidien et réflexes
respiratoires, II. Influences respiratoires réflexes de l'acidose, de l'alcalose, de
l'anhydride carbonique, de l'ion hydrogène et au dela des poumons. Arch. Int.
Pharmacyn. Ther., 39, 400-408.
Loeschcke, H. H, H. P. Koepchen and K. H. Gertz (1958). Über den Einflub der
Wasserstoff-ionenkonzentration und CO_2-Druck im Liquor cerebrospinalis auf die Atmung.
Pflügers Arch., 266, 569-585.
Marino, P. L. and T. W. Lamb (1975). Effects of CO_2 and extracellular H^+ iontophoresis on
single cell activity in the cat brainstem. J. Appl. Physiol., 38, 688-695.
Miles, R. (1983). Does low pH stimulate central chemoreceptors located near the ventral
medullary surface? Brain Res., 271, 349-353.

Coupling Between Respiratory and Stepping Rhythms During Locomotion

Y. Miyamoto, K. Kawahara and
Y. Nakazono

Department of Information, Faculty of Engineering,
Yamagata University, Yonezawa 992, Japan

ABSTRACT

For the purpose to elucidate the characteristics of coupling between respiratory and stepping rhythms, following experiments were carried out on healthy humans and decerebrated cats. First, human subjects stepped on a treadmill moving at a constant speed in such a way to synchronize his stepping rhythm with a metronome rhythm. It was found that the ratio, respiratory interval/stepping interval, approached closely to 1 or 2. An entrainment of respiratory rhythm to stepping rhythm was also observed during free voluntary stepping though the strength of coupling was rather weak. In the next, to determine whether and how the strength of coupling varies depending on locomotor patterns, correlation analysis was done of diaphragmatic and gastrocnemius muscle activities in decerebrated, spontaneously breathing cats. Tonic electrical stimulation was delivered to the mesencepharic locomotor region (MLR) to induce locomotion on a treadmill. Various locomotor patterns were elicited by changes in the belt speed of the treadmill and in the intensity of the MLR stimulation. Cross-correlograms showed that coupling was absent or weak when the animals walked slowly. The strength of coupling varied depending on the locomotor pattern elicited. When the animals were galloping, the respiratory rhythm was entrained 1:1 with the stepping rhythm. There is a possibility that the locomotor-respiratory coupling may improve the efficiency of ventilation and thereby reduce the work of breathing during exercise.

KEYWORDS

Respiratory rhythm; exercise ryhthm; entrainment; decerebrated cat

It has generally been recognized both in human and animal experiments that respiratory rhythm entrains to the rhythm of exercise under some conditions (Iscoe and Polosa, 1976; Bechbache and Duffin, 1977; Jasinskas et al., 1980; Iscoe, 1981). One factor affecting the entrainment is certainly chemical stimuli mediated by the central and peripheral chemoreceptors (Paterson et al., 1987; Kawahara et al., 1989b). However, it has been believed that the coupling strength is primarily modified by activities originating either in the central nervous system (Haas et al., 1986; Kawahara et al., 1989a and 1989b) or in the peripheral reflex (Iscoe and Polosa, 1976; Iscoe, 1981; Kawahara et al., 1988). The purpose

of the present paper is to clarify the role of these neurognic factors to   couple
breathing rhythm with stepping rhythm during exercise.

ENTRAINMENT OBSERVED IN EXERCISING HUMAN SUBJECTS

As   a   preliminary   test   we measured in human subjects   both   the   intervals   of
breathing   and   walking   during   two different   conditions   of   exercise   using   a
treadmill.   The   treadmill   speed was increased linearly from 2 km/h upto 6   km/h
within   15   min.   At first,   the subject was allowed to walk with   his   favorable
rhythm.   As shown in Fig.1 (a),   no significant correlation was observed   between
walking and breathing intervals. In the second, the subject was asked to listen a
train   of   metronome   beats,   of   which   frequency   was   adjusted   to   vary   in
synchronization with the treadmill speed.   He tried to fit his walking rhythm   to
the   metronome   rhythm   as   close as possible.   As shown in   Fig.1   (b),   a   good
correlation   was   observed between walking and breathing rhythms.   When   walking
speed is slow,   breathing rhythm was equal to walking interval, that is to say, an
entrainment   of 1:1 was observed.   Breath interval was twice as long   as   walking
interval when tradmill speed was increased,   entrainment being now 2:1. It should
be   noted,   however,   that   there was a considerable difference among   individual
responses.

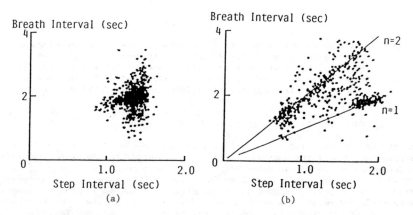

Breath Interval (sec)   **Breath Interval (sec)**

Step Interval (sec)   Step Interval (sec)

(a)   (b)

Fig.1. Relationships between stepping interval and breathing
interval   obtained   from   a   subject   during   free
walking(a)   and   synchronized   (forced)   walking   with
metronome(b). Treadmill speed varied from 2 to 6 km/h.

The   probability   of   occurrence of entrainment   between   breathing   and   stepping
rhythms observed in above conditions are given in Fig.2.   The upper diagrams show
the results obtained during free wlaking.   The ratio,   breathing interval/walking
interval,   showed   a   trend being in focus around 2.   The lower diagrams show   the
same   ratio   during   synchronized (forced) walking with metronome   rhythm.   The
interval ratio   was   in focus sharply around 2.   In a few cases   the   ratio   was
discrete   in 1 and 2.   As an index indicating the coupling strength between   both
the   rhythms,   we   compared variances from the mean value of the   interval   ratio
between free and synchronized walkings. The variance was significantly smaller in
6   out of 8 subjects in the synchronized walking than that in free walking.   The
human   experiments   showed obviously that the peripheral feedback signal and   the
feedforward   central   command   was additive in effect to link the   respiratory   and
stepping   rhythms tightly.   These observations agreed well with those reported by
Bechbache and Duffin (1977).

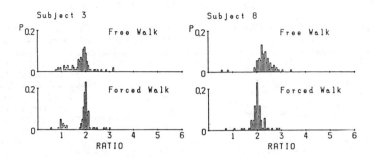

Fig.2. Relationships between the breathing interval/stepping interval ratio (abscissa) and the probability of its occurrence (ordinate) obtained from two human subjects during free walking (upper panel) and synchronized (forced) walking with metroneome (lower panel).

COUPLING STRENGTH BETWEEN RESPIRATORY AND STEPPING RHYTHMS

In the next, we studied whether and how the strength of coupling between respiratory and stepping rhythms might vary depending on the locomotor pattern in decerebrated and spontaneously breathing cats (Kawahara et al., 1989a). The animal was decerebrated at the precollicular-postmammillary level (mesencephalic preparation) under halothane anesthesia. The head of the animal was fixed in a stereotaxic frame, and the mesencephalic locomotor region (MLR) was stimulated by an AC current of 50 Hz (0.2 msec in duration, 30–70 μ A in intensity) through a tungsten microelectrode. Electromyograms (EMG) were recorded from the bilateral gastrocnemius muscles to monitor locomotion activity. Electromyograms of diaphragm were also recorded to monitor respiratory activity. The mesencephalic cat breathed spontaneously and could keep normal standig position on a treadmill. The various locomotor patterns, such as walking, trotting, and galloping could be induced by adjusting the intensity of the MLR stimulation and by changing treadmill speed.

Figure 3 (a) shows the EMG activities of diaphragm and gastrocnemius during locomotion induced by MLR stimulation (50μA) at a treadmill speed of 1 km/h. The integrated EMG of left and right gastrocnemius, IG(L) and IG(R), showed alternative rhythmic activities in response to MLR stimulation after a short delay, suggesting that the animal was walking. In contrast, the amplitude and frequency of rhythmic activity of diaphragm, ID, increased immediately after the stimulation of MLR. PETCO$_2$ tracing showed a significance of slight hyperventilation. Figure 3 (b) shows the EMG activities of the same cat during galloping. The galloping was induced by increasing treadmill speed upto 3.5 km/h and the intensity of MLR stimulation upto 60μA. Rhythmic changes in the EMG of left and right gastrocnemius, IG(L) and IG(R), were in phase, suggesting the locomotor pattern was galloping. PETCO$_2$ tracing showed a significant reduction caused by hyperventilation.

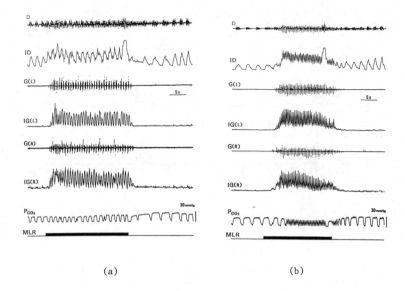

(a)   (b)

Fig. 3. EMG activities in a decerebrate cat during
locomotion   elicited by stimulation of MLR at a
treadmill   speed   of 1.0 km/h (a) and 3.5 km/h (b).
D, diaphragmatic EMG; ID, integration of D; G(L), left
gastrocnemius EMG; IG(L), integration of G(L); G(R), right
gastrocnemius EMG; IG(R), integration of G(R); PCO_2, end-
tidal tension of CO_2.

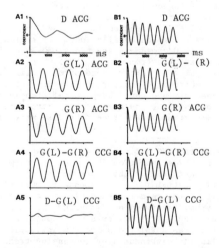

Fig.4. Autocorrelograms (ACG) and cross-correlograms (CCG)
obtained during waking (A1-A5) and galloping (B1-B5) in a
cat. See Fig.3 legend for definition of abbreviations.

Correlation analysis of diaphragmatic and gastrocnemius activities was then done
to detect their periodicity and to evaluate quantitatively the strength of
locomotor-respiratory coupling. Figure 4 A1-A5 showed the results during walking
and B1-B5 showed those during galloping. The autocorrelograms of diaphragmatic
activities indicated that the mean respiratory intervals were 1.5 sec for walking
(A1) and 0.43 sec for galloping (B1). The progressive decrease in the amplitude
of the oscillation reflected irregularities in respiratory rhythm during
trotting. The autocorrelograms of left and right gastrocnemius activity indicated
that the mean stepping intervals were 0.73 sec for trotting (A2 and A3) and that
for galloping was 0.43 sec (B2 and B3). The cross-correlograms between left and
right gastrocnemius activities were given in A4 and B4. In A4, the difference in
time between the peaks of the oscillation in A2 or A3 and the peak in A4 was
about half the mean stepping interval, reflecting the alternative activities of
left and right legs during walking. In contrast, the almost coinciding
oscillation between B2 or B3 and B4 reflected a synchronized activity during
galloping. The flat cross-correlogram in A5 showed that diaphragmatic and
gastrocnemius activities were not correlated with each other, although the
respiratory interval was twice that of the stepping interval. The clear
oscllation in B5 with the same intervals between peaks as those in both B2 and B3
indicated 1:1 entrainment of the respiratory rhythm to the stepping rhythm. These
results showed that coupling between the respiratory and locomotor rhythm
generator was weak or absent during walking but became stronger during galloping.

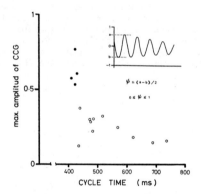

Fig.5. Relationship between cycle time (mean stepping
interval) and maximum amplitude of cross-correlogram between
diaphragmatic and left gastrocnemius activities. Closed
circles, results obtained during galloping; open circles,
those obtained during walking and trotting.

Figure 5 shows the relationship between the cycle time (mean stepping interval)
and the maximal amplitude of the cross-correlograms between respiratory and
stepping rhythms obtained from a cat. This parameter was adopted to evaluate the
strength of coupling between respiratory and locomotor rhythms. The strength of
locomotor-respiratory coupling increased slightly as the cycle time decreased
during walking and trotting (open circles). The coupiling became suddenly strong
when the gait of locomotion was altered from trotting into galloping (closed
circles), although the cycle time remained unchanged. This result raised the
possibility that the strength of locomotor-respiratory coupling would vary
depending primarily on whether the gait of the animal was a gallop.

The role of the central command on entrainment was also studied in cats by Kawahara et al. (1989 b). The animal was decerebrated, immobilized with gallamine triethiodide, bilaterally vagotomized and artficially ventilated. In normocapnia (32 mmHg), a MLR stimulation increased the frequency of the phrenic nerve discharge significantly, and induced a rhythmic efferent discharge of the medial gastrocnemius nerve, but no entrainment was observed betwen these two rhythms. In hypocapnia (18 mmHg), the MLR stmulation of the same intensity elicited fictive locomotion and resulted in the 1:1 entrainment of rhythms between the phrenic and gastrocnemius activities. It has also been demonstrated in conscious cats (Iscoe, 1981) and in anesthetized cats (Iscoe and Polosa, 1976; Kawahara et al., 1988) that repetitive somatic afferent stimulations produced a 1:1 entrainment of respiratory frequency to the stimulus frequency. Thus, conclusion can be drawn that in cats as well as in humans both neural inputs, one coming from the central nervous system and the other from the walking muscles, can cause independently entrainment between breathing and stepping rhythms.

THE ROLE OF ENTRAINMENT IN THE REGULATION OF BREATHING DURING EXERCISE

We designed a special type of static exercise for human subjects so that strong muscular tension could be induced rhythmically (Miyamoto et al., 1987). Figure 6 shows typical ventilatory responses to various types of cycle exercise obtained from a subject. Respiratory frequency (f) was fixed at 30 breaths/min during rhythmic static exercise (RSE) of 30 and 60 stepps/min (C and D). This suggested that an entrainment of 1:1 (C) or 2:1 (B) was formed. Since no entrainment was observed in dynamic cycle exercise (DE) of the same frequency (E), it seems obvious that afferent stimulation originating in exercising limbs would intensify the coupling strength between respiratory and stepping rhythms. When entrainment was formed, minute ventilation ($\dot{V}E$) increased significantly and the kinetics thereof was accelerated, although oxygen consumption ($\dot{V}O_2$) remained at almost the same level as that in dynamic exercise (E). It may be assumed that

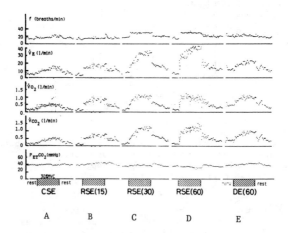

Fig.6. Respiratory and metabolic responses of a human subject to A: continuous static (CSE), B–D: rhythmic static (RSE), and E: dynamic (DE) exercises of a moderate level. Numbers in parentheses indicate the frequency of exercise rhythm per min. f, respiratory frequency; $\dot{V}E$, minute ventilation; $\dot{V}O_2$, oxygen consumption; $\dot{V}CO_2$, CO_2 output; $PETCO_2$, end-tidal CO_2 tension.

entrainment contributes to improve the efficiency of ventilation and minimizes the respiratory work during exercise. It should be noted however that in humans individual difference in the ventilatory response is considerablly great. In some subjects entrainment did not always produce an increase in ventilation since an incarease in respiratory frequency was canceled out by a concomitant decrease in tidal volume. Further studies should be nescessary to evaluate the physiological meaning of entrainment in the regulation of breathing during exercise.

REFERENCES

Bechbache,R.R. and J.Duffin (1977). The entrainment of breathing frequency by exercise rhythm. J.Physiol. (London) 272,553-561.
Haas,F., S.Distenfeld and K.Axen (1986). Effects of perceived musical rhythm on respiratory pattern. J.Appl.Physiol., 61,1185-1191.
Iscoe,S., and C.Polosa (1976). Synchronization of respiratory frequency by somatic afferent stimulation. J.Appl.Physiol., 40,138-148.
Iscoe,S. (1981). Respiratory and stepping frequencies in conscious exercising cats. J.Appl.Physiol., 51,835-839.
Jasinskas,C.L., B.A.Wilson and J.Hoare (1980). Entrainment of breathing rate to movement frequency during work at two intensities. Respir.Physiol., 42,199-209.
Kawahara,K., S.Kumagai, Y.Nakazono and Y.Miyamoto (1988). Analysis of entrainment of respiratory rhythm by somatic afferent stimulation in cats using phase response curves. Biol.Cybern., 58,235-242.
Kawahara,K., S.Kumagai, Y.Nakazono and Y.Miyamoto (1989a). Coupling between respiratory and stepping rhythms during locomotion in decerebrate cats. J.Appl.Physiol., 67,110-115.
Kawahara,K., Y.Nakazono, Y.Yamauchi and Y.Miyamoto (1989b). Coupling between respiratory and locomotor rhythms during fictive locomotion in decerebrate cats. Neuroscience Letters, 103,326-332.
Miyamoto,Y., Y.Nakazono and K.Yamakoshi (1987). Neurogenic factors affecting ventilatory and circulatory responses to static and dynamic exercise in man. Jpn. J.Physiol., 37,435-446.
Paterson,D.J., G.A.Wood, R.N.Marshall, A.R.Morton, and A.B.C.Harrison (1987). Entrainment of respiratory frequency to exercise rhythm during hypoxia. J.Appl.Physiol., 62,1761-1771.

Spinal Generation of Respiratory Rhythm: a Study in an *in vitro* Brainstem-Spinal Cord Preparation of New-born Rat

M. Aoki and A. Mizuguchi

Department of Physiology, Sapporo Medical College,
Sapporo 060, Japan

ABSTRACT

In vitro preparations of the brainstem-spinal cord from neonatal rats were used for investigation of the respiratory rhythm generating mechanism. The respiratory thorax movement synchronized with the periodic phrenic nerve activity was observed in a brainstem-spinal cord preparation perfused with Krebs solution. When a transection was made at the medulla-cervical cord junction just above C1 segment, we could still observe the rhythmic thorax movement and the synchronous phrenic nerve discharge with a frequency of about 5/min. in about 19% of the preparations. It is suggested that a respiratory neuronal circuit capable of generating spinal respiratory rhythm is localized within the upper cervical cord.

KEYWORDS

Respiratory rhythm; Brainstem-spinal cord preparation; Spinal respiratory rhythm; New-born rat.

INTRODUCTION

Previous experiments by us (Aoki et al., 1980) and others (Coglianese et al., 1977) have demonstrated that spontaneous respiratory movements corresponding to normal breathing could be induced in high spinalized animals. Recently we discovered a group of respiratory neurons in the upper cervical segments of the spinal cord in cats, rats, monkeys (Aoki et al., 1984, 1987, 1988) and rabbits (Kubin and Romaniuk, 1988). This group of cervical respiratory neurons form a longitudinal column which extends from C1 to C3 segments. They send descending projections to lower cervical and thoracic segments (Aoki et al., 1984, 1987, Duffin and Hoskin, 1987, Lipski and Duffin, 1986) and receive descending inputs from the brainstem (Aoki et al., 1987, 1990, Hoskin and Duffin, 1987). These observations strongly suggested the existence of a respiratory rhythm generating circuit within the spinal cord. In the present study, we examined whether spontaneous spinal respiratory rhythm could be produced in neonatal rats, using in vitro brainstem-spinal cord preparations. It is suggested that a spinal respiratory generator is likely to exist within the upper cervical cord.

METHODS

The head and the thorax were isolated from 2 to 4 day-old neonatal rats anesthetized with halothane or chloroform. The preparation was placed in a 30 $m\ell$ dissection bath and perfused with modified Krebs solution at 27 ℃. The procedures are essentially the same as described in previous papers (Smith and Feldman, 1987a, 1987b, Suzue, 1984). After a craniotomy, the cerebellum was removed by suction and the cerebrum was also removed by transection at the level of the rostral pons using a pair of fine scissors and a corneal knife. The spinal cord was exposed along the spinal column by midline section. The thorax was divided along the sternum, and the rib cage was movable during contraction of the intercostal muscles. The lungs were removed bilaterally and the phrenic nerves were left intact for recording neural activity. The preparation was fixed, ventral side upwards at the head and ribs (Th10 - Th12) to the bottom of the perfusion bath with needles. The respiratory thoracic movements were recorded by connecting a probe of a force displacement transducer to a rib (Th10) by a thread. For recording respiratory neural activity from the phrenic nerve a glass capillary suction electrode was used. Conventional equipment was used for monitoring and recording the thorax movement and the neural activity.

RESULTS

Spontaneous respiratory movement in the brainstem-spinal cord preparation

Immediately after decerebration at the rostral pons, spontaneous respiratory movement of the thorax occurred with a somewhat irregular frequency of about 5/min. The frequency of the movement then reached a stable level of

Thorax movement

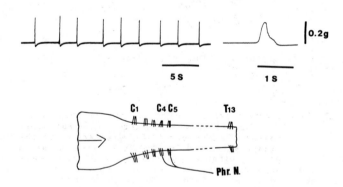

Fig. 1.   Spontaneous respiratory movement of the thorax obtained from a brainstem-spinal cord preparation of a 2 day-old rat. Upward deflexion represents the upward movement of the thorax. A record with expanded time scale is shown to the right. Simultaneous recordings of the phrenic nerve discharge was attempted from the left phrenic nerve.

10-15/min. in about 10 min. In the present experimental condition, the preparation gradually deteriorated and the frequency of the respiratory movement decreased. It became irregular again in 40 min. to 1.5 hr. and the movement finally stopped (Fig. 1). Such spontaneous respiratory movement after decerebration was observed in most of the preparations examined (63/70). One cycle of the rhythmic motor pattern consisted of a short inspiratory phase of about 0.2 ~ 0.3 sec when the phrenic nerve discharges, and a prolonged expiratory phase.

When the brainstem was transected at the level of the caudal medulla in decerebrated preparations, the spontaneous thorax movement could be still maintained in 40% of the animals (2/5). The thorax movement was synchronized with phrenic nerve discharges recorded from a peripheral cut-end with a suction electrode (Fig. 2). The frequency of the spontaneous rhythm was 5 - 7/min., lower than that of the decerebrated preparation. One cycle of the respiratory rhythm was composed of a short inspiratory phase of the phrenic nerve discharge, and a prolonged expiratory phase, as observed in the decerebrated preparation. The phrenic nerve bursts consisted of a decrementing discharge lasting approximately 200 ms.

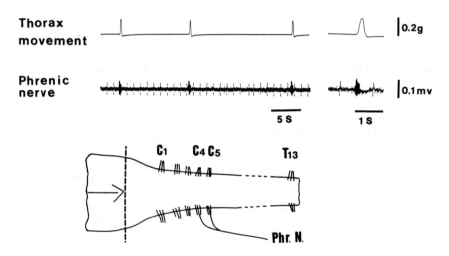

Fig. 2.   Synchronization of the thorax movement with the phrenic nerve discharge in a brainstem-spinal cord preparation, transected at the caudal medulla. The format is the same as in Fig. 1. ECGs are superimposed on the nervous record.

Spontaneous respiratory activity in the spinal preparation

When a transection was made at the medulla-spinal junction just above the C1 dorsal root, we could still obtain the spontaneous rhythmic thorax movement and the synchronized phrenic nerve discharge in some preparations (Fig. 3). This spinal respiratory rhythm was observed in about 19% (3/16) of the preparations examined. Routinely, spinal transection was made stepwise from the dorsal part of the cord to the ventral part. When the transection was completed, the spontaneous respiratory movement of the rib cage was

abolished. In the successful preparations, spontaneous respiratory activity
was resumed in 5 - 10 sec. The frequency of the movement was about 5/min.
similar to that of the caudal medulla preparation, although the amplitude of
the thorax movement was much smaller. This spontaneous spinal resiratory
activity quickly deteriorated and stopped in about 10 to 30 min. after
transection. In one experiment, we could observe both the medullary
respiratory rhythm (rhythmic respiratory jaw movement) and spinal rhythm
(rib cage movement and the phrenic nerve discharge), persisiting with
different independent frequencies.

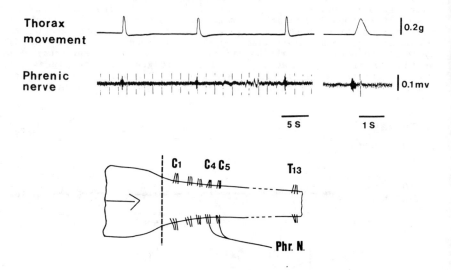

Fig. 3.   Spontaneous respiratory activity in a spinal
           preparation of a 4 day-old rat. Transection
           was made at the medulla-cervical junction
           above the C1 segment. Records were obtained
           about 10 min. after total transection.

DISCUSSION

The present experiments demonstrated, in agreement with previous studies
(Morin-Surun and Denavit-Saubié, 1989, Murakoshi et al. 1985, Smith and
Feldman, 1987a, 1987b, Suzue, 1984), that spontaneous respiratory rhythm
can be maintained in the in vitro brainstem-spinal cord preparation. The
frequency of the spontaneous respiratory rhythm, under the present in vitro
condition, was 6 - 12/min. (0.1 - 0.2 Hz). The low frequency of the rhythm
could be partly attributable to the greatly reduced afferent inputs, the
relatively insufficient supply of oxygen, and the lower temperature in
vitro. This slow respiration may correspond to gasping (Suzue, 1984).

With regard to the origin of the respiratory rhythm, we could confirm an
existence of the medullary respiratory generator, since a "facial
respiration", i.e., rhythmic respiratory jaw movements, persisted after the
medulla-spinal transection in the present preparation. This observation
agrees with the previous reports that periodic nervous discharges were

present on cranial nerves such as glossopharyngeal and hypoglossal, in the brainstem-spinal cord preparation (Smith and Feldman, 1987a, 1987b, Suzue, 1984).

Concerning the spinal respiratory generator, we could observe the spontaneous respiratory activity after spinal transection at C1 - C2 levels in about 19% of the preparations examined. This spinal respiratory rhythm was slower than in the isolated brainstem. These observations imply that probably the activity of the spinal respiratory generator is normally driven by the medullary generator, causing the respiratory motoneurons to discharge. After transection at the medulla-cervical junction, the spinal respiratory generator may regain the ability to discharge spontaneously in some preparations. However, the low occurrence (19%) of the spontaneous respiratory rhythm of spinal origin may, at least in part, explain the results of previous transection experiments which failed to demonstrate the spinal respiratory activity in neonatal rats (Smith and Feldman, 1987b, Suzue, 1984). A pharmacological activation could disclose, and facilitate, the spinal capabilities for respiratory rhythm generation after medulla-spinal transection, as demonstrated in acute high spinal rabbit preparations (Viala et al., 1979, Viala and Freton, 1983). The spinal respiratory generator could display chemosensitivity. The discharge frequency could be changed by reduced PH or certain perturbation of the ionic composition of the solution in a bath.

Thus, the brainstem-sinal cord preparation of the new-born rat seems quite useful in clarifying the mechanisms of medullary and spinal respiratory rhythm generation. Our results suggest that the basic properties of the respiratory rhythm generation are similar in the spinal and the brainstem preparations. We believe that the respiratory neuronal substrate localized in the upper cervical cord has a complete capability of generating spinal respiratory rhythm, at least under certain conditions.

REFERENCES

Aoki, M., Mori, S., Kawahara, K., Watanabe, H. and Ebata, N. (1980). Generation of spontaneous respiratory rhythm in high spinal cats. Brain Res., 202, 51-63.

Aoki, M., Kasaba, T., Kurosawa, Y., Ohtsuka, K. and Satomi, H. (1984). The projection of cervical respiratory neurons to the phrenic nucleus in the cat. Neurosci. Lett., Suppl. 13, S9.

Aoki, M., Y. Fujito, Y. Kurosawa, H. Kawasaki and I. Kosaka (1987). Descending inputs to the upper cervical inspiratory neurons from the medullary respiratory neurons and the raphe nuclei in the cat. In: Respiratory Muscles and Their Neuromotor Control (G.C. Sieck, S.C. Gandevia and W.E. Cameron, Eds.), pp.75-82. Alan R. Liss, New York.

Aoki, M., Kosaka, I., Fujito, Y. and Kobayashi, N. (1988). Distribution pattern of the cervical respiratory neurons in the cat, rat and monkey. Neuroscience Res., Suppl. 7, S89.

Aoki, M., Y. Fujito, I. Kosaka and N. Kobayashi (1990). Supraspinal descending control of propriospinal respiratory neurons in the cat. In: Respiratory Control: A Modeling Perspective (G.D. Swanson and F.S. Grodins, Eds.), pp.451-459. Plenum, New York.

Coglianese, C.J., Peiss, C.N. and Wurster, R.D. (1977). Rhythmic phrenic nerve activity and respiratory activity in spinal dogs. Resp. Physiol., 29, 247-254.

Duffin, J. and Hoskin, R.W. (1987). Intracellular recordings from upper cervical inspiratory neurons in the cat. Brain Res., 435, 351-354.

Hoskin, R. and Duffin, J. (1987). Excitation of upper cervical inspiratory neurons by inspiratory neurons of the nucleus tractus solitarius in the cat. Exp. Neurol., 95, 126-141.

Kubin, L. and J.R. Romaniuk (1988). Propriospinal inspiratory neurons in the upper cervical spinal cord of the rabbit: location and efferent spinal projections. In: Control of Breathing During Sleep and Anesthesia (W.A. Karczewski, P. Grieb, J. Kulesza and G. Bonsignore, Eds.), pp.197-201. Plenum, New York.

Lipski, J. and Duffin, J. (1986). An electrophysiological investigation of propriospinal inspiratory neurons in the upper cervical cord of the cat. Exp. Brain Res., 61, 625-637.

Morin-Surun, M.P. and Denavit-Saubié, M. (1989). Rhythmic discharges in the perfused isolated brainstem preparation of adult guinea pig. Neurosci. Lett., 101, 57-61.

Murakoshi, T., Suzue, T. and Tamai, S. (1985). A pharmacological study on respiratory rhythm in the isolated brainstem-spinal cord preparation of the newborn rat. Br. J. Pharmac., 86, 95-104.

Smith, J.C. and J.L. Feldman (1987a). Central respiratory pattern generation studied in an in vitro mammalian brainstem-spinal cord preparation. In: Respiratory Muscles and Their Neuromotor Control (G.C. Sieck, S.C. Gandevia and W.E. Cameron, Eds.), pp.27-36, Alan R. Liss, New York.

Smith, J.C. and Feldman, J.L. (1987b). In vitro brainstem-spinal cord preparations for study of motor systems for mammalian respiration and locomotion. J. Neurosci. Methods, 21, 321-333.

Suzue, T. (1984). Respiratory rhythm generation in the in vitro brain stem-spinal cord preparation of the neonatal rat. J. Physiol., 354, 173-183.

Viala, D., Vidal, C. and Freton, E. (1979). Coordinated rhythmic bursting in respiratory and locomotor muscle nerves in the spinal rabbit. Neurosci. Lett., 11, 155-159.

Viala, D. and Freton, E. (1983). Evidence for respiratory and locomotor pattern generators in the rabbit cervico-thoracic cord and for their interactions. Exp. Brain Res., 49, 247-256.

The Role of a Putative Excitatory Amino Acid Transmitter in the Generation of Respiratory Rhythm in Medulla Isolated From Newborn Rat

H. Onimaru, A. Arata and I. Homma

Department of Physiology, Showa University School of
Medicine, 1-5-8 Hatanodai, Shinagawa-ku, Tokyo 142,
Japan

ABSTRACT

We examined the role of excitatory amino acid (EAA) receptors in generation of
respiratory rhythm in in vitro preparations from newborn rats. EAA antagonists
(NMDA and non-NMDA) depressed activity of rhythm generating neurons, Pre-I
neurons in the medulla. EAA receptors are important in synchronized Pre-I burst
generation, hence in respiratory rhythm generation in the medulla.

KEYWORDS

excitatory amino acid; respiratory rhythm; medulla; in vitro.

INTRODUCTION

Brainstem-spinal cord preparations isolated from newborn rats generate stable
respiratory rhythm for several hours in perfusate after complete removal of
inputs from peripheral structures (Suzue, 1984). We have demonstrated that
respiratory rhythm is probably produced primarily by Pre-I neurons located in
the rostral ventrolateral medulla (RVL) (Onimaru et al., 1988a). Pre-I neurons,
whose firing precedes inspiratory neuronal activity, are considered to
periodically trigger an inspiratory pattern generator (IPG) in the medulla. We
proposed that synchronized Pre-I bursts are generated in a neuronal network
connected through excitatory synapses, including Pre-I pacemaker cells as the
main elements (Onimaru et al., 1989). A role of EAA receptors in respiratory
rhythm generation in the brainstem was recently suggested (Feldman and Smith,
1989). To assess the contribution of EAA to excitatory synaptic transmission
between Pre-I neurons and to Pre-I burst generation, we examined effects of some
EAA antagonists on Pre-I and inspiratory neuron activity.

METHODS

The methods used have been previously reported (Onimaru et al.,1988; Suzue,
1984). Briefly, the brainstems and spinal cords of 22 newborn (0-to 4-day-old)
Wistar rats were isolated under deep ether anesthesia. The preparation was
continuously perfused in a 2 ml chamber with the following standard solution
(mM): NaCl, 124; KCl, 5.0; KH_2PO_4, 1.2; $CaCl_2$, 2.4; $MgSO_4$, 1.3; $NaHCO_3$, 26;

Advances in the Biosciences Vol. 79
© 1991 Pergamon Press plc.
Printed in Great Britain.

57

glucose, 30; equilibrated with 95% O_2 and 5% CO_2; at 25-26°C, pH 7.4. The unit activity of neurons was recorded extracellularly from the right and/or left RVL. Motoneuronal activity corresponding to inspiration was monitored at the C4 or C5 ventral root. EAA antagonists used were: kynurenic acid (KYN), a broad spectrum amino acid antagonist; 2-amino-5-phosphonovaleric acid (2-APV), a specific N-methyl-D-aspartate (NMDA) antagonist; γ-D-glutamylglycine (γ-DGG), an antagonist relatively selective to non-NMDA receptors; 6-cyano-7-nitro-quinoxaline-2,3-dione (CNQX), a specific non-NMDA receptor antagonist.

RESULTS AND DISCUSSION

KYN in lower doses (20-500 μM) reduced the intraburst firing frequency and the burst duration of Pre-I neurons (14 units in 7 preparations) without significantly decreasing the burst rate. Then, right and left Pre-I firing tended to be desynchronized (Fig. 1). These were followed by intermittence of C4 bursts, hence reduction of C4 burst rate with no significant reduction of amplitude or duration, probably due to failure of Pre-I neurons to periodically trigger the IPG. In higher doses (0.5-1 mM), KYN reduced the rate of Pre-I bursts or caused their complete disappearance. 2-APV (50-100 μM; 12 units in 8 preparations), γ-DGG (50-100 μM; 10 units in 6 preparations), and CNQX (0.2-1 μM; 9 units in 5 preparations) produced effects similar to those of KYN. Figure 2 shows that 50 μM γ-DGG reduced the intraburst firing frequency of Pre-I neurons and decreased C4 burst rate without significantly reducing inspiratory burst duration. The excitatory effect of 5 μM NMDA on rhythm generation was blocked by 50 μM 2-APV, but not by 50 μM γ-DGG.

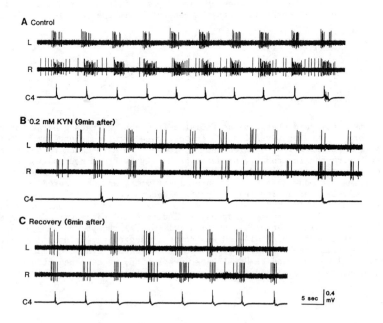

Fig. 1. Effects of 0.2 mM KYN on Pre-I neurons. A: left and right Pre-I and C4 activity in a standard bath. B: activity after 9 min perfusion with 0.2 mM KYN. C: activity 6 min after perfusate was returned to standard solution.

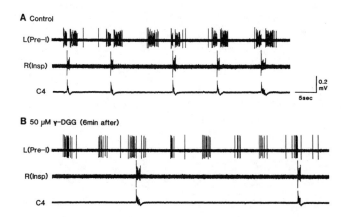

Fig. 2. A: Pre-I activity from left RVL (L), inspiratory
activity from right RVL (R) and C4 activity in standard bath.
B: activity after 6 min perfusion with 50 μM γ-DGG.

EAA antagonists depressed rhythm generation more potently than they depressed
synaptic transmission from bulbospinal inspiratory neurons to spinal motoneurons
(McCrimmon et al., 1989). Reduction of intraburst firing frequency of Pre-I
neurons and disturbance of their synchronism by blockade of EAA receptors are
consistent with possible involvement of EAA transmitter(s) in synaptic connections between the Pre-I neurons. Tonic activation of EAA receptors is probably
essential to intrinsic Pre-I burst generation, since higher doses of the
antagonists reduced the rate of Pre-I bursts or blocked the bursts completely.
Blockade of EAA receptors may cause an increase of tonic inhibition via
inhibitory amino acid (IAA) receptors (Onimaru et al., 1988b) on Pre-I neurons
by removing tonic excitatory inputs. Thus, Pre-I burst generation can be
regulated by balance between activation of EAA and IAA receptors. Both NMDA and
non-NMDA receptors are considered to contribute to Pre-I burst generation, while
differences in the roles of these receptor subtypes are not clear at present.

REFERENCES

Feldman, J.L. and J.C. Smith (1989). Cellular mechanisms underlying modulation
    of breathing pattern in mammals. In: Modulation of defined vertebrate neural
    circuits, Ann. N.Y. Acad. Sci. (M. Davis, B.L. Jacobs and R.I. Schoenfeld,
    Eds), Vol. 563, pp. 114-130. N.Y. Acad. Sci., New York.
McCrimmon, D.R., J.C. Smith and J.L. Feldman (1989). Involvement of excitatory
    amino acids in neurotransmission of inspiratory drive to spinal respiratory
    motoneurons. J. Neurosci., 9, 1910-1921.
Onimaru, H., A. Arata and I. Homma (1988a). Primary respiratory rhythm
    generator in the medulla of brainstem-spinal cord preparation from newborn
    rat. Brain Res., 445, 314-324.
Onimaru, H., A. Arata and I. Homma (1988b). Inhibitory synaptic inputs to
    respiratory rhythm generator in medulla isolated from newborn rats. J.
    Physiol. Soc. Jpn., 50, 584.
Onimaru, H., A. Arata and I. Homma (1989). Firing properties of respiratory
    rhythm generating neurons in the absence of synaptic transmission in rat
    medulla in vitro. Exp. Brain Res., 76, 530-536.
Suzue, T. (1984). Respiratory rhythm generation in the in vitro brain stem-
    spinal cord preparation of the neonatal rat. J. Physiol. Lond., 354, 173-183.

GABA-Mediated Inhibitory Mechanisms in Control of Respiratory Rhythm

A. Haji*, R. Takeda* and J.E. Remmers[†]

*Department of Pharmacology, Faculty of Medicine,
Toyama Medical and Pharmaceutical University,
Toyama, Japan
[†]Department of Medicine, University of Calgary,
Calgary, Alberta, Canada

ABSTRACT

The present study provides evidences that gamma-aminobutyric acid (GABA) mediates postsynaptic inhibitions in the ventral respiratory group neurons. This mechanism seems to play a crucial role in the respiratory pattern formation and control of respiratory rhythm.

KEYWORDS

Respiratory neuron; GABA; bicuculline; benzodiazepines; inhibitory postsynaptic potentials; control of breathing

Several populations of neurons with discharge patterns in synchrony with the respiratory motor activity can be recorded in the medulla oblongata. The membrane potential of these neurons are largely regulated by excitatory (E) and inhibitory (I) postsynaptic potentials (PSPs) occurring during the precise interval of the respiratory cycle (Richter, 1982). Microiontophoretic studies combined with an extracellular recording of a respiratory unitary activity suggest that GABA and glycine are primary candidates for mediators of postsynaptic inhibitions in the bulbar respiratory neurons (Champagnat et al., 1982; Kirsten et al., 1978; Toleikis et al., 1979). Recently, we obtained more direct evidences for GABA-mediated postsynaptic inhibitions in the respiratory neurons of the ventral respiratory group (VRG) using a coaxial compound multi-barrelled microelectrode. This electrode is suitable for intracellular recording of membrane potential and extracellular iontophoresis of the inhibitory amino acid and its antagonist close to the recording site (Haji et al., 1987). Additionally, we examined the effects of benzodiazepines, the specific enhancers for the GABA-A receptor-mediated response, on these inhibitory potentials.

Experiments were carried out on decerebrate, vagotomized and paralyzed cats. End-tidal CO_2 concentrations were held at 4-5%. Tracheal pressure, blood

pressure and rectal temperature were continuously monitored and maintained at
normal conditions by appropriate means.   The efferent activity of the phrenic
nerve was used for monitoring the central respiratory rhythm.   Inspiratory (I)
and post-inspiratory (PI) neurons (Richter, 1982) were impaled in the VRG.   The
center recording pipette of the multi-barrelled electrode was filled with 3 M
KCl or 2 M potassium citrate.   The peripheral six drug pipettes were filled with
NaCl (165 mM), GABA (1 M), flurazepam (0.2 M), bicuculline (5 mM), strychnine (5
mM) and tetrodotoxin (0.5 mM), with their tips recessed 20-40   μm from the tip
of the recording electrode.   In some experiments, glycine (1 M) was used in
place of flurazepam.   All drugs were ejected with cationic currents.   Diazepam
was applied intravenously.

RESULTS

Iontophoresis of GABA decreased the spike activity and hyperpolarized the
membrane in all respiratory neurons examined.   It consistently reduced the input
resistance and respiratory fluctuations of membrane potential.   Intracellular
injection of Cl ions inverted the hyperpolarization produced by GABA to
depolarization together with a reversal of the spontaneous IPSP wave.   The
reversal potential for GABA-induced hyperpolarization was measured with a
current clamp method and ranged between -80 and -90 mV.   These values
corresponded to the reversal potential for the spontaneous IPSPs.   Figure 1
shows an example of a PI-neuron where the extrapolated reversal potential for
the GABA-response was -88 mV similar for the inspiratory IPSPs.

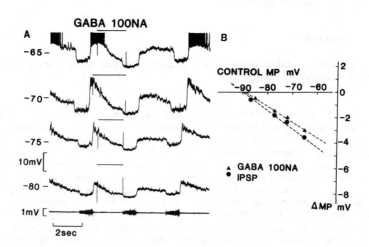

Fig. 1.   Current clamp measurements of the reversal potential
for the GABA-response and for the inspiratory IPSP wave in a
PI-neuron.   A: membrane potential responses to intracellular
current injection.   GABA was applied during the bar at 100
nA.   B: plots of the amplitudes (ordinates) of the GABA-
induced responses (triangles) and of the inspiratory IPSPs
(dots) against the membrane potential (abscissa).

Iontophoresis of bicuculline selectively blocked the action of GABA but not the action of glycine. Bicuculline itself produced a sustained depolarization associated with an increase in input resistance of both I- and PI-neurons during the entire respiratory cycle. Bicuculline, but not strychnine, decreased the spontaneous IPSP waves and initiated the repetitive action potentials during the inactive phase in these neurons (Haji et al., 1987). Iontophoresis of flurazepam augmented the spontaneous IPSP waves and the hyperpolarization induced by GABA. Bicuculline suppressed the action of flurazepam (Takeda and Haji, 1989). Intravenous injection of diazepam (0.05-0.10 mg/kg) potentiated specifically the periodic IPSP waves occurring during the inactive phase in both types of neurons and consistently shortened the respiratory cycle (Takeda et al., 1989).

CONCLUSION

The present results document that the inhibitory response of the VRG neurons to iontophoretically applied GABA was consistent with this amino acid being a trans-synaptic mediator for the periodic IPSPs. Benzodiazepines augmented both the GABA-induced response and the IPSP waves in these neurons. Bicuculline specifically antagonized the inhibitory actions induced by iontophoretically applied GABA and flurazepam. In addition, systemic application of diazepam enhanced the phasic IPSPs and altered the respiratory rhythm. These results suggest that GABA mediates the postsynaptic inhibition during expiration in I-neuron and during inspiration in PI-neuron. This inhibitory mechanism appears to play a crucial role in pattern formation of the bulbar respiratory neurons and, hence, control the respiratory rhythm.

REFERENCES

Champagnat, J., M. Denavit-Saubie, S. Moyanova and G. Rondouin (1982). Involvement of amino acids in periodic inhibitions of bulbar respiratory neurones. Brain Res., 237, 351-365.
Haji, A., C. Connelly, S.A. Schultz, J. Wallace and J.E. Remmers (1987). Postsynaptic actions of inhibitory neurotransmitters on bulbar respiratory neurons. In: Neurobiology of the Control of Breathing. (C. von Euler and H. Lagercrantz, Eds.), Raven Press, New York, pp.187-194.
Kirsten, E.B., J. Satayavivad, W.M. St.John and S.C. Wang (1978). Alteration of medullary respiratory unit discharge by iontophoretic application of putative neurotransmitters. Br. J. Pharmacol., 63, 275-281.
Richter, D.W. (1982). Generation and maintenance of the respiratory rhythm. J. exp. Biol., 100, 93-107.
Takeda, R. and A. Haji (1989). Microiontophoresis of flurazepam on inspiratory and postinspiratory neurons in the ventrolateral medulla of cats: an intracellular study in vivo. Neurosci. Lett., 102, 261-267.
Takeda, R., A. Haji and T. Hukuhara (1989). Diazepam potentiates postsynaptic inhibition in bulbar respiratory neurons of cats. Resp. Physiol., 77:173-186.
Toleikis, J.R., L. Wang and L.L. Boyarsky (1979). Effects of excitatory and inhibitory amino acids on phasic respiratory neurons. J. Neurosci. Res., 4:225-235.

Respiratory Pattern Generation in the Ventral Respiratory Group Neurons

R. Takeda*, A. Haji*, J.E. Remmers[†] and T. Hukuhara[‡]

*Department of Pharmacology, Toyama Medical and
Pharmaceutical University, Toyama, Japan
[†]Department of Medicine, University of Calgary,
Calgary, Canada
[‡]Department of Pharmacology, Jikei University School
of Medicine, Tokyo, Japan

ABSTRACT

Microiontophoresis of tetrodotoxin abolished the respiratory fluctuations of
membrane potential in virtually all inspiratory, post-inspiratory and expiratory
neurons recorded in the ventral respiratory group. This suggests that the
respiratory patterns in these neurons are shaped exclusively by synaptic drives.

KEYWORDS

Respiratory neuron; VRG; membrane potential; postsynaptic potentials;
respiratory pattern; tetrodotoxin

The neurons constituting the mechanism for the generation of respiratory rhythm
are still uncertain. This mechanism is thought to locate in the lower brain
stem including the two main regions, dorsal and ventral respiratory groups (DRG
and VRG), where respiration-related neurons relatively aggregate. It is assumed
that the respiratory patterns of the VRG and DRG neurons are generated not by an
intrinsic pacemaker mechanism but by periodically arriving excitatory and
inhibitory synaptic drives (Richter, 1982). In order to assess this hypothesis,
we attempted to functionally isolate a VRG neuron from the presynaptic neuronal
activities by locally applying tetrodotoxin (TTX) in vivo. We employed a
coaxial multi-barrelled microelectrode for intracellular recording and
extracellular microiontophoresis (Haji et al., in press). The present results
demonstrated that iontophoretic application of TTX effectively blocked the
synaptic inputs onto a VRG neuron and eliminated the respiratory fluctuations in
membrane potential (MP).

MATERIALS AND METHODS

Experiments were performed on decerebrate, paralyzed and artificially ventilated
cats after vagotomy. End-tidal CO_2 concentrations were maintained at 4-5%. The

mean arterial blood pressure was kept more than 80 mmHg. Tracheal pressure was kept between 8 and 2 cmH_2O, and rectal temperature at 36-38 °C. The efferent activity of the phrenic nerve was recorded to monitor the central respiratory rhythm. Respiratory neurons were penetrated with the center pipette (2 M potassium citrate, 20-30 MΩ) of a coaxial multi-barrelled microelectrode while TTX (0.5 mM, pH 6.5) was applied by extracellular iontophoresis 20-40 μm from the recording site (Haji et al., in press). Augmenting inspiratory (I), decrementing expiratory or post-inspiratory (PI) and augmenting expiratory (E) neurons were classified. Further, according to the response to electrical stimulation to the ipsilateral vagus nerve and the spinal cord, neurons were identified as the laryngeal motor (LM), bulbospinal (BS) or not-antidromically-activated (NAA) neurons (Richter, 1982). They were located 3.0-4.0 mm lateral to the midline, 0-3.0 mm rostral to the obex and 2.7-4.5 mm below the dorsal surface.

RESULTS

With a continuous iontophoresis at current strength of 25-50 nA, TTX produced a complete arrest of action potential generation and a sustained depolarization of the membrane within 30 sec. This was followed by hyperpolarization that progressively increased to a final value of approximately -90 mV. The respiratory fluctuations in MP were consistently reduced in I-, PI- and E-neurons (Fig. 1).

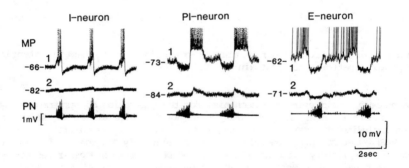

Fig. 1. Effects of iontophoretically applied TTX on the membrane potential fluctuations in an I- , PI- and E-neuron. MP; membrane potential, PN; phrenic nerve activity. MP records were taken before (1) and after (2) iontophoresis of TTX (50 nA for 15 min). Voltage calibrations reveal the hyperpolarizing shift of MP after TTX.

In most of the VRG neurons, the respiratory undulation in MP disappeared and the MP profile became flat in a whole respiratory cycle following TTX application. The input resistance increased during the period of membrane hyperpolarization. These effects of TTX on the MP trajectory were observed similarly in LM, BS and NAA neurons. In some neurons (about 10% of all neurons examined), prolonged application of TTX (50 nA, 25 min) did not abolish, though markedly depressed, the MP fluctuations particularly in the depolarizing phase of the respiratory cycle, i.e., during inspiration of I-neuron, stage I expiration of PI-neuron and stage II expiration of E-neuron.

DISCUSSION AND CONCLUSION

TTX, a specific blocker of the fast sodium channel (Ritchie, 1980), blocks action potentials pre- and post-synaptically. Iontophoretically applied TTX had no influence on the hyperpolarizing effect of iontophoretically applied GABA but eliminated the effect of iontophoresed bicuculline antagonizing the inhibitory postsynaptic potentials (IPSPs) in the VRG neurons (Haji et al., in press). These results show that TTX does not suppress the sensitivity to an inhibitory neurotransmitter postsynaptically and blocks the axonal conduction and release of the transmitter presynaptically. That TTX virtually eliminated the respiratory fluctuations of MP in I-, PI- and E-neurons may provide an evidence that the respiratory oscillation of MP in the VRG neurons results from the periodic synaptic activities among the respiratory neuronal network (Richter, 1982). Additionally, a small dose of halothane (a 90 sec infusion at 2%) and of thiopental (2.5 mg/kg i.v.) produced a depression of action potential firing, reduction of the respiratory MP fluctuations and increase of input resistance in the VRG neurons, the effects being similar to those caused by TTX (Takeda et al., in press). This suggests that anesthetic agents also disrupted the synaptic transmission and suppressed the respiratory fluctuations of MP in the VRG neurons. However, in some neurons the respiratory MP fluctuations diminished but not disappeared after iontophoresis of TTX. This can be explained by postulating that the adequate concentration of TTX was not achieved at the presynaptic nerve terminal. Since the hyperpolarizing phase of MP fluctuations was preferentially blocked by TTX, the loci of the inhibitory synaptic inputs seem to be closer to the recording site than the excitatory synapses. This may be consistent with the result that TTX initially produced a sustained depolarization and later a profound hyperpolarization of the membrane. The latter result also leads to a concept that the VRG neurons receive not only phasic synaptic inputs but also tonic inhibitory and tonic excitatory synaptic drives.

REFERENCES

Haji, A., J.E. Remmers, C. Connelly and R. Takeda (1990). Effects of glycine and GABA on bulbar respiratory neurons in the cat. J. Neurophysiol., in press.

Richter, D.W. (1982). Generation and maintenance of the respiratory rhythm. J. Exp. Biol., 100, 93-107.

Ritchie, J.M. (1980). Tetrodotoxin and saxitoxin and the sodium channels of the excitable tissues. Trends Pharmacol. Sci., 1, 275-279.

Takeda, R., A. Haji and T. Hukuhara (1990). Selective actions of anesthetic agents on membrane potential trajectory in bulbar respiratory neurons of cats. Pflugers Arch., in press.

Correlation of Inspiratory Unit Activity in the Brain Stem With Phrenic High-frequency Oscillation of Rabbits

K. Takano, F. Kato, N. Kimura and
T. Hukuhara, Jr.

Department of Pharmacology II, Jikei University School
of Medicine, Minato-ku, Tokyo 105, Japan

ABSTRACT

High-frequency oscillation (HFO), synchronization of the motoneuronal discharges at a high-frequency range, is observed in the inspiratory discharges of the phrenic efferent nerve activity. The physiological significance of the HFO-correlated reticular inspiratory unit activities in terms of respiratory rhythmogenesis was examined in anesthetized and normoventilated rabbits. The results suggest that the neural mechanism primarily responsible for the generation of respiratory rhythm makes little functional contribution to the HFO generation.

KEYWORDS

High-frequency oscillation; respiratory center; respiratory rhythmogenesis; brain stem; reticular formation; neurons; correlation analysis; phrenic nerve.

INTRODUCTION

The neural mechanism responsible for generation and formation of high-frequency oscillation (HFO) in a range from 70 to 130 Hz has been proposed to be located in the brain stem (Cohen, 1973; Berger et al., 1978). The HFO is a characteristic component of the activities of the efferent nerves which innervate skeletal muscles associated with respiratory movements (Kato et al., 1978). We have proposed, on the other hand, that respiratory neurons with a highly stable respiratory rhythm would be "primary respiratory neurons" responsible for respiratory rhythmogenesis as confirmed by quantitative measurements (Hukuhara, 1973, 1988a). Hukuhara (1984) confirmed that the candidates of the primary respiratory neurons were highly resistant to a respiratory depressant action of thiamylal. Present investigation was performed to examine the physiological significance of the HFO-correlated inspiratory neurons in terms of the rhythmogenesis.

METHODS

Experiments were performed on 49 rabbits of either sex weighing 2.0-3.5 kg. Animals were anesthetized with diethyl ether and paralyzed with gallamine triethiodide (3-6 mg/kg,i.v.). Vagus, sympathetic and depressor nerves were cut bilaterally at the neck under artificial ventilation. End-tidal carbon dioxide gas concentration was kept at 3.7±0.4 %. Spontaneous reticular inspiratory unit discharges in the brain stem and efferent discharges of the phrenic nerve were simultaneously recorded. Each unit spike potential was confirmed to be originated from the somadendritic part of a neuron with a conventional method. Spike-triggered averaging technique was employed in order to estimate the degree of the correlation of individual spikes of inspiratory unit activities with each wave of phrenic HFO ("HFO-correlation", H-Cor) according to the methods previously described (Hukuhara et al., 1988b). To identify the candidates for primary respiratory neurons, correlation analysis and estimation of coefficient of variation were used (Hukuhara, 1984). Statistical comparisons were made by means of Student's t-test. Values are expressed as means±SD.

RESULTS

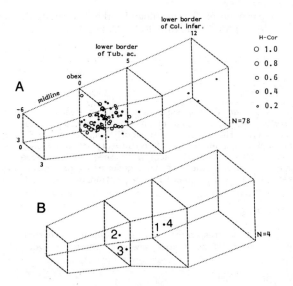

Fig. 1. Distribution of HFO-correlated neurons plotted in the three-dimensional representation of hemisphere of the brain stem. 0, obex; 5, the lower border of the tuberculum acusticum; 12, the lower border of the colliculus inferior; -6, lower border of the medulla oblongata. The figures of 5, 12, and -6 indicate the distance from the obex in mm. Right, rostral; Left, caudal direction. A: Inspiratory activities (n=78) recorded in the brain stem. B: Four candidates for primary respiratory neurons (units 1-4). The area of each circle is proportional to the H-Cor of each unit.

Seventy-eight inspiratory unit activities were recorded in the bulbar and pontine reticular formation of the brain stem of rabbits (12.0 mm rostral to the obex; 2.0 mm caudal to the obex; 0.5-3.5 mm lateral to the midline; 0.4-5.0 mm below the dorsal surface; Fig. 1, A). Estimated H-Cors varied with the individual reticular inspiratory unit activities (0.04 to 0.92, 0.35±0.24, n=78). Thirty-eight unit activities (49 %, 0.54±0.18, n=38) out of 78 were fulfilled the previously reported criteria (Hukuhara et al., 1988b) of the HFO-correlated activities. The mean H-Cor of these correlated unit activities was significantly higher than that of little correlated ones (51 %, 0.15±0.05, n=40). Most of the neurons with high H-Cor were concentrated in the reticular formation in the vicinity of the obex near to the corresponding region to DRG (dorsal respiratory group) and VRG (ventral respiratory group) defined in cats (Fig. 1, A). The respiratory discharges of four inspiratory unit activities recorded in the lateral region of the bulbar reticular formation (units 1-4 in Fig. 1, B) were found to be highly stable and they were quantitatively identified as the candidates for primary respiratory neuron. These four unit activities had little H-Cor (0.14±0.07), whose value was significantly smaller than that of HFO-correlated unit activities. The mean value of H-Cors of three pontine inspiratory unit activities was 0.14±0.03 and none of them were identified as HFO-correlated.

DISCUSSIONS

We found that the inspiratory neurons existing in the brain stem had functional heterogeneity in respect to the HFO-correlation and that the highly correlated neurons were thought to belong to the neural mechanisms involved in the generation of the HFO or the synchronization of the respiratory premotor- and cranial motor neuron population in the brain stem. These findings may indicate that the respiratory neurons with high H-Cor are involved in the output system in the central respiratory mechanisms and that some members of neurons of the DRG and the VRG are functionally related to the respiratory output system in rabbits. Moreover, the unit activities of four neurons, identified as the candidates for the primary respiratory neurons, were found to be little correlated to the HFO. This result indicates that the neural mechanism primarily responsible for the generation of respiratory rhythm has little functional contribution to the HFO generation.

Supported partly by the Ministry of Education, Science and Culture, Japan, Grant-in-Aid for Developmental Scientific Research, No. 01870012 and by the Science Research Promotion Fund of Japan Private School Promotion Foundation (1988).

REFERENCES

Berger, A. J., D. A. Herbert and R. A. Mitchell (1978). Properties of apneusis produced by reversible cold block of the rostral pons. Respir. Physiol., 33. 323-337.

Cohen, M.I. (1973). Synchronization of discharge, spontaneous and evoked, between inspiratory neurons, Acta Neurobiol. Exp., 33. 189-218.

Hukuhara, T. Jr. (1973). Neuronal organization of the central respiratory mechanisms in the brain stem of the cat. Acta Neurobiol. Exp., 33, 219-244.

Hukuhara, T. Jr. (1984). Discharge properties of respiratory-modulated brainstem reticular neurons and their relation to slow arterial pressure fluctuations in the rabbit. In: Mechanisms of Blood Pressure Waves (K. Miyakawa, H. P. Koepchen and C. Polosa, eds.), pp. 305-316, Springer-Verlag, Berlin.

Hukuhara, T. Jr. (1988a). Organization of the brain stem neural mechanisms for generation of respiratory rhythm-Current problems. Jpn. J. Physiol., 38. 753-776.

Hukuhara, T. Jr., K. Takano, F. Kato and N. Kimura (1988b). Medullary inspiratory neurons with a stable respiratory rhythm and little correlation to phrenic high-frequency oscillation. Tohoku J. Exp. Med., 156(Suppl.). 11-19.

Kato, F., N. Kimura, K. Takano and T. Hukuhara, Jr. (1987). Quantitative spectral analysis of high frequency oscillations in efferent nerve activities with respiratory rhythm. In: Respiratory Muscles and Their Neuromotor Control (G. C. Sieck, S. C. Gandevia and W. E. Cameron, eds.), pp. 263-267, Alan R. Liss, New York.

Effects of Localized Cooling of the Ventral Medullary Surface (VMS) on Expiratory Muscle Activity

T. Chonan, S. Okabe, W. Hida,
T. Izumiyama, M. Satoh, M. Sakurai,
Y. Kikuchi, N. Iwase, O. Taguchi,
H. Miki and T. Takishima

First Department of Internal Medicine, Tohoku
University School of Medicine, Sendai 980, Japan

ABSTRACT

Focal cooling of the ventral medullary surface (VMS) produces respiratory
depression. The cooling effects of the VMS, particularly the intermediate area,
on the activity of some respiratory motoneurons and respiratory muscles have
been reported to be inhomogeneous. We assessed the effects of VMS cooling on
the activity of the chest wall and abdominal expiratory muscles in six
anesthetized and artificially ventilated dogs after denervation of the vagus and
carotid sinus nerves. Electromyograms (EMG) of the triangularis sterni (TS),
internal intercostal (II), external oblique (EO), internal oblique (IO), and
transversus abdominis (TA) muscles were measured during localized cooling (2x2
mm) of the thermosensitive area, with the EMG of the diaphragm (DI) as an index
of inspiratory activity. Bilateral cooling of the thermosensitive area produced
temperature-dependent reduction of both inspiratory and expiratory muscle
activity. However, the amount of reduction was different among the expiratory
muscles. The EMG of the TS decreased consistently less than other expiratory
EMGs at a constant degree of VMS cooling. With moderate to severe cooling (<20
°C) DI activity disappeared, but TS activity remained and became tonic; this
tonic activity of the TS was reciprocally inhibited when the activity of the DI
resumed during rewarming of the VMS. These results indicate that the effects of
cooling the VMS differ between the activity of inspiratory and expiratory
muscles, and among the expiratory muscles. This variability may be due to
inhomogeneous inputs from the VMS to respiratory motoneurons or to a different
responsiveness of various respiratory motoneurons to the same input from the
VMS.

KEYWORDS

Cold block; expiratory muscles; inhomogeneous respiratory control;
ventral medullary surface

It has been reported that the superficial layer of the ventrolateral medulla
contains neural structures which participate in the shaping of respiratory
rhythm and vasomotor tone (Bruce and Cherniack, 1987). Focal cooling of the
thermosensitive area of the ventral medullary surface (VMS) produces respiratory

depression in cats, rats and dogs (Schlaefke and Loeschcke, 1967; Mitra et al., 1988; Chonan et al., 1989). However, it has been reported that the cooling-induced decrease in respiratory activity is inhomogeneous among some respiratory motoneurons and muscles (Haxhiu et al., 1985). In this study we examined the effects of cooling of the thermosensitive areas on the activity of chest wall and abdominal expiratory muscles in anesthetized dogs.

METHODS

Experiments were carried out in six dogs anesthetized with pentobarbital sodium. Following bilateral thoracotomy, vagotomy and denervation of carotid sinus nerves, the animal was fixed in a prone position using a stereotaxic holder (Narishige) and artificially ventilated with a hyperoxic gas mixture ($Fo_2 > 0.5$) under 10 cmH_2O threshold load. Bilateral localized cooling of the ventral medullary surface (VMS) was performed with a double footed 2x2 mm thermoprobe. The regions cooled were within the thermosensitive areas which are located 4-9 mm caudal from the foramen cecum and lateral to the pyramids (Chonan et al., 1989). Electromyograms (EMG) of the triangularis sterni (TS), internal intercostal (II), external oblique (EO), internal oblique (IO) and transversus abdominis (TA) muscles were measured with pairs of stainless steel wire electrodes. EMG of the diaphragm (DI) was recorded as an index of inspiratory activity. The electrical signals were amplified, band-pass filtered (100-2 kHz), full wave rectified and processed by "leaky" integrators (100 ms time constant).

RESULTS

Bilateral localized cooling of the thermosensitive areas produced temperature dependent depression of all the respiratory muscle activity. However, the degree of depression differed between the DI and expiratory muscles, and among the expiratory muscles. Table 1 shows the amplitude of integrated EMG of each muscle at the VMS temperatures of 25 and 15°C. Expiratory activity of chest wall muscles was less susceptible to cold block of the TSA than was that of the abdominal muscles. Especially, the EMG of the TS decreased consistently less than other expiratory EMGs at a constant degree of VMS cooling. TS activity remained and became tonic even when the DI activity disappeared at low VMS temperatures (<20°C); this tonic activity of TS was reciprocally inhibited with the resumption of DI during rewarming of the VMS.

DISCUSSION

The results of this study indicate that localized cooling of the thermosensitive areas of the VMS reduces expiratory as well as inspiratory muscle activity, but the effect of cold block is inhomogeneous among the expiratory muscles and TS shows tonic activity with the disappearance of DI.

Schwanghart et al.(1974) reported that the activity of both inspiratory and expiratory neurons was depressed when the ventral brain stem was perfused with a mock cerebro-spinal fluid which contained novocaine, and that the majority of expiratory neurons began to discharge continuously as soon as the inspiratory neurons ceased firing. This is consistent with the findings of this study and suggest that the VMS has an important role in determining expiratory amplitude. It is also suggested that there is a discrepancy between inspiratory and expiratory activity in response to functional block of the VMS.

Recently, Smith et al.(1989) reported that different expiratory muscles respond differently to chemical stimuli. This study provides additional evidence which

Table 1. EMG amplitudes of respiratory muscles during graded
          cooling of the thermosensitive areas

	VMS Temperature	
	25 °C	15 °C
Triangularis sterni (% control)	84 + 18	68 + 35
Internal intercostal	70 + 26	40 + 40
External oblique	49 + 35	32 + 18
Internal oblique	39 + 16	14 + 22
Transversus abdominis	47 + 19	14 + 11
Diaphragm	60 + 18	10 + 15

Data are means + SD.

suggests inhomogeneous characteristics among the expiratory muscles.

The variability in responsiveness of expiratory EMGs to VMS cooling may be due
to inhomogeneous inputs from the VMS to the expiratory motoneurons or differing
responsiveness of expiratory motoneurons to the same input from the VMS.
Alternatively, the VMS may modulate expiratory activity indirectly by affecting
the inspiratory motoneurons, and the differential responsiveness of expiratory
activity may reflect variability in the level of inhibition from the inspiratory
to the expiratory motoneurons.

References

Bruce, E.N. and N.S. Cherniack (1987). Central chemoreceptors.   J. Appl.
    Physiol., 62, 389–402.
Cherniack, N.S., C. von Euler, I. Homma and F.F. Kao (1979).   Graded changes
    in central chemoreceptor input by local   temperature changes on the ventral
    surface of medulla. J. Physiol.(London), 287, 191–211.
Chonan, T., W. Hida, S. Okabe, T. Izumiyama and T. Takishima (1989). Effects of
    localized cooling of the ventral surface of medulla in dogs. Proc. IUPS,,
    XVII, 171.
Haxhiu, M.A., J. Mitra, E. van Lunteren, N.P. Prabhaker and N.S. Cherniack
    (1985). Am. J. Physiol., 249, R266–R273.
Mitra, J., N.R. Prabhaker, J.L. Overholt and N.S. Cherniack (1988). Respiratory
    and vasomotor responses to focal cooling of the ventral medullary surface
    (VMS) of the rat. Respir. Physiol., 74, 35–48.
Schlaefke, M.E. and H.H. Loeschcke (1967). Lokalisation eines an der Regulation
    von Atmung und Kreislauf beteiligten Gebietes an der ventralen Oberfläche der
    Medulla oblongata durch Kälteblockade. Pflügers Archiv, 297, 201–220.
Schwanghart, F., R. Schröter, D. Klüssendorf and H.P. Koepchen (1974). The
    influence of novocaine block of superficial brain stem structures on
    respiratory and reticular neurons. In: Central Rhythmic and Regulation (W.
    Umbach and H.P. Koepchen, Eds.), pp. 104–110. Hippokrates Verlag, Stuttgart.
Smith, C.A., D.M. Ainsworth, K.S. Henderson and J.A. Dempsey (1989).
    Differential responses of expiratory muscles to chemical stimuli in awake
    dogs. J. Appl. Physiol., 66, 384–391.

Differential Respiratory Effects of HCO_3 and CO_2 Applied on the Ventral Medullary Surface of the Rat

H. Tojima*, T. Kuriyama* and Y. Fukuda[†]

*Department of Chest Medicine, School of Medicine,
Chiba University, 280 Chiba;
[†]Department of Psychology II, School of Medicine,
Chiba University, 280 Chiba, Japan

ABSTRACT

To estimate whether the H^+ is a unique stimulus to the medullary chemosensor ventilatory effects of HCO_3 and CO_2 applied on the ventral medullary surface with using an improved superfusion technique and of CO_2 inhalation were compared in the halothane anesthetized spontaneously breathing rat. Superfusion with acidic, low $[HCO_3^-]$ solution at a constant Pco_2 increased ventilation compared to normal CSF. Superfusion with high $[HCO_3^-]$ solution decreased ventilation. Increase or decrease of Pco_2 of the superfusing fluid at a constant $[HCO_3^-]$ produced no significant change of respiratory parameters. Superfusion with solution containing the cholinergic blocking agent, mecamylamine, decreased ventilation and depressed ventilatory response to inhalaed CO_2. We conclude that the examined area of the rat ventral medulla contains HCO_3^- (or H^+) sensitive neural substrates which may be, however, little affected by CO_2 in the subarachnoid fluid. CO_2-H^+ sensitive components exist elsewhere apart functionally from the surface chemosensor.

KEYWORDS

Ventral medullary surface; superfusion; $CO_2-HCO_3^--H^+$; central chemosensitivity; mecamylamine; rat.

METHODS

Fourteen male Wistar rats weighing 300-400g were used. The animal was anesthetized with halothane (maintanance during experiment 0.8-0.9%) and was placed in the supine position. Techniques for measuring respiratory parameters, end-tidal Pco_2, and blood gases in the anesthetized rat have been described in previous papers (Fukuda et al.,1982, Tojima et al.,1988). All experiments were performed in spontaneously breathing rats under hyperoxic condition with intact carotid sinus and vagus nerves. To expose the ventral surface of the medulla oblongata, we removed the larynx, the esophagus, and the muscles covering the occipital bone. The basis-occipital bones were chipped away and the dura-arachnoid membranes covering over the ventral medulla were exposed from the lower edge of the pons to just caudal to the junction of the vertebral arteries. Superfusion cannulae were inserted into the subarachnoidal space through a small hall in the midline of the membrane

at the level of the hypoglossal nerve roots (Fig.1). Superfusing fluid (mock
CSF) was overflowed through the same hole and removed by continuous suction.
The rate of superfusion was limited at 0.2-0.4 ml/min for selective superfusion
of the ventral medulla. It was confirmed that there was no leak of CO_2 from
the pump-cannula system and Pco_2 of of the overflowed fluid dropped only less
than 2 mmHg from that inflow fluid.

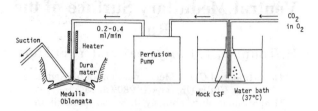

Fig.1. Scheme of experimental set-up used for superfusing
the ventral surface of the rat medulla oblongata

RESULTS

Identification of superfused areas

It was confirmed that superfused areas were restricted to the ventral medullary
surface at the level from the caudal portion of the XIIth cranial nerve root
and the trapezoid body by adding methylene blue in the solution at the end
of each experiment.

Superfusion with mock CSF of varied [HCO_3^-] or Pco_2

As shown in Fig.2, the superfusion with low [HCO_3^-] - acid pH (7.1-7.2) mock
CSF caused a significant increase in ventilation. In contrast, high [HCO_3]
- alkaline pH (7.7-7.9) solution produced a reduction in ventilation. Changes
in ventilation began immediately on the arrival of acid or alkaline solution
and reached steady state condition within 5 min. Changes in ventilation were
produced mainly by alteration of V_T. When CO_2 gas was injected into the
inspiratory line to maintain end-tidal Pco_2 during the superfusion with acid
solution, a further marked increase in ventilation was seen. The increase
or decrease of pH by changing Pco_2 of the solution at maintained [HCO_3] (22mM)
on the other hand, produced no significant changes in ventilation although
superfusion was continued at least for a period of 15 min (or more) even at
a higher flow rate (up to 1.2 ml/min).

Superfusion with solution of changing [HCO_3] and Pco_2 simultaneously

When the superfusion was performed by low [HCO_3^-] - low Pco_2 solution, there
was a marked increase in V_T, f and V_E which accompanied reduction in end-tidal
Pco_2. In contrast, high [HCO_3^-] - high Pco_2 solution depressed ventilation
and elevated end-tidal Pco_2. Since end-tidal Pco_2 level was not the same
in both conditions, comparison was made at the same end-tidal Pco_2 level by
breathing CO_2 gas during superfusing with low [HCO_3^-] - low Pco_2 solution.
As shown in Fig.3, respiration was stimulated markedly during superfusing
with [HCO_3^-] - low Pco_2 solution but was depressed by high [HCO_3^-] - high Pco_2
solution despite both the end-tidal Pco_2 and pH of the superfusing solution
were nearly identical.

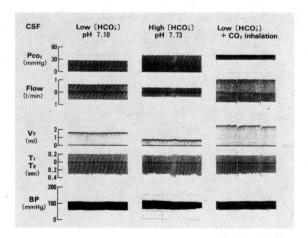

Fig.2. Effects of ventral medullary superfusion with mock
CSF of different [HCO$_3^-$].

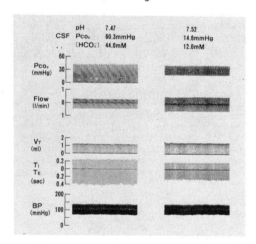

Fig.3. Effects of superfusing the ventral medulla with
solutions in which [HCO$_3^-$] and Pco$_2$ were changed
simultaneously to maintain pH.

Superfusion with solution containing the cholinergic blocking agent

Ventilation was depressed during superfusing with mecamylamine containing
solution. Furthermore, ventilatory response to CO$_2$ inhalation was depressed
by mecamylamine.

REFERECES
Fukuda,Y.,W.R.See and Y.Honda (1982). Effect of halothane anesthesia on end-
tidal Pco$_2$ and pattern of respiration in the rat. Pflugers Arch.,392,244-250.
Tojima,H. et al.(1988). Jpn.J.Physiol.,38,445-457

Stereotyped Phrenic Responses to Mechanical Stimulation of the Epiglottal Mucosa

Y. Sakai and T. Hukuhara, Jr

Department of Pharmacology, Saitama Medical School,
Saitama, 350-04, and Department of Pharmacology II,
The Jikei University School of Medicine, Tokyo, 105,
Japan

ABSTRACT

Each of single or trains of vibratory stimulation of the epiglottis in both the adult cat and rabbit was followed by a brief fast-conducting afferent volley in the superior laryngeal nerve (SLN) and then by biphasic (excitatory to inhibitory) phrenic responses. These had almost the same pattern and characteristics as those of the well-known stereotyped phrenic responses to electrical stimulation of the internal branch of the SLN. We conclude that the stereotyped responses are probably produced by central neural procession of myelinated afferent impulses from dynamic mechanoreceptors in the larynx; they may have an important role in respiratory slowing during phonation or snoring.

KEYWORDS

Epiglottis; Vibratory stimulation; Dynamic mechanoreceptors; Myelinated afferent fibers; Phrenic nerve; Histogram; Stereotyped responses; Adult animals.

Using peristimulus time histogram (PSTH), Iscoe *et al.* (1979) first described the stereotyped phrenic response to afferent stimulation of the SLN. While the excitatory response is repeated even at 100 Hz, the inhibitory one is rarely repeated at 30 Hz (Sakai, 1988). Because of the short latency, the responses may be mediated by myelinated afferents. In this study, we tried to ascertain if the epiglottal mucosal or capsular receptors with high dynamic sensitivity (Davies and Nail, 1987) are involved in producing the stereotyped responses.

METHODS

Experiments were performed on twenty cats of either sex (2.2-5 kg) and five male rabbits (2.7-3.5 kg), which were vagotomized, paralyzed with pancuronium bromide and ventilated with a mixture of nitrous oxide and oxygen (55:45). Anesthesia was often deepened by adding halothane (1-1.5 %). The laryngeal surface of the epiglottis (3 mm x 2 mm on each side of the midline) was stimulated with a plexiglass probe, which was driven by a stimulator-controlled moving-coil vibrator or galvanometer. The histograms of laryngeal afferent and phrenic discharge were computed. Almost similar results were obtained in both species.

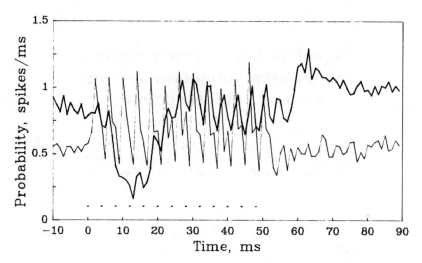

Fig. 1.   Superimposed histograms to show laryngeal afferent
          volleys (thin) and stereotyped phrenic responses
          (bold) evoked by a train of weak epiglottal shocks
          in a cat. The vibrator driven at dots. Note a kind
          of adaptation of the inhibitory response, enhanced
          excitatory ones and a rebound excitation.

RESULTS

Weak Stimulation. Since the movement of vibrator-driven probe (0.2-0.3 mm) was
repeatable even at 200 Hz, the device was suitable for single or trains of weak
vibratory stimulation of the epiglottis.   Each single shock evoked a brief (2-3
ms) afferent volley along the SLN, which was followed by a biphasic stereotyped
phrenic response.   The latencies, measured between the onsets, from the afferent
volley to both excitatory and inhibitory responses of the phrenic nerve were 4-5
ms and 7-8 ms, respectively. The inhibitory response lasted about 10 ms.   When a
long train of high frequency shocks (>100 Hz) was given, as shown in Fig. 1, the
initial excitatory response was followed by a more powerful and prolonged
inhibitory one, which never exceeded 30 ms even though afferent volleys could be
further evoked in response to each epiglottal shock.   With paired train test, a
full extent of the potent inhibitory response was at most repeatable at 20 Hz.
The phrenic responses to single shocks, at least the inhibitory duration,   were
reduced by deepening anesthesia, while the inhibitory response to a train of
shocks was enhanced.   Using the conduction velocity determination along the SLN,
the relevant afferent fibers were ascertained to belong mainly to group II.

Stronger Stimulation.   The movement of galvanometer-driven probe (2-3 mm)   was
hardly repeated at 30 Hz.   Each epiglottal shock elicited two large afferent
volleys as on and off responses and biphasic phrenic responses; the inhibition
was especially marked and was enhanced by deepening anesthesia (Fig. 2).   The
inhibitory duration rarely exceeded 30 ms even when the width of drive pulse was
increased up to 40 ms or more.   Without any significant reduction, the second
inhibitory response to paired shocks occurred only after 50 ms.   The conduction
velocity of volleys along the SLN was those of groups II and III afferents.

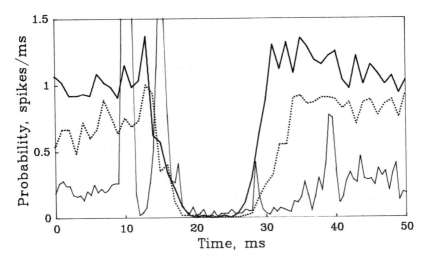

Fig. 2.   Superposed histograms to show two afferent volleys
(thin) and stereotyped phrenic responses in light
(bold) and deep anesthesia (dotted) after single
stronger shocks given to the epiglottis in a cat.
The movement of stimulating probe, driven by 5-ms
pulses at zero, causes the actual indenting shock
at 8 ms and the second volley on retraction.

DISCUSSION

We found that vibratory epiglottal stimuli cause the same stereotyped phrenic
responses as those to electrical afferent stimulation of the SLN (Sakai, 1988).
The responses to two types of stimulation were similar in respect to the dual
pattern, latency, duration, property to undergo adaptation, refractory period,
mediation by myelinated afferent fibers and anesthetic sensitivity.   Therefore,
we conclude that the stereotyped phrenic responses would be caused by   a
simultaneous activation of highly dynamic epiglottal receptors (Davies and Nail,
1987).   Thus, this reflex may be involved in the respiratory slowing during
phonation or snoring, when a similar epiglottal stimulation, if any, occurs.   In
contrast to the inhibitory response, the excitatory one to mucosal stimulation
was not so potent as that to afferent stimulation. This is probably due to the
receptor volley to exhibit a greater temporal dispersion, both at the onset in
the larynx and along the pathway before invading the afferent terminals.

REFERENCES

Davies, P.J. and B.S. Nail (1987). Quantitative analysis of laryngeal mechano-
    sensitivity in the cat and rabbit. *J. Physiol.*, 388, 467-485.
Iscoe, S., J.L. Feldman and M.I. Cohen (1979).   Properties of inspiratory
    termination by superior laryngeal and vagal stimulation. *Respir. Physiol.*,
    36, 353-366.
Sakai, Y. (1988). Stereotyped phrenic response to laryngeal afferent volleys:
    the mechanism and anesthetic sensitivity. *Tohoku J. Exp. Med.*, 156, 33-41.

Hypoxic Ventilatory Response During Recovery Period from Sustained Hypoxia

Motoo Sato, Sohei Kagawa, Masayuki Kamide, Yasumasa Tanifuji and Kenichi Kobayashi

Department of Anesthesiology, The Jikei University School of Medicine 3-19-18 Nishi-shinbashi, Minato-ku, Tokyo, Japan

ABSTRACT

Healthy volunteers were exposed to a hypercapnic hypoxic state ($PEO_2=44$ torr)for 30 min. Then,after 15 min of hypercapnic hyperoxic interlude (PEO_2 more than 200 torr), a second 15 min of hypercapnic hypoxic state was established. $PECO_2$ was kept constant at 44 torr throughout the experiment. Minute ventilation during the 15 min interlude, before the 2nd hypoxic exposure, was significantly higher than the resting ventilation before the 1st hypoxic exposure. There was no significant change in the peak minute ventilation between the 1st and 2nd hypoxia. It is possible that the origin of the increment in ventilation shown after 30 min of hypoxic exposure and the origin of 2nd hypoxic ventilatory response are the same.

KEYWORDS

Hypoxia; ventilatory response;acclimatization

INTRODUCTION

It is well known that in the normal adult the isocapnic hypoxic ventilatory response is biphasic, an initial increase in minute ventilation followed by gradual decline (i.e. hypoxic ventilatory depression) during the first 5-30min of hypoxia. Ventilation then stabilizes a little higher level than the resting value (Kagawa et al.,1982). When hypoxia is removed, on the other hand, the stimulation of carotid body will disappears rapidly, but the hypoxic ventilatory depression has been shown to persist for 5-10min. One might expect that normoxic minute ventilation should be depressed for a while and would gradually return to control. We conducted the following experiment in order to measure in detail the ventilatory response after cessation of hypoxia, and hypoxic ventilatory response during this recovery period from hypoxia.

METHOD

The subjects were four normal male adult volunteers. They breathed spontaneously through a one way valve and a face mask. A mixture of oxygen, nitrogen and carbon dioxide was delivered into a reservoir bag which was attached to the one way valve. Expired CO_2 and O_2 concentrations, sampled at the nostril, were

Table . PEO2, SPO2, PECO2 and V̇I during steady state,hypoxia,
interlude and second hypoxia. Values are means ± SD.

n=4	Steady state	Hypoxia		Interlude		Hypoxia
		Initial	Final	Initail	Final	
	A	B	C	D	E	F
PEO2(mmHg)	211±5	44±1	44±1	211±9	216±9	44±2
SPO2 (%)	98±1	75±4	75±5	97±1	98±1	77±4
PECO2(mmHg)	44±0	44±1	44±1	44±1	44±1	44±1
V̇I (L/min)	9.5±0.6	22.4±3.4	14.5±2.2	8.5±1.5	14.6±1.3	26.3±2.3

measured.   Arterial oxygen saturation was measured with an ear pulse oximeter.
Respiratory flow was measured with a hot wire spirometer and minute ventilation
was caculated.   The subjects were exposed to 30min of hypoxia and 15 min second
hypoxia which were separated by an interlude of 15 min hyperoxia. The level of
hypoxia was represented by PEO2 44±2 torr, and SpO2 76±4%. We kept PEO2 at above
200 torr to remove hypoxic drive during the steady state and 15 min interlude.
In order to prevent the rise in PECO2 accompanied by a decrease in minute
ventilation after sessation of   30 min of hypoxia we maintained PECO2 at 44±1
torr throughout the experiment by administering CO2 ahead of the time of
exposure to hypoxia.

RESULTS

The ventilatory response to 30 min of hypoxia was biphasic with an initial
increase in minute ventilation and followed by gradual decline.   Soon after the
cessation of 30 min of hypoxia, minute ventilation declined below control level,
then gradually increased and stabilized higher than the prehypoxic steady state
level.This change was statistically significant.In the second hypoxic challenge,
the pattern of the change of minute ventilation was the same as the first one.
The peak ventilation during the second hypoxia was little higher than that of
the first hypoxia,but this was not statistically significant.

DISCUSSION

To understand the changes in ventilation resulting from repeated hypoxic
challenge, we postulated two elements which are facilitatory and inhibitory
elements as shown in the figure.   Inhibitory element is the origin of hypoxic
ventilatory depression.Two potential factors have been implicated in the genesis
of this inhibitory element.One consists in the interrelation of brain tissue CO2
level and pH ; it has been postulated that increased blood flow in the medulla
induced by hypoxia may lead to CO2 washout from the cerebral tissue with
consequent alkalosis, thereby giving this inhibitory element   (Feustel et al.,
1984). Secondly, possible participation of neurotransmitters and neuromodulators
such as GABA or adenosine have also been postulated (Easton et al.,1988;Millhorn
et al.,1984).   The facts that the onset of hypoxic ventilatory depression lags
briefly on exposure to hypoxia and that this depression persists for some time
even after termination of hypoxia would suggest possible

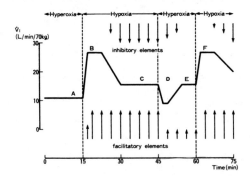

Fig. Inhibitory and facilitatory elements of ventilation

involvement of some alteration of metabolic process. A facilitatory element may be separated into two parts. One originates in carotid body stimulation and causes hypoxic ventilatory response. Another one is the origin of increment in ventilation after sessation of 30 min hypoxia. As we show that there is no significant change in the degree of ventilatory response between 1st and 2nd hypoxic challenge, the latter facilitatory element may originate somewhere in the same neural pathway of respiratory control. This facilitatory element may play a role in high altitude acclimatization.

REFERENCES

Easton, P.A.and N.R. Anthonisen(1988)   Ventilatory response to sustained hypoxia after pretreatment with aminophylline. J. Appl. Physiol. 64,1445-1450

Feustel, P. J., M.J. Stafford, J.S. Allen and J.W. Severinghaus (1984) Ventrolateral medullary surface blood flow determined by hydrogen clearance. J.Appl. Physiol. 56,150-154

Kagawa, S.,M.J. Stafford, T.B. Waggener and J.W. Severinghaus(1982) No effect of naloxone on hypoxia-induced ventilatory depression in adults . J.Appl Physiol. 52,1030-1034

Millhorn, D.E., F.L. Eldridge,J.P. Kiley and T.G. Waldrop(1984)   Prolonged inhibition of respiration following acute hypoxia in glomectomized cat.Respir. Physiol. 57,331-340

Ventilatory Response to Pseudorandom Work Rate Exercise in Man

S. Usui*, Y. Fukuba[†], M. Munaka[†],
T. Tsuji[‡], K. Iwanaga[§], T. Koba[§] and S. Koga[¶]

*Laboratory of Exercise Physiology Biomechanics,
Faculty Integrated Arts and Science, Hiroshima
University, Hiroshima 730;
[†]Department of Biometrics, Research Institute of Nuclear
Medical Biology, Hiroshima University;
[‡]Laboratory of Biology Engineering, Faculty
Engineering, Hiroshima University;
[§]Saga Research Institute, Otsuka Pharmaceutical Ltd;
[¶]Department Physical Education Ergonomics, Kobe
Design University, Japan

ABSTRACT

The dynamics of the ventilatory response to moderate exercise on a bicycle ergometer was studied in two healthy males. The work rate was varied between 0 and 100 W as a pseudorandom binary sequence (PRBS). Four possible models were applied to describe the ventilatory dynamics. The dynamics of response was well represented by model III, which is characterized by parallel components of two first order dynamics. One was a fast component and accounted for a much smaller proportion of the total response. The other was a slow component with a large gain which followed after a delay.

KEYWORDS

Ventilatory response; Exercise hyperpnea; Pseudorandom binary sequence; Dynamic system; System identification;

INTRODUCTION

The ventilatory response to dynamic exercise in human subject provides a basis to identify the physiological system and to diagnose the clinical abnormality involved in the control of ventilation. To identify the ventilatory response, step, ramp, sinusoidal wave, or short-duration pulse have been utilized as exercise input in previous studies. Although these inputs are easy to implement, some repetitions of forcing are needed to estimate the model parameters with high S/N ratio of measurement (Lamarra et al., 1987). Moreover, the subjects can anticipate the variation in exercise and may adjust their ventilation voluntarily .

Recently, a system identification technique by white noise forcing has applied to the research in the dynamics of ventilatory response during exercise (Bennett el al., 1981, Greco et al., 1986, Eβfeld et al., 1987). The purpose of this study is to obtain the dynamics of ventilatory response to random exercise on a bicycle ergometer from two healthy subjects.

METHODS

Models

Four possible models (Laplace transform notation) for describing the dynamics of the
ventilatory response to random work rate exercise are shown in Fig. 1. Model I and II
are the first-order dynamics and characterized by a time constant (Tc) and a gain (K).
Moreover, model II contains a dead time (Td). Model III consists of two components, a
fast component and a slow component which follows after a delay. Model IV is a second-
order dynamics, which contains of two first-order dynamics in series.

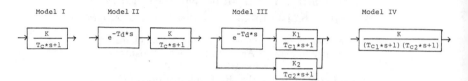

Fig. 1.   Schematic representation of the model hypotheses for the
          relation of the ventilatory response to the input exercise.
          K:gain; Td:dead time; Tc:time constant; s:Laplace notation
          of complex frequency variable.

Input work rate

To minimize the contributions of nonlinearities, the work load should not exceed
the anaerobic threshold. The anaerobic threshold was determined during a 1-minute
incremental work test and is presented as ventilatory threshold (VT) in Table 1. Based
on VT of two subjects, the PRBS was switched between 0 and 100 W in this study.

The work rate was changed as a PRBS while subjects pedaled on a bicycle ergometer.
The sequence was generated by an m-stage shift register. The sequence is characterized
by Δt, the interval at which the sequence is updated, and N, the number of intervals in
a sequence. Therefore, the duration of a sequence is $N\Delta t$. At the end of Δt second,
the algorithm decides whether the work load will be high or low for the next Δt second.
During the sequence the work load may remain in a given state for a number of
consecutive intervals.

Experimental protocol

Subjects used in this study were two healthy males. Their physical characteristics
data are presented in Table 1. The subject exercised on a bicycle ergometer and was
instructed to maintain pedaling rate constant at 50 rpm. The work rate was at 0 W
during warm-up period, and then varied as a PRBS. The experimental procedure was
divided into four experiments. The differences between experiments were Δt and N
in PRBS and the work rate (Table 2).

Data acquisition and model fitting

Throughout the exercise period, the ventilatory response data were collected by a
respiratory gas analyzer (Magna88, Morgan, and Aerobic processor-391, NEC Sanei) at
every 10 seconds. The fitting of models to experimental data was performed on a
Nyquist plot using nonlinear least squares method (Fig. 2).

Table 1.   Physical characteristics of subjects.

subject	age		ht		wt		$\dot{V}o2$-max		VT $(\dot{V}o2)$	
Y	32	(yrs)	176	(cm)	68.5	(kg)	38.8	(ml/kg/min)	18.3	(ml/kg/min)
S	35		169		65.0		46.2		29.5	

Table 2.   Protocols of four experiments.

experiment number	work rate	PRBS Δt	N	exercise duration
1	0 - 50 w	30 sec	63	31 min 30 sec
2	0 - 50 w	20 sec	127	42 min 20 sec
3	0 - 100 w	20 sec	127	42 min 20 sec
4	50 - 100 w	20 sec	127	42 min 20 sec

RESULTS AND DISCUSSION

Fig. 2 displays an example of ventilatory response and its Nyquist plot.   Table 3 indicates the estimates for the model parameters for each of two subjects and each of four experiments.   The values of AIC, one of the criteria for the goodness of fit, suggests that model Ⅲ, that is parallel two first order models, can simulate most adequately the dynamics of the ventilatory response.

It should be noted that the time constant parameter Tc1 is larger than Tc2 in model Ⅲ, then Tc1 indicates a slow component and Tc2 does a fast mode.   The fast component takes place immediately after the onset of exercise stimulus and followed by the slow component in some dead time. Since K2, gain of the fast component, represents much smaller portion of total gain, the over all response is mainly determined by the slow component.   The results obtained from this study are consistent with previous investigators suggesting the hypothesis of exercise hyperpnea, that is the initial fast component caused by a neural factor and slow component was in response to a humoral stimulus.

To identify the ventilatory response, comparing the usual input such as step, ramp, or sinusoidal work, the stochastic exercise input according to PRBS has two main advantages; 1) to stimulate the fast component adequately without the effect of volitional factor such as anticipation, and 2) to be able to estimate the parameters of fast component in a single measurement. The estimated parameters, however, have some variations in this experiments.

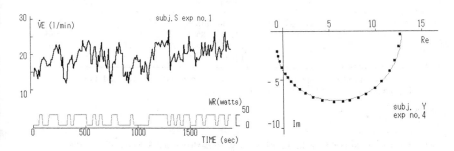

Fig. 2.   An example of ventilatory response and Nyquist diagram.
          left :ventilation response (upper solid curve) to PRBS
                exercise work rate (lower dotted line).
          right:Nyquist plot of measured dynamics (closed squares)
                and its predicted dynamics (dotted curve) by model Ⅲ.

S. Usui *et al.*

Table 3.   Parameters estimated by four models.

subj	exp. no.	work rate [0 - 1]	model	K1 (1/min)	Tc1 (sec)	Td1 (sec)	K2 (1/min)	Tc2 (sec)	AIC
Y	1	0 - 50 w	I	9.11	61.3				1995
			II	8.42	49.9	6.1			1698
			III	6.60	51.7	17.0	1.95	12.9	1644
			IV	8.40	47.5			6.9	1608
Y	2	0 - 50 w	I	12.71	90.0				2337
			II	11.57	69.3	11.2			1480
			III	8.84	66.3	26.9	2.81	20.7	962
			IV	11.43	59.5			14.9	986
Y	3	0 - 100 w	I	15.95	105.2				2046
			II	12.92	62.5	6.7			1359
			III	9.96	58.2	22.8	2.99	12.0	631
			IV	12.83	58.6			8.1	1047
Y	4	50 - 100 w	I	14.05	74.1				2883
			II	11.95	43.5	17.4			1580
			III	10.11	39.3	25.4	1.95	15.3	972
			IV	12.44	28.2			28.2	1803
S	1	0 - 50 w	I	10.11	53.6				2548
			II	8.86	35.6	12.1			2089
			III	6.36	21.5	30.5	2.64	5.65	922
			IV	8.99	22.0			22.0	1806
S	2	0 - 50 w	I	15.93	105.2				2046
			II	15.62	100.4	2.8			2002
			III	13.36	84.7	20.6	2.17	0.003	872
			IV	15.45	97.0			4.4	1974
S	3	0 - 100 w	I	17.37	90.4				1642
			II	16.87	84.3	3.3			907
			III	15.81	82.9	9.1	1.05	2.5	850
			IV	16.85	83.6			3.5	860
S	4	50 - 100 w	I	15.76	113.8				2256
			II	14.71	95.6	9.6			1666
			III	11.86	88.3	29.2	2.90	16.5	505
			IV	14.52	86.5			12.6	1247

K:gain modified corresponding to 50 w, Tc:time constant, Td:dead time,
AIC:Akaike's information criterion.

REFERENCES

Bennett, F.M., P. Reischl, F.S. Grodins, S.M. Yamashiro and W.E. Fordyce (1981).
Dynamics of ventilatory response to exercise in humans. J. Appl. Physiol., 51, 194-203.
E β feld, D., U. Hoffmann and J. Stegemann (1987). $\dot{V}$o2 kinetics in subjects differing
in aerobic capacity: investigation by spectral analysis. Eur. J. Appl. Physiol., 56,
508-515.
Greco, E.C., H. Baier and A.Saez (1986). Transient ventilatory and heart rate responses
to moderate nonabrupt pseudorandom exercise. J. Appl. Physiol., 60, 1524-1534.
Lamarra, N., B.J. Whipp, S.A. Ward and K. Wasserman (1987). Effect of interbreath
fluctuations on characterizing exercise gas exchange kinetics. J. Appl. Physiol., 62,
2003-2012.

A Dynamical Analysis of the Respiratory System by the Optimal Principle — Analysis of the Inspiratory Phase

H. Hirayama, T. Kobayashi and H. Yasuda

Department of Cardiovascular Medicine, Hokkaido
University School of Medicine, Sapporo, Japan

Abstract

The pressure-flow-volume relation of the respiratory system was ana
lyzed based on the optimal control theory. The performance functon
was defined as to minimize the instantaneous changes in the flow
rate and the mechanical work produced by the inspiratory muscle.
The reconstructed pressure, flow and the volume loops were compara
ble with those usually observed.

Key words.

Optimal control. inspiratory phase. performance function.

Search for the optimality in the respiratory system

Several studies had been reported of the mechanical efficiency for
the respiratory system (Otis, 1956, Mead, 1968) However those studies were carried out on the stand point of necessary conditions.
In the present study we searched and analyzed the trajectory of the
pressure-flow-volume which satisfy the assumed optimal conditions
which seems to be most reasonable to control the respiratory system.

Mathematical expansions.

The dynamics of the lung-ribcage system was expressed as

$$P(t) = K \cdot V(t) + R \cdot \dot{V}(t)$$

where $P(t)$; driving pressure. $V(t)$:
changes of the lung volume from the resting level. K : total elas
tance of the lungand thoracs. R : viscous resistance of the total
respiratory system. The performance function to be minimized is

$$J(ti) = \int^{ti} [\ddot{V}(t)^2 + \alpha \cdot P(t) \cdot \dot{V}(t)] \, dt$$

where ti is the duration of the inspiratory phase. α is the weigh
tening coefficient. The initial and the boundary conditions are

$$V(0) = Vi, \quad \dot{V}(0) = 0, \quad V(ti) = V0 + Vt, \quad \dot{V}(ti) = 0$$

where the $V0$ is the end expiratory lung volume, Vt is the tidal vo
lume. Substituting $P(t)$ into $J(ti)$, the Euler Lagrange equation is

$$Q = (\ddot{V}(t)^2 + \alpha (R \cdot \dot{V}(t)^2 + K \cdot V(t) \dot{V}(t))$$

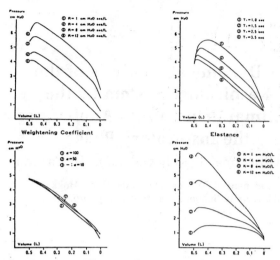

Fig I. The effects of changes in the system parame
ters on the pressure-volume relation under the op
timal conditions.

$$\frac{d\,Q}{d\,V} \;-\; \frac{d}{dt}\,\frac{d\,Q}{d\,\dot{V}} \;+\; \frac{d^2}{dt^2}\,\frac{d\,Q}{d\,\ddot{V}} \;=\; 0$$

Then a linear forth order ordinary differential equation can be ob
tained as $V(t)^{(4)} \;-\; \alpha\,R\,V(t)^{(2)} = 0.$
By utilyzing the initial and the boundary conditions, the solution
of the above euqation can be expressed as

$V(t)=$ CI exp(at)+C2exp(-at)+C3 t + C4 where $\qquad a=\sqrt{\alpha\cdot R}.$

Results.

I. Pressure-Volume relations. (Fig I).
The increase of the R induced a parallel shifts of each loops. The
changes in the Ti caused the increase of the curvatures of the para
bolic loops with having an identical pressure and flow rate at the
beggining and the end of the inspiration. The changes in the K induced a remarkable deviation between each other while the initial
portions of the loops were almost coinsided. However changes in the
α did not bring an evident changes in those relations.

II. Pressure-Flow relations. (Fig 2).
The basic pattern was parabolic although not completely symmetric.
The changes in the K increased the end inpiratory pressure while
the peak flow rate did not change. The increase of the R caused the
increase of the end inspiratory pressure and the flow while the
peak flow rate decreased. The duration of the plateau flow has been
prolonged. The increase of the Vt enhanced the total Pressure-flow
loops almost symmetrically and the duration of the peak flow part
has been increased. The changes in the α induced the decrease of
the plateau flow rate and flatten the peak flow part. On the other
hand the pressure and flow rate at the end and beggining of the inspiratory phase did not change definitely.

III. The instantaneous Pressure-Volume ratios. (Fig 3).
As in the case of the cardiovascular system, the P/V ratios was

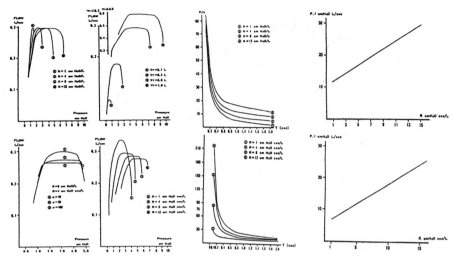

Fig 2. The effects of changes in the system parame
ters on the pressure-flow relation. Fig 3. on the
instantaneous pressure-volume ratios.Fig 4. the be
haviour of the performance functions.

analyzed. The P/V vs time shows a hyperbolic pattern. The increase
of the K caused an upward shifts of the P/V curves. Those changes
appered at later half of the inspiratory phase (T $>$ 0.6 sec) while
P/V ratios at the beggining of the inspiratory phase were almost
identical. For the case of the R on the contrary the P/V changed
remarkably at the beggining of the inspiration while there are no
evident changes in the later half of the inspiration (T $\searrow$ 0.4 sec).

IV. The behaviour of the performance function. (Fig 4)
The relation between the values of the performance function vs K
and R were linear. It seems to be possible to evaluate the state of
the system under the condition of the optimal control.

[Conclusion]. The pressure-flow-volume relations were almost compa
tible with those of usually observed ones within the physiological
range. It is possible to evaluate and analyze the inspiratory phase
and dynamic characters of the respiratory system either it is opera
ted under the optimal conditions or not.

References

I. Otis, A., Mckerrow,C.B.,Mead,J et al(I956). J.   Mechanical
factors in distribution of pulmonary ventilation. J. Appl. Physiol.
8, 427.
2. Grimby,G., Takishima,T., Graham,W., Mackelem.P., Mead, J. Frequ
ency dependency of flow resistance in patients with obstructive
lung disease. J. Clinical. Inv. 47. I455. (I968).
3. Hamalainen, R.P., Viljianen, A.A. (I978). Modeling the respirato
ty airflow pattern by optimization criterion. Biol. Cybernetics. 29
I43.

Section 2

ABNORMALITY OF
RESPIRATORY CONTROL

Possible Role of the Awake Ventilatory Chemosensitivity in Sleep-disordered Breathing

Y. Honda

Department of Physiology, School of Medicine, Chiba
University, Chiba, 280 Japan

ABSTRACT

Since termination of sleep apnea is usually preceded by the arousal state in EEG,
the awake chemosensitive ventilatory drive is assumed to play an important role
in resumption of breathing from apnea.
We found that sleep arterial oxygen desaturation was significantly correlated
with awake hypercapnic ventilatory response (HCVR) in interstitial pulmonary
disease (IPD), with awake hypoxic ventilatory response (HVR) in sleep apnea syndrome (SAS), and with both HCVR and HVR in chronic obstructive pulmonary disease
(COPD) and during sleep-disordered breathing in the climbers at high altitude.
Thus, hypercapnic and hypoxic ventilatory chemosensitivities were related
differently with abnormal breathing during sleep in different respiratory diseases and environment.
It was further noted that the female patients maintained the chemosensitivity
better and suffered less disturbance than the male. In this connection, progesterone therapy and its limitation were investigated. For this purpose, we used a
synthetic progesterone, chlormadinone acetate (CMA), which has 150 times luteinizing action of progesterone. Administration of CMA was inevitably induced
augmentation of HCVR and HVR in most patients. However, not all the patients
improved the level of arterial blood gases. Ameliorated patients, called the
correctors, were 9 out of 12 in COPD and 7 of 9 SAS. We noted that concomitant
enhancement of both ventilatory chemosensitivity and load compensation response
appeared important to obtain therapeutic success.

KEYWORDS

Sleep-disorders; ventilatory chemosensitivities; hypercapnic response; hypoxic
response; arterial desaturation; gender difference; progesterone.

INTRODUCTION

Since termination of sleep apnea is usually preceded by arousal state in EEG,
awake chemosensitive ventilatory drive is assumed to play an important role in
resumption of breathing and thus prevents further arterial desaturation during
sleep (Phillipson et al., 1986). In this paper, therefore, the magnitude of
sleep-disordered breathing in terms of oxygen desaturation was evaluated in
association with hypercapnic and hypoxic ventilatory responses observed during

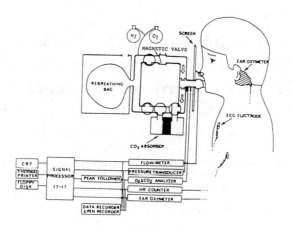

Fig. 1.   Experimental setup.   For CO_2 response test, ca. 7 %
          CO_2 in O_2 was rebreathed and for hypoxic response,
          room air was rebreathed while maintaining end-tidal
          Pco_2 constant. All the parameters were fed in a
          signal processor and treated on line.

wakefulness.

METHOD

Figure 1 illustrates the experimental setup used in this study. Due to limitation
in time to examine patients, rebreathing method was used. For hypercapnic response, approximately 7 % CO_2 in O_2 was rebreathed and the data were analyzed as
a linear Pco_2-stimulus-response relationship. For hypoxic response, progressive
isocapnic test was conducted. The result was analyzed as a linear Sao_2-ventila-
tion relationship. Both hypoxic and hypercapnic ventilatory drives were also
assessed by the occlusion pressure response which was measured by closing inspiratory airway at the beginning of inspiration. In some hypercapnic tests, respiratory resistive loading in an amount of 10 - 20 cmH_2O pressure per 1/sec of airflow was also applied, thus the degree of load compensation of the CO_2-ventila-
tion feedback system was evaluated.

RESULTS AND DISCUSSION

Influence of Body Weight-loading on Ventilatory Chemosensitivities

Figures 2 and 3 show the influence of body weight elevation on ventilatory responses (Nishibayashi et al., 1987). In comparing normal healthy male subjects
and judo athletes, normalized hypercapnic ventilatory response slope was significantly correlated with body weight in the former whereas no correlation was
found in the latter. Furthermore, we found that the difference in the magnitude
of body fat percentage is linearly related with the change in response slope in
the control group. No such mass loading effect was clearly demonstrated in
hypoxic chemosensitivity. Figure 4 shows the relationship between body weight and

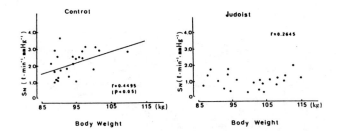

Fig. 2. Relationship between normalized hypercapnic ventilatory response, S_N, and body weight. Significant
correlation was seen in the obese control but not
in the judoist group. From Nishibayashi et al.,
1986, reproduced by permission.

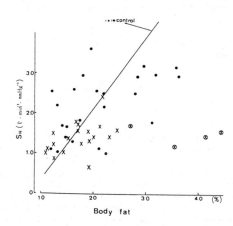

Fig. 3. Relationship between S_N and body fat as % of body
weight. Significant correlation was found in the
obese control group as indicated by closed circles
whereas in judoists (x and circled x symbols) no
such correlation was found. From Nishibayashi
et al., 1987, reproduced by permission.

hypercapnic and hypoxic chemosensitivities in patients with eucapnic obesity
(Kunitomo et al., 1988). Two characteristic features are seen. First, in contrast
to the normal subjects hypercapnic response in terms of both ventilation and
occlusion pressure response slopes are mostly not increased with increasing body
weight, whereas hypoxic chemosensitivities are mostly elevated with weight.
Second, when compared male and female patients as indicated broken and solid
lines, respectively, augmented chemosensitivity, particularly in hypoxia, with
increasing body weight, is well preserved in the female than the male. Thus, we
tended to believe that hypercapnic ventilatory chemosensitivity is more easily
affected by physiological and patho-physiological conditions. This finding may

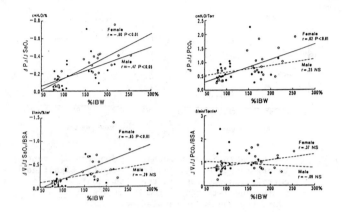

Fig. 4. Relationship of percentage of ideal body weight
(%IBW) to occlusion pressure and ventilatory
responses to hypoxia and hypercapnia in female
(open circles) and male (closed circles) subjects.
From Kunitomo et al., 1988, reproduced by permission.

well be in accord with the reports in the literatures (Kronenburg
et al., 1975, Kronenburg et al., 1977) that after weight reduction in
obesity hypoventilation syndrome (OHS) blunted hypercapnic ventilatory
response was restored but not in hypoxic response. It may be speculated
that hypercapnic response has phylogenetically developed lately and
thus easily affected than the hypoxic response.

Sleep-disordered Breathing and Ventilatory Chemosensitivities in Patho-physiological Conditions

Next, the relationship between sleep arterial desaturation and ventilatory chemosensitivities in pathological and abnormal physiological conditions were investigated. In chronic obstructive pulmonary disease (COPD) (Tatsumi et al., 1986)
both hypercapnic and hypoxic sensitivities are sifnificantly correlated with desaturation while in interstitial pulmonary disease (IPD) (Tatsumi et al., 1989)
sleep desaturation was mostly well related with hypercapnic sensitivity, only.
We assumed that the difference may have been ascribed to higier CO_2 response in
the latter than the former.
Masuyama et al., (1988) conducted sleep study at altitude 5360 m in Kunlun Moun-
tains. Sleep desaturation was found to correlate positively with both hypercapnic
and hypoxic chemosensitivities. On the other hand, in the patients with sleep
apnea syndrome (SAS) (Kunitomo et al., 1988) main finding was a significant relationship between hypoxic chemosensitivity and desaturation. The extent of oxygen
desaturation in high altitude and SAS are severe, so the role of hypoxic response
may be greater than the hypercapnic. The loss of CO_2 response – desaturation
relationship in the SAS patients may be associated with blunted hypercapnic
ventilatory drive in this pathological condition.
Thus, we found that hypercapnic and hypoxic ventilatory chemosensitivities were
related differently with sleep desaturation in different respiratory disorders
and environment.

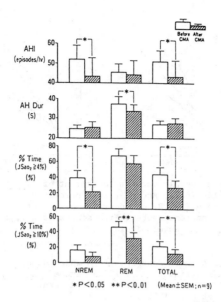

Fig. 5.   Effect of CMA on apnea-hypopnea index (AHI), apnea-
          hypopnea duration (AHDur) and oxygen desaturation.
          Open columns show mean ± SEM value before CMA, and
          hatched column during CMA. From Kimura et al.,
          1989, reproduced by permission.

<u>Effect of Synthetic Progesterone, CMA, on Sleep-disordered Breathing</u>

As presented previously, females maintain ventilatory chemosensitivity better
than males in the patients with eucapnic obesity. It is also known that sleep
disorders are less in females up to menopause (Block et al., 1979, Block et al.,
1980), less during pregnancy than after delivery (Brownell et al., 1986), number
of patients with chronic respiratory disease is less in the female (Block et al.,
1979) and administration of progesterone agent resulted in concomitant augmentation in both phrenic and hypoglossal nerve activities, suggesting its usefulness
to prevent airway obstruction during sleep (St. John et al., 1986). These advantages in the female appear to be mainly ascribed to the influence of progesterone.
With these reasoning in mind, we investigated usefulness and limitation of progesterone therapy. The progesterone agent used by us was chlormadione acetate
(CMA) which has 150 times luteinizing action of progesterone.
Beneficial effect administrating CMA for sleep disorders is presented in terms of
apnea-hypopnea index, apnea-hypopnea duration and sleep desaturation in SAS patients (Kimura et al., 1989) (Fig. 5).
However, CMA therapy was not always effective in improving the respiratory condition. Ameriolated patients, called the correctors, were 9 out of 12 in COPD
(Tatsumi et al., 1987) and 7 of 9 SAS (Kimura et al., 1989). Failure in success
was sometimes seen in the patients exhibited shallow and rapid breathing and thus
resulted in further desaturation despite of enhanced ventilatory drive.
Enhancement of ventilatory chemosensitivity is also not always successful after
CMA therapy. Lack of progesterone effect may, at least in part, be explained by

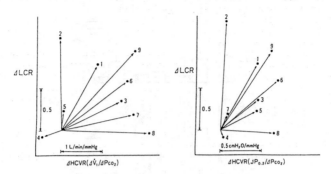

ΔLCR ... ΔHCVR($\Delta\dot{V}_{i}/\Delta$Pco$_2$)

ΔLCR ... ΔHCVR(JP$_{0.2}/\Delta$Pco$_2$)

Fig. 6. Relationship between the amount of load compensation
ratio (ΔLCR) and that in hypercapnic ventilatory response (ΔHCVR) demonstrated by a vector. Numbers
are patient number. From Kimura et al., 1989, reproduced by permission.

the number of existing progesterone receptors which depend on esterogen level
(Brodeur et al., 1986, Bayliss et al., 1987). Indeed, in most of mammals except
humans estrogen priming is prerequisite to obtain ventilatory augmentation by
progesterone (Dempsey et al., 1988).
In our recent experience (Kimura et al., 1989), we noted that not only augmented
ventilatory drive, but also concomitant enhancement in exogenous loading response, i.e., augmented load compensation response was necessary to obtain therapeutic success (Fig. 6).

REFERENCES

Bayliss, D.A., D.E. Milhorn, E.A. Gallman and J.A. Gidlawski (1987). Progesterone stimulates respiration through a central nervous system steroid receptor-
mediated mechanism in cat. Proc. Natl. Acad. Sci., 84, 7788-7792.
Block, A.J., P.G. Boysen, J.W. Wynne and L.A. Hunt (1979). Sleep apnea, hypopnea, and oxgen desaturation in normal subjects. A study male predominance.
N. Eng. J. Med., 300, 513-517.
Block, A.J., J.W. Wynne and P.G. Boysen (1980). Sleep disordered breathing and
nocturnal oxygen desaturation in postmenopausal women. Am. J. Med., 69, 75-79.
Blodeur, P., M. Mockus, R. McCullough and L.G. Moore (1986). Progesterone recep-
tors and ventilatory stimulation by progestin. J. Appl. Physiol., 61, 590-595.
Brownell, L.G., P. West and M.H. Kryger (1986). Breathing during sleep in normal
pregnant women. Am. Rev. Respir. Dis., 133, 38-41.
Dempsey, J.A., E.B. Olson Jr. and J.B. Skatrud (1988). Hormones and neurochemi-
cals in the regulation of breathing. In: Handbook of Physiology, Sect. 3. The
Respiratory System, Vol. II. Control of Breathing (N.S. Cherniack and J.G.
Widdicombe, ed.), Part 1, pp. 181-221. American Physiological Society,
Bethesda, MD.
Kimura, H., K. Tatsumi, F. Kunitomo, S. Okita, H. Tojima, S. Kouchiyama, S.
Masuyama, T. Shinozaki, Y. Honda and T. Kuriyama (1988). Progesterone therapy
for sleep apnea syndrome evaluated by occlusion pressure response to exogenous
loading. Am. Rev. Respir. Dis., 139, 1198-1206.
Kronenburg, R.S., R.A. Gabel and J.W. Severinghaus (1975). Normal chemoreceptor
function in obesity, before and after ileal bypass surgery to force weight
reduction. Am. J. Med., 59, 349-353.

Kronenburg, R.S., C.W. Drage and J.W. Severinghaus (1977). Acute respiratory failure and obesity with normal ventilatory response to carbon dioxide and absent hypoxic drive. Am. J. Med., 62, 772-776.

Kunitomo, F., H. Kimura, K. Tatsumi, T. Kuriyama, S. Watanabe and Y. Honda (1988). Sex differences in awake ventilatory drive and abnormal breathing during sleep in eucapnic obesity. Chest, 93, 968-976.

Kunitomo, F., H. Kimura, K. Tatsumi, S. Okita, H. Tojima, T. Kuriyama and Y. Honda (1989). Abnormal breathing during sleep and chemical control of breathing during wakefulness in patients with sleep apnea syndrome. Am. Rev. Respir. Dis., 139, 164-169.

Masuyama, S., K, Hasako, H. Kimura, T. Kuriyama and Y. Honda (1988). Periodic breathing during sleep at high altitude and ventilatory chemosensitivities to hypoxia and hypercapnia. Jpn. J. Mt. Med., 8, 130-146.

Nishibayashi, Y., H. Kimura, R. Maruyama, Y. Ohyabu, H. Masuyama and Y. Honda (1987). Differences in ventilatory responses to hypoxia and hypercapnia between normal and judo athletes with moderate obesity. Er. J. Appl. Physiol., 56, 144-150.

Phillipson, E.A. and G. Bowes (1986). Control of breathing during sleep. In: Handbook of Physiology, Sect. 3. The respiratory System, Vol. II (Fishman, A.P., N.S. Cherniack, J.G. Widdicombe and S.R. Geiger, ed.), pp.669-689. American Physiological Society, Bethesda.

St. John, W.M., D. Bartlett, Jr., K.V. Knuth, S.L. Knuth and J.A. Daubenspeck (1986). Differential depression of hypoglossal nerve activity by alcohol. Protection by pretreatment with medroxyprogesterone acetate. Am. Rev. Respir. Dis., 132, 46-48.

Tatsumi, K., H. Kimura, F. Kunitomo, T. Kuriyama, S. Watanabe and Y. Honda (1986). Sleep arterial oxygen desaturation and chemical control of breathing during wakefulness in COPD. Chest, 90, 68-75.

Tatsumi, K., H. Kimura, F. Kunitomo, T. Kuriyama, S. Watanabe and Y. Honda (1986). Effect of chlormadinone acetate on sleep arterial oxygen desaturation in patients with chronic obstructive pulmonary disease. Am. Rev. Respir. Dis., 133, 552-557.

Tatsumi, K., H. Kimura, F. Kunitomo, T. Kuriyama and Y. Honda (1989). Arterial oxygen desaturation during sleep in interstitial pulmonary disease. Correlation with chemical control of breathing during wakefulness. Chest, 95, 962-967.

Ventilation, Chemosensitivity and Ventilatory Load Compensation During Sleep

Clifford W. Zwillich, Laurel Wiegand and
Kevin Gleeson

Division of Pulmonary/Critical Care Medicine,
Pennsylvania State University College of Medicine,
Hershey, Pennsylvania, USA

ABSTRACT

Increasing interest in the control of breathing during sleep has resulted from the fact that clinically significant respiratory disorders limited to the sleeping state are very common. Deranged gas exchange limited to the sleeping state is frequently seen in individuals with obstructive sleep apnea and chronic obstructive lung disease. The reasons for abnormal gas exchange during sleep are multifactorial: following sleep onset, inspiratory airflow resistance rises two to three fold. This increased ventilatory impediment results from pharyngeal narrowing which appears to be more marked during sleep in men and particularly those with obstructive sleep apnea. During sleep, most normals demonstrate alveolar hypoventilation with resultant arterial hypercapnia. Is this the result of increased pharyngeal resistance or diminished ventilatory drive? Recent studies have demonstrated that ventilatory chemsensitivity is diminished during sleep as the breathing responses to both hypoxia and hypercapnia are lower in all sleep stages when compared to wakefulness. However, the diminished ventilatory response may result from the increase impediment of high pharyngeal resistance while asleep. A few studies have evaluated sleeping ventilatory drive utilizing the mouth occlusion technique. This measure of central ventilatory drive demonstrates preservation of the awake level of sensitivity during all sleep stages except during REM where attenuated ventilatory and mouth occlusion pressure responses to hypercapnia are seen. Therefore, the depression in ventilation seen during sleep appears to result from increased resistance to airflow with maintained but not augmented inspiratory drive.

Most recently investigators have evaluated the impact of inspiratory resistive loading on alveolar ventilation during wakefulness and sleep. Most studies demonstrate that normals exposed to increasing inspiratory loads develop progressively severe alveolar hypoventilation. Interestingly, ventilation falls immediately following the application of a load. However, alveolar ventilation thereafter increases but never returns to the unloaded value. The decrement in ventilation during sleep following loading results from a fall in tidal volume with resultant hypercapnia. During wakefulness no such decrement is found because, unlike during sleep, inspiration is prolonged and tidal volume is maintained with loading. The influence of naturally occurring loading present for prolonged time in man is unknown.

In conclusion, the interaction between ventilatory control and the sleeping state appears to be complex. Factors such as pharyngeal resistance, ventilatory timing, and the various sleep stages themselves impact upon man's responses and suggests that breathing during sleep may be different from that which occurs while awake.

KEY WORDS

Ventilatory Control, Breathing During Sleep, Loaded Breathing, Chemosensitivity, Hypoventilation During Sleep, Ventilatory Drive During Sleep, Mouth Occlusion Pressure

INTRODUCTION

Interest in breathing during sleep results from an increasing appreciation that clinically significant respiratory disorders limited to the sleeping state are very common. For example, individuals with obstructive sleep apnea, chronic obstructive lung disease, and those with congestive heart failure may develop very severe blood gas derangements only during sleep. This suggests that the sleeping state is associated with fundamental changes in the operational integrity of the respiratory system that result in a predisposition for abnormal gas exchange. The following chapter will focus on some of what has recently been learned about alterations in breathing during sleep in normal man. Changes that occur during sleep in normal individuals may help explain the severe derangements in gas exchange which occur in the clinical setting of disease states will be emphasized.

The Influence of Sleep on Upper Airway Airflow Resistance:

Ventilatory resistance increases during sleep in normal men. Inspiratory airflow resistance may be two to three fold higher during sleep than during wakefulness. This increased resistance to airflow is thought to reside in the pharynx and not the intrathoracic airways Fig. 1 (Hudgel, 1984). Although still somewhat controversial, the higher pharyngeal resistance resulting from the sleeping state may be related to a sleep-induced decrement in pharyngeal dilator muscle tone which in turn may cause partial collapse of the pharyngeal airway in response to negative intrapharyngeal pressures accompanying inspiration. Individuals who snore or suffer from obstructive sleep apnea have a greater increase in pharyngeal resistance during sleep than is found in those without these abnormalities. Interestingly, women who are known to have a much lower frequency of disordered breathing during sleep, have lower pharyngeal resistance than man when measured during wakefulness (White et al, 1985), and have recently been shown to have smaller sleep-induced increments in pharyngeal resistance when compared to men (Wiegand and Wiegand, 1990).

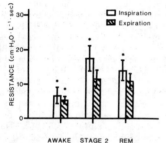

FIG. 1. Inspiratory and expiratory airflow resistance during sleep in normal humans. There is significant difference in inspiratory resistance between all phases, wakefulness, stage 2, and REM sleep. Expiratory resistance is similar in stage 2 and REM but higher than wakefulness. Inspiratory resistance is higher than expiratory resistance in all phases; this difference is greater during sleep. $P < 0.05$ between stages.

Metabolic rate and ventilation during sleep:

During wakefulness there is a tight link between metabolic rate (oxygen consumption and CO_2 production), and alveolar ventilation such that arterial pCO_2 is maintained within very narrow boundaries in normals. This "finely tuned" respiratory system is modified by intra-arterial and central nervous system chemoreceptors as well as other reflex systems. The resultant and rapid change in alveolar ventilation which occur in response to alterations in metabolic rate effectively maintain arterial blood gas tensions. During sleep, metabolic rate decreases approximately 20%. Minute ventilation also declines during sleep due to a decrease in tidal volume. However, the decrement in alveolar ventilation during sleep appears to be greater than the decrement in carbon dioxide production and results in a small degree of arterial hypercapnia and a small fall in arterial oxygen tension. The 3 to 5 mm Hg rise in pCO_2 and minor fall in PaO_2 seen in normals during sleep is apparently of little consequence. However, in those with lung disease or in normal individuals residing at altitude who display arterial hypoxemia during wakefulness, the expected decrement in arterial blood gas values which occur during sleep may have pathological consequences.

Respiratory drive during sleep:

The extent to which the respiratory system responds to ventilatory stimuli during sleep has generated a great deal of interest recently when it was recognized that normal humans hypoventilate during sleep, and many abnormal individuals develop blood gas derangements in excess of those found during the awake state. Are there alterations in the respiratory control system during sleep which might explain the predisposition for hypercapnia and hypoxemia seen in sleeping man? Tests of ventilatory chemosensitivity (the respiratory response to arterial hypercapnia and hypoxemia) are traditional means of assessing autonomic ventilatory reflexes. During wakefulness arterial hypoxemia is a major ventilatory stimulant that will result in alveolar hyperventilation whenever arterial pO_2 falls below 60 mm Hg. This ventilatory response is mediated by stimulation of the carotid chemoreceptors. Arterial hypercapnia with its resultant acidemia also stimulates alveolar ventilation mostly through its influence on the central medullary chemoreceptor. During alveolar hypoventilation both hypoxemia and arterial hypercapnia occur, which together are very powerful ventilatory stimuli. A few recent studies

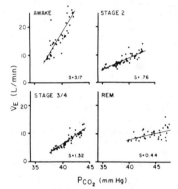

(Douglas, White, Picket et al, 1982; Douglas, White Weil et al, 1982; White, 1986) have measured ventilatory chemosensitivity in normals while awake and during sleep. There is general agreement among investigators that the sleep state induces a decrement in the ventilatory responses to both hypoxemia and hypercapnia. In general, these studies have demonstrated an attenuation in the minute ventilation responses to chemical stimuli which appear to be most marked during rapid eye movement (REM) sleep (Fig. 2).

As mentioned earlier, there is an expected increase in inspiratory pharyngeal resistance present during the sleeping state. Therefore, it may be argued that the lower ventilatory response to chemical stimuli found during the sleeping state may result from the added impediment of pharyngeal resistance rather than an intrinsic decrement in ventilatory drive. White (1986) recently used the technique of mouth occlusion pressure (P.1) as a measure of

FIG. 2. Representative hypercapnic ventilatory response in Subject 5 showing decreased hypercapnic ventilatory response in sleep most marked during REM sleep.

central respiratory drive in an attempt to determine the impact of the sleeping state on ventilatory reflexes in normals. As has been shown in previous reports, normals had a decrement in minute ventilation with accompanying hypercapnia during sleep. Men who snored (exhibited the highest impediment) demonstrated a greater fall in minute ventilation when compared to non-snoring men and women (Fig. 3). However, central ventilatory drive, measured as mouth occlusion pressure, increased during sleep in all groups studied and was highest in the snoring men (Fig. 3). This suggests that during unstimulated breathing ventilatory drive increases during sleep and responds further to naturally occurring inspiratory resistive loading (snoring) by further augmentation of inspiratory drive. However, the increment in drive in response to this load appears to be incomplete during sleep since hypoventilation and hypercapnia are present.

In order to further evaluate central ventilatory drive during sleep, arterial hypercapnia was induced by a rebreathing technique. Although the ventilatory response to hypercapnia was shown to be less than that found during wakefulness, the mouth occlusion pressure response to hypercapnia was not different during non REM sleep from that found during wakefulness. This data suggests that central ventilatory drive is maintained during sleep. However, during rapid eye movement sleep (REM), ventilatory and the mouth occlusion pressure responses to laboratory-induced hypercapnia were clearly less than that found during wakefulness. In summary, it appears that ventilatory drive increases in response to chemical stimuli and intrinsic resistive loading (higher pharyngeal resistance) during sleep. However, the response appears to be incomplete in that hypercapnia occurs in the unstimulated state during sleep while the ventilatory response to chemical stimuli appears to be less than that found during wakefulness. This is particularly marked during REM sleep.

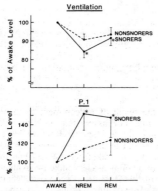

FIG. 3. Comparisons of percent changes ± SE from wakefulness to non-rapid-eye-movement (NREM) and rapid-eye-movement (REM) sleep for ventilation and occlusion pressure ($P_{0.1}$) in snorers and non-snorers are depicted. * $P < 0.05$ different from awake value.

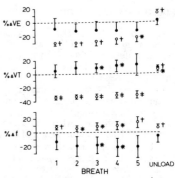

FIG. 4. Percent change (%Δ) in minute ventilation ($\dot{V}_E$), frequency (f), and tidal volume (V_T) from control over 5 consecutive loaded breaths and subsequent 1st unloaded breath. *Closed circles* are awake data, *open circles* NREM sleep in 5 subjects. See RESULTS for absolute mean values of preload control. Significant changes from control (preload) are shown: * $P < 0.05$, † $P < 0.01$, ‡ $P < 0.001$.

The impact of inspiratory resistive loading on breathing during sleep:

Investigators have been increasingly interested in the influence of ventilatory loading on breathing during sleep because of the high resistive loads found in men who snore and in those with obstructive sleep apnea. What is the impact of inspiratory resistive loading on breathing during sleep in normal human subjects? Immediately following the application of inspiratory loads of about 20 cm $H_2O/L/sec$, most normals demonstrate a significant fall in tidal volume Fig. 4 (Iber *et al*, 1982) associated with an increase in arterial pCO_2. This is markedly different from that which occurs during wakefulness where the imposition of an inspiratory load is accompanied by maintenance of alveolar ventilation and blood gas tensions. Smaller loads applied and evaluated over prolonged periods of time generally demonstrate that sleeping man may compensate adequately while demonstrating normal tidal volume and blood gas tension maintenance.

Careful and systematic comparison of ventilatory load compensation during wakefulness and sleep in normal man has demonstrated interesting findings. When resistive loads varying

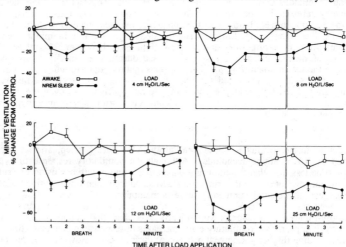

FIG. 5. Mean (±SE) values for all subjects for minute ventilation expressed as percent change from control over the first five consecutive breaths and *min 1–4* after application of each resistive load during wakefulness and non-rapid-eye-movement (NREM) sleep. Note that minute ventilation was well maintained after resistive load application during wakefulness but decreased significantly from control values at all points after resistive load application during NREM sleep. □—□, awake subjects; ●—●, NREM subjects. * $P < 0.05$ different from control.

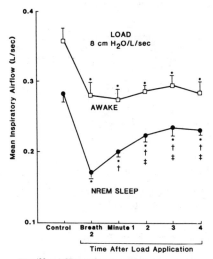

FIG. 6. Mean (±SE) values for all subjects for mean inspiratory flow rate (VT/TI) for the unloaded control period and at *breath 2* and *min 1–4* after the application of a representative resistive load (8 cmH₂O·l⁻¹·s) during wakefulness and non-rapid-eye-movement (NREM) sleep. Although VT/TI decreased after resistive load application during both wakefulness and sleep, all NREM sleep values were significantly decreased (*P* < 0.05) from awake values. During NREM sleep, VT/TI improved significantly over the sustained load period. * *P* < 0.05 different from control. † *P* < 0.05 different from *breath 2*. ‡ *P* < 0.05 different from *min 1*.

between 4 and 25 cm H₂O/L/sec were applied for 4 minute loading periods, sleeping normals demonstrated increasingly severe hypoventilation as the inspiratory loads were increased in size Fig. 5 (Wiegand *et al*, 1988). In contrast, minute ventilation was preserved following resistive loads during wakefulness throughout the loading period. The decline in ventilation seen during loading during sleep was the result of a decrement in inspiratory flow rate not associated with an adequate prolongation of inspiratory time (Fig. 6). As a decrement in inspiratory flow rate was also found during wakefulness it appears that the lack of a compensatory increase in inspiratory time differentiates the incomplete ventilatory load compensatory response during sleep from that of the complete loading response found during wakefulness where inspiratory time was significantly prolonged. Under all loading conditions during sleep some ventilatory load compensation was demonstrated such that the most severe hypoventilation in response to any load was always found during the first few breaths following the application of the load. Thereafter, minute ventilation improved over the sustained loading period such that between 1 and 4 minutes after the load was applied, ventilation had increased significantly from the first few loaded breaths (Fig. 5). These data suggest that the adequacy of ventilatory load compensation is time-dependent as improvement is seen over the first several minutes. However, load compensation is never complete as the level of ventilation during loading during sleep is less than that seen in the sleeping unloaded state, and less than that present during loading in wakefulness. How man responds during prolonged loading periods (weeks, months, and years) is yet unknown.

Conclusion:

In summary, normals demonstrate a decrease in alveolar ventilation during sleep which is greater than the decrement in metabolic rate and results in mild arterial hypercapnia. Alveolar hypoventilation during sleep appears to be multifactorial in origin and results from (1) ventilatory impediment resulting from a sleep induced increase in pharyngeal resistance which occurs with sleep onset and (2) an inadequate increase in inspiratory drive in response to this load.

Ventilatory responses to hypoxemia and hypercapnia are attenuated during the sleeping state and appear to be at their lowest during rapid eye movement sleep. This decrement in ventilatory responses appears in part to be related to the higher impediment to breathe that results from increased pharyngeal resistance. Central ventilatory drive as measured by the mouth occlusion pressure response to arterial hypercapnia is maintained during non REM sleep when compared to wakefulness but is clearly lowest during REM sleep. Therefore, a complex picture emerges relating ventilatory responses and drive during sleep.

External resistive load compensation is incomplete during sleep. Hypoventilation resulting from decreased inspiratory flow without compensatory prolongation of inspiratory timing is most marked during the first few breaths following the application of a resistive load. Larger inspiratory loads are associated with greater decrements in alveolar ventilation. Following the application of inspiratory loads the immediate fall in ventilation appears to improve over several minutes such that at four minutes following load application ventilation has significantly increased. However, load compensation during sleep is always significantly attenuated when compared to that which occurs during wakefulness.

The interaction between ventilatory control and the sleeping state appears to be complex. Factors such as pharyngeal resistance, ventilatory timing, and the various sleep states themselves appear to impact upon man's responses and strongly suggests that breathing during sleep may be a good deal different from that which occurs during wakefulness.

REFERENCES

Douglas, N.J., D.P. White, C. Picket, et al (1982). Hypercapnic ventilatory response in sleeping adults. *Am Rev Respir Dis* 126:758-762.

Douglas, N.J., D.P. White, J.V. Weil, et al (1982). Hypoxic Ventilatory response decreases durng sleep in normal man. *Am Rev Respir Dis* 125:286-289.

Iber, C., A Berssenbrugge, J Skatrud, et al (1982). Ventilatory adaptation to resistive loading during wakefulness in non-REM sleep. *J Appl Physiol* 64:1186-1195.

Hudgel, D.J., R.J. Martin, B. Johnson, et al (1984). Mechanics of the respiratory system and breathing pattern during sleep in normal humans. *J Appl Physiol* 56:133-137.

White D.P. (1986) Occlusion pressure and ventilation during sleep in normal humans. *J Appl Physiol* 61:1279-1287.

White D.P., R.M. Lombard, R. Cadiuex, et al (1985). Pharyngeal resistance in normal humans. *J Appl Physiol* 58:365-371.

Wiegand, L., D.A. Wiegand, C.W. Zwillich (1990) Minimal upper airway collapsibility during sleep in normal women. *Am Rev Respir Dis* In press.

Wiegand, L., C.W. Zwillich, D.P. White (1988). Sleep and the ventilatory response to resistive loading in normal men. *J Appl Physiol* 64:1186-1195.

Treatment of Obstructive Sleep Apnea with Airflow Demand-type Submental Stimulator

Wataru Hida, Hiroshi Miki,
Yoshihiro Kikuchi, Tatsuya Chonan
and Tamotsu Takishima

First Department of Internal Medicine, Tohoku
University School of Medicine, Sendai 980, Japan

ABSTRACT

Among the upper airway muscles, the genioglossus (GG) appears to
be of particular importance in maintaining the upper airway since
it is responsible for pulling the tongue forward. We therefore,
expect that GG stimulation improves upper airway patency. First,
we examined the relationship between the frequency of electrical
stimulation of GG and upper airway resistance (Rua) in
anesthetized dogs and found that GG stimulation decreased Rua with
increase in frequency (f); below 50 Hz Rua decreased markedly, but
above 50 Hz Rua plateaued at a minimum value. Secondly, we
developed an airflow demand-type electrical stimulator, which was
triggered by apneic episodes, detected by tracheal sound or nasal
and oral airflow. Stimulation was performed via the skin of the
submental region with 0.5 msec pulses (repetition rate 50 Hz), 15-
40 volts, when apnea lasted more than 5 sec and was stopped
immediately after breathing resumed, or after 10 sec at maximum.
We then examined the effects of this device on apnea episodes in
patients with obstructive sleep apnea syndrome (OSAS)
polysomnographically in the supine position during all-night
sessions. With submental stimulation, apnea index and apnea
time/total sleep time decreased, and desaturation and sleep stage
were improved. These studies suggest that a stimulation frequency
of more than 50Hz is necessary to maintain the airway patency, and
that submental stimulation with an airflow demand-type stimulator
may be a non-invasive and effective treatment for OSAS.

KEYWORDS

Obstructive sleep apnea syndrome; genioglossus muscle; electrical
stimulation; upper airway patency.

INTRODUCTION

Sleep apnea syndrome is one of the respiratory disorders of sleep.
The recurrent apnea episodes which occur during sleep in patients
with this condition can lead to hypoxia and hypercapnia, which
affect cardiopulmonary and brain function, and may lead to severe

cardiopulmonary consequences including sudden death.   An apneic
episode is defined as a cessation of airflow for at least 10
seconds (Guilleminault et al., 1976).   Obstructive apnea is
characterized by absence of respiratory airflow despite the
persistence of thoracoabdominal movements, and this type of sleep
apnea is the most common, compared with central and mixed types
(Guilleminault et al., 1976).   The pathogenesis of obstructive
sleep apnea is as follows: (1) anatomical disorders of the upper
airway, such as adenoids, hypertrophy of the tonsils, micrognathia
or deposit of fatty tissue on oropharyngeal submucosa and (2)
functional disorders of the upper airway, such as hypotonia of the
upper airway muscles, oropharyngeal mucosal adhesion, or
hypersecretion.   The appropriate therapy for obstructive apnea
depends on which of these conditions is present.

The present report focuses on hypotonia of the upper airway
muscles, especially the genioglossus.   This condition would lead
the tongue to fall back due to the negative intraluminal pressure
generated by inspiratory muscle contractions, resulting in upper
airway obstruction (Remmers et al., 1978).   Therefore, it is
expected that an increase in the geniogloassal activity due to
electrical stimulation opens the upper airway by pulling the
tongue forward and may be applicable to the treatment of
obstructive apnea.

In the present study, we first investigated the effects of
electrical stimulation of the genioglossus on upper airway
resistance in anesthetized dogs.   Second, we examined the effects
of submental stimulation on the frequency of apneic episodes in
patients with obstructive sleep apnea syndrome (OSAS), using an
airflow demand-type stimulator which we have developed.

METHODS

Animal Studies

Six spontaneously breathing mongrel dogs were anesthetized.
Anesthetic level was maintained stable.   The upper airway was
isolated from the lower airway and chest wall by transecting the
cervical tracheal about 5 cm below the larynx.   The vagus and
recurrent laryngeal nerves were carefully identified so as not to
be injured.   A stiff polyethylene tube (8 mm inner diameter and 10
cm in length) connected to a pneumotachometer (Fleisch no.2) with
a pressure transducer was inserted in the rostral direction.   A
vacuum source was attached to the proximal end of this tube.
Driving pressure defined as lateral pressure in the tube,
referenced to atmosphere, was measured with a differential
pressure transducer between the pneumotachometer and the isolated
upper airway, and controlled manually by changing the power of the
vacuum.   The pressure flow relationship of the upper airway was
obtained by applying constant driving pressures of 5, 10 and 20 cm
H_2O, while the genioglossus was stimulated by a pair of specially
designed electrodes at different frequencies from 5 to 100 Hz
during five consecutive breaths.   Stimulation at each frequency
was performed at 10 to 20 volts and a duration of 0.2 msec with an
electrical stimulator and isolator.   The head of the animal was
fixed in place 40 to 50 degrees from the horizontal plane in the
supine position, and the tongue was left free so as not to prevent
prolapse into the pharynx.   The nose and mouth were not sealed.

Secretions and mucus that could affect upper airway patency were removed using a bronchofiberscope. Upper airway resistance (Rua) during both inspiration and expiration was calculated from the upper airway flow and driving pressure at each frequency.

Human Studies

Sixteen patients with sleep apnea syndrome (SAS) previously diagnosed by polysomnography, none of whom had cardiopulmonary disease, were studied. Average age, height and body weight were 50.9 ± 11.1 yr, 166.3 ± 5.4 cm and 83.4 ± 15.5 kg (mean $\pm$ SD), respectively. Apnea was defined as the cessation of airflow at the nose and mouth, and of breath sound at the trachea lasting longer than 10 seconds. On the basis of the inductive plethysmography (Respitrace; Ambulatory Monitoring, Ardsley, NY) and airflow signals, apnea was classified as central, obstructive or mixed apnea as described in our previous report (Miki et al., 1989a). Thus, sixteen patients with SAS were grouped into 12 with obstructive apnea, 3 with mixed apnea and one with central apnea. Two of twelve OSAS patients had hypertrophy of the tonsils and the other ten patients with OSAS had no clearly definable upper airway abnormality on clinical examination.

Details of the submental electrical stimulator which we have developed are given in a previous paper (Miki et al., 1989a). In brief, airflow signals were recorded by thermistors placed near the nose and mouth, and tracheal breath sounds were monitored by a microphone attached to the skin overlying the cervical trachea. Tracheal sounds were displayed as bandpass filtered sound envelopes. The presence of apnea was defined as any point where both the thermistor and tracheal sound signals fell to less than 15% of their respective intensities during tidal breathing. Two silver electrodes were attached 10 mm apart to the skin in the submental region. Stimulation was performed with 0.5 msec pulses, repeated at 50 Hz and an intensity of 15 to 40 volts, using the airflow demand-type stimulator. Electrical stimulation was started when apnea lasted for five seconds. This is half the duration used to define an apneic episode. Stimulation was stopped immediately after breathing resumed or after ten seconds at the longest. The intensity of stimulation was previously determined for each patient while awake, by choosing an intensity just below the threshold of mild pain. The timing of stimulation was not dependent on the respiratory cycle.

Overnight sleep studies were performed using polysomnographic techniques (Miki et al., 1989a). All patients had underwent polysomnography initially. Subsequent control and stimulation nights were randomly ordered with more than 3 days between two test nights. Here, "control night" was defined as a night studied polysomnographically without submental electrical stimulator. "Stimulation night" was defined as a night of sleep studied with an airflow demand-type submental electrical stimulator. We compared apneic episodes on control nights with those on stimulation nights.

RESULTS

Animal Studies

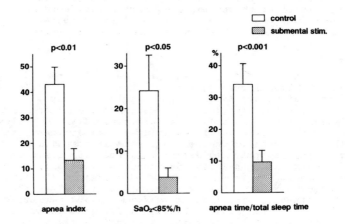

Fig. 1. Comparison of sleep apnea episodes between
control night (open column) and stimulation
night (shaded column). Apnea index = apneic
episodes per hour; $SaO_2 < 85\%/h$ = the number
of times per hour that oxygen saturation
dropped below 85%.

Upper airway flow showed phasic changes corresponding to the
respiratory cycle and increased during the inspiratory phase.
Therefore, we could obtain the upper airway resistance at both
maximally opened and minimally narrowed points for each of the
stimulation frequencies from zero to 100 Hz. At each driving
pressure, opened and narrowed upper airway resistances were
largest when the genioglossus was not stimulated. From 10 to 40
Hz, these resistances decreased rapidly and reached a plateau at
about 50Hz (Miki et al., 1989b). This indicates that genioglossus
muscle tone may play an important role in maintaining the patency
of the upper airway. Furthermore, frequency-resistance curves
were shifted significantly upwards as driving pressure increased
from 5 to 20 cm H_2O (analysis of variance, $p < 0.01$). This suggests
that the upper airway resistance increases with the negativity of
intraluminal pressure in the upper airway.

Human Studies

Figure 1 shows average values of the frequency of apneic episodes
expressed per hour, the number of times per hour that oxygen
saturation dropped below 85%, and the fraction of time spent in
apnea on control and submental stimulation nights obtained from
ten patients with OSAS, who had no definable upper airway
abnormality. The values of these three parameters decreased
significantly on submental stimulation nights.
In three patients with SAS who had mixed apneic episodes, the

submental stimulator decreased the apneic episodes slightly.
However, in two OSAS patients with hypertrophy of the tonsils and
one SAS patient with central apneic episodes, submental stimulator
did not improve apneic episodes. These finding suggest that
submental electrical stimulation is effective in reducing
obstructive episodes caused by functional apneic disorders of the
upper airway, such as hypotonia of the upper airway muscles.

DISCUSSIONS

In the first part of this study, we examined the relationship
between the frequency of electrical stimulation of the
genioglossus and upper airway resistance in anesthetized dogs, and
found that stimulation of the genioglossus decreased upper airway
resistance with increase in frequency during both inspiratory and
expiratory phases; below 50 Hz Rua decreased markedly, but above
50 Hz Rua plateaued at a minimum value. These animal studies
provide information additional to that of Gottfried et al. (1983)
who reported that electrical stimulation of hyoid muscles reduced
Rua in anesthetized dogs, and observed a decrease in Rua dependent
on the amplitude of electrical stimulation at a given frequency
(40 Hz). Our animal experiments suggest that increase in the
genioglossus activity has an important role in maintaining upper
airway patency and that a stimulation frequency of more than 50 Hz
is necessary to effectively open the upper airway.

In the second part of this study, we examined whether genioglossus
stimulation also improves upper airway patency in patients with
OSAS who had no definable upper airway abnormalities. We found
that submental stimulation using an airflow demand-type stimulator
which we have developed decreased the incidence of apneic episodes
in these patients. We found the differential effects of submental
stimulation on the frequency of central, mixed and obstructive
apnea types in ten patients with OSAS. Submental stimulation
greatly reduced the frequency of obstructive apneic episodes.
However, the frequency of central apneas was not reduced, and
mixed apnea showed only marginal benefit from submental
stimulation. Moreover, submental stimulation was not effective
for OSAS patients with hypertrophy of the tonsils or patients with
central apnea.

There are several factors affecting the effectiveness of submental
stimulation on apneic episodes in terms of stimulating conditions
such as stimulation frequency, timing of onset of stimulation,
stimulation duration or intensity of stimulation. In the present
study, we used a stimulation frequency of 50 Hz based on our
animal experiments. Also in a pilot study, stimulation with
frequencies higher than 50 Hz was found to be painful.
Stimulation was started 5 sec after the onset of apnea. This
prevented desaturation significantly more than stimulation
beginning after 10 sec at the longest. Continuous stimulation was
less effective than intermittent stimulation. The intensity of
stimulation for each patient was set below the pain threshold
while awake. Under these stimulating conditions, the quality of
sleep stage seemed to be improved, since stages I and II
decreased, whereas stages III and IV increased on stimulation
nights. No arousal effect in the electroencephalogram was found.
None of the subjects was awakened by the stimulation, and none
complained of skin pain or any other feeling of discomfort the

following morning. Sleep stage or skin thickness in the submental area may also affect the effectiveness of stimulation. During some obstructive apneic episodes, submental stimulation did not open the upper airway. These obstructive apneas tended to occur in rapid eye movement stages. Submental skin thickness in obese patients was thicker than in other patients. The intensity of stimulation set while awake, was greater in the former than in the latter. There are possibly other factors, e.g., mucosal secretion and surface adhesion in the oropharynx.

We found that similar stimulation of the arms or legs had no effect on the frequency of apneic episodes. Therefore, the mechanisms of the effectiveness of the submental stimulator is likely to be due to stimulation via the skin that augments genioglossus and geniohyoid muscle activity. The effects of submental stimulation on two or three separate night were reproducible (Miki et al.,1989a). Further studies will be necessary to establish the long-term clinical efficacy of submental stimulation.

In summary, we observed that the genioglossus is of importance in maintaining upper airway patency, and suggest that an airflow demand-type submental stimulator may be effective in treatment of patients with obstructive sleep apnea.

REFERENCES

Gottfried,S.B., K.P.Strohl, W.Van de Graaff, J.M.Fouke and A.F.DiMarco (1983). Effects of phrenic stimulation on upper airway resistance in anesthetized dog. J. Appl. Physiol., 55, 419-426.

Guilleminault,C., A.Tilkian and W.C.Dement (1976). The sleep apnea syndrome. Ann. Rev. Med., 27, 465-484.

Miki,H., W.Hida, T.Chonan, Y.Kikuchi and T.Takishima (1989a). Effects of submental electrical stimulation during sleep on upper airway patency in patients with obstructive sleep apnea. Am. Rev. Respir. Dis., 140, 1285-1289.

Miki,H., W.Hida, C.Shindoh, Y.Kikuchi, T.Chonan, O.Taguchi, H.Inoue and T.Takishima (1989b). Effects of electrical stimulation of the genioglossus on upper airway resistance in anesthetized dogs. Am. Rev. Respir. Dis., 140, 1279-1284.

Remmers,J.E., W.J.DeGroot, E.K.Sauerland and A.M.Anch (1978). Pathogenesis of upper airway occlusion during sleep. J. Appl. Physiol., 44, 931-938.

Alteration of Ventilatory Pattern and Ventilatory Responsiveness to CO_2 with Growth and Aging in the Rat

Y. Fukuda

Department of Physiology II, School of Medicine, Chiba
University, 1-8-1 Inohana, Chiba 280, Japan

ABSTRACT

Ventilatory pattern, metabolic rates, blood gases and ventilatory response to CO_2
inhalation were determined in halothane anesthetized spontaneously breathing male
Wistar rats of various ages; 1.5, 3, 6, 12, and 20-24 (aged) months after birth.
Minute expiratory volume (V_E), tidal volume (V_T) and metabolic rates ($\dot{V}o_2$, $\dot{V}co_2$)
corrected for body weight and respiratory frequency (f) during the breathing of
air decreased sharply at the age of 1.5-3.0 months, which was followed by further
gradual decline. However, the ratio of $\dot{V}_E$ to $\dot{V}co_2$ remained almost constant
throughout life. The slope of CO_2-ventilation response line decreased progressively with age accompanying a significant reduction in CO_2-f response. Young rats
responded to CO_2 with a high f, whereas the aged animal showed a relatively
large V_T with low f responses. The ratio of the maximum increase in $\dot{V}_E$ during CO_2
inhalation to the control (without CO_2 inhalation) $\dot{V}_E$, however, remained unchanged among different ages. We conclude that a relative reserve capacity for
increasing ventilation during CO_2 loading can be well maintained throughout life
despite significant reductions in $\dot{V}_E$ and in the sensitivity of ventilatory
control system to CO_2 stimulus with growth and aging.

KEY WORDS

Rat; growth and aging; ventilatory pattern; blood gases, sensitivity to CO_2;
ventilatory increasing capacity.

INTRODUCTION

During neonatal and developing phase of all mammals there are dramatic changes
in structure of the respiratory system (Brody and Thurlbeck, 1986). In the aged,
on the other hand, pathophysiological changes in the airway, lungs and thorax
have been observed (Cohn et al., 1963; Cotes, 1979; Nunn, 1987). All these
morphological changes accompany some functional alterations of respiratory control
system. However, systematic longitudinal studies concerning the respiratory
function throughout entire life is difficult in humans because of differences in
individual life circumstances, genetics, nutrition and longer longevity. The
present experiment aimes to know changes in respiratory control function during
growth and aging with using the rat of a defined strain, short life span and
with well controlled external environment and nutrition.

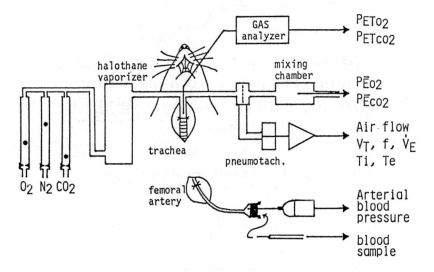

Fig. 1.   Schematic representation of experimental setup.
The trachea was cannulated with a polyethylene
tubing and connected to a respiratory gas circuit
consisted of halothane vaporizer and flow meters.
End-tidal Po_2 and Pco_2 were monitored by a respiratory gas analyzer. A small Fleisch type resistance head was placed in series with respiratory
gas circuit. A mixing chamber was placed to obtain
mixed expiratory O_2 and CO_2 concentrations.

METHODS

Male Wistar rats were housed in a standard rat cage with controlled room temperature (20–22 C) and humidity (60–80%). Animals were given food and water ad
libitum. The rat of various ages (1.5, 3, 6, 12, and 20–24 months after birth)
were anesthetized with halothane. The depth of anesthesia was kept constant at
1.1–1.2 MAC for halothane in every experiment. The femoral artery was catheter-
ized for blood sampling. The animal breathed spontaneously normoxic gas delivered
from a respiratory gas circuit (Fig. 1). The rectal temperature was kept constant
at 37.2 ± 0.1 C. Tidal volume (V_T), respiratory frequency (f), and minute
expiratory volume ($\dot{V}_E$) were obtained by computing respiratory flow signal
measured with pneumotachograph. End-tidal and arterial Po_2 and Pco_2 (P_{ETo_2}, PET-
co_2, Pao_2 and $Paco_2$ respectively) were measured (Fukuda et al., 1982). O_2
consumption ($\dot{V}o_2$) and CO_2 production ($\dot{V}co_2$) were calculated with using baseline
gas flow through the respiratory circuit, and fractional concentrations of O_2 and
CO_2 in inspiratory and mixed expiratory gases (Fig. 2).

The ventilatory response to CO_2 inhalation was performed in hyperoxic condition
(F_{Io_2} 0.4). The animal was exposed to gas mixtures containing 3–4 different
levels of high CO_2 concentration for a period of 5–7 min and the ventilation was
measured in steady state condition. The slope of CO_2-ventilation response line
was calculated. The ratio of ventilation during the breathing of high CO_2 (P_{ETco_2}
upto about 65mmHg) to the baseline (before CO_2 inhalation in hyperoxia) value
was calculated to estimate a relative capacity for increasing ventilation during
CO_2 loading.

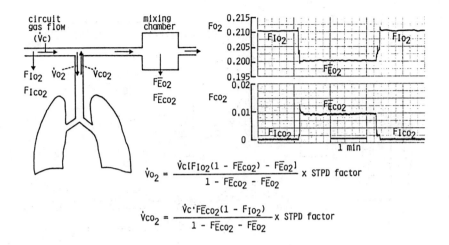

$$\dot{V}_{O_2} = \frac{\dot{V}_c[F_{IO_2}(1 - F\bar{E}_{CO_2}) - F\bar{E}_{O_2}]}{1 - F\bar{E}_{CO_2} - F\bar{E}_{O_2}} \times STPD\ factor$$

$$\dot{V}_{CO_2} = \frac{\dot{V}_c \cdot F\bar{E}_{CO_2}(1 - F_{IO_2})}{1 - F\bar{E}_{CO_2} - F\bar{E}_{O_2}} \times STPD\ factor$$

Fig. 2.   Measurement of O_2 consumption ($\dot{V}_{O_2}$) and CO_2
production ($\dot{V}_{CO_2}$). $\dot{V}_c$, baseline gas flow through
respiratory circuit; F_{IO_2}, F_{ICO_2}, $F\bar{E}_{O_2}$, $F\bar{E}_{CO_2}$,
fractional concentration of O_2 and CO_2 in inspira-
tory and mixed expiratory gases respectively.

Though the longevity of the rat differs with different ways of nutrition or
animal cares, the rat of 20-24 months old without macroscopic abnormality in
general autopsy findings was defined as the healthy aged rat in the present
experiment. The mortality increased apparently after 24 months.

RESULTS

Changes in ventilation, metabolism and blood gases

Changes in body weight, metabolic rates ($\dot{V}_{O_2}$, $\dot{V}_{CO_2}$) and minute expiratory volume
(∇_E) during the breathing of air at various ages are shown in Fig. 3. The body
weight reached a steady value of about 700 g at 12 months. Metabolic rates and
$\dot{V}_E$ corrected by body weight fell sharply at the age of 1.5-3 months, which was
followed by further gradual decline with increasing age. The ratio of $\dot{V}_E$ to V_{CO_2},
however, remained fairly constant at different ages, i.e., 33, 28, 28, 32, and 36
at 1.5, 3, 6, 12, and 20-24 months respectively. This means that an adequate and
necessary ventilation for metabolism would be maintained throughout entire life.
The arterial blood P_{O_2} (Pa_{O_2}) ranged from 75 to 85 mmHg until 12 months old but
decreased to about 64 mmHg in the aged group (20-24 months). Pa_{CO_2} was about
38-40 mmHg until 12 months old, but it increased slightly at the aged (43 mmHg).
The tidal volume (V_T) corrected by body weight decreased progressively with age
from 0.47 ± 0.08 at 1.5 months to 0.27 ± 0.06 (mean $\pm$ SD, mlBTPS/100g body weight)
at 20-24 months. Respiratory frequency (f) decreased also progressively from
117 ± 18 at 1.5 months to 83 ± 9 (mean $\pm$ SD, breaths/min) at 12 months. The f
turned to increase slightly at the age of 20-24 months (89 ± 16, mean $\pm$ SD,
breaths/min).

Ventilatory response to CO_2 inhalation

The ventilatory response to hypercapnia was performed by injecting CO_2 gas into
inspiratory line to raise $P_{ET_{CO_2}}$ up to about 65 mmHg with 3-4 steps in hyperoxic

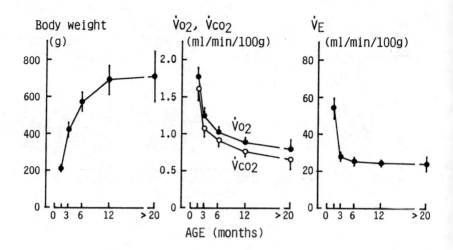

Fig. 3. Changes in body weight, metabolic rates ($\dot{V}_{O_2}$, $\dot{V}_{CO_2}$),
and minute expiratory volume ($\dot{V}_E$) with age. Values
are mean $\pm$ SD (n = 9-12); $\dot{V}_{O_2}$ and $\dot{V}_{CO_2}$, STPD; $\dot{V}_E$,
BTPS; Volumes are corrected by 100g body weight.

condition ($F_{I_{O_2}}$ 0.4). Averaged response lines at various ages are shown in
Fig. 4. The figure indicates also the mean values of ventilatory parameters
before CO_2 inhalation (BASE, open triangle) and the maximum values during CO_2
inhalation (MAX, open triangle). $\dot{V}_E$ and V_T values are corrected by 100 g body
weight. The mean CO_2-$\dot{V}_E$ response slope was the steepest at the age of 1.5 months
and became flattened with increasing age. A reduction in the slope with age was
also seen in CO_2-V_T or CO_2-f response line. However, changes in the slope were
smaller in CO_2-V_T than in CO_2-f response line. The slope of CO_2-V_T response at
1.5 and 20-24 months was 0.0133 $\pm$ 0.005 and 0.009 $\pm$ 0.004 (mean $\pm$ SD) mlBTPS/100g
/mmHg P_{CO_2} respectively (about 30% reduction). However, CO_2-f response slope was
2.47 $\pm$ 1.0 and 0.84 $\pm$ 0.49 (mean $\pm$ SD, breaths/min/mmHg P_{CO_2}) at 1.5 and 20-24
months respectively (66% reduction). Therefore an increase in f during CO_2
inhalation was clearly limited at higer ages. The ratio of the maximum ventilation to the baseline value, which may represent the relative increasing capacity
of ventilation during CO_2 inhalation, did not show significant decrease with
increasing age (Fig. 5). Similarly calculated ratio for V_T increased slightly
in the aged group, whereas the ratio for f decreased progressively with age.
Therefore reciprocal changes in the ratio for V_T and f seem to contribute to the
maintenance of max/base ratio of $\dot{V}_E$ even at the highest age. In other words,
reduction in f-response was at least partly compensated by relative increase in
V_T response despite the overall sensitivity of respiratory control system to
CO_2 stimulation as judged by the CO_2-$\dot{V}_E$ response slope decreased progressively
with increasing age.

DISCUSSION

Previous may reports describe changes in lung volumes, forced expiratory volume,
elasticity and other mechanical properties of the lung and thorax during development, growth and aging (Begin et al., 1977; Brody and Thurlbeck, 1986; Bryan et
al., 1977; Bryan and Wohl, 1986; Cohn et al., 1963). Change in the control
mechanism of breathing have been extensively studied in fetal, neonatal and early

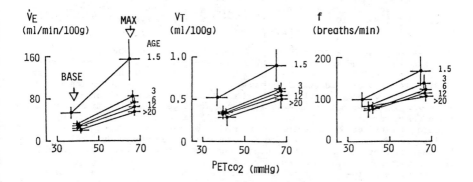

Fig. 4.   Ventilatory response to CO_2 inhalation. Mean response
lines of $\dot{V}_E$, V_T and f in different age groups are
shown. Baseline values before CO_2 inhalation (BASE,
mean ± SD) and the maximum values during CO_2 inhalation (MAX, mean ± SD) are also shown. $\dot{V}_E$ and V_T are
corrected for body weight (100g). Experiments were
performed in hyperoxic condition.

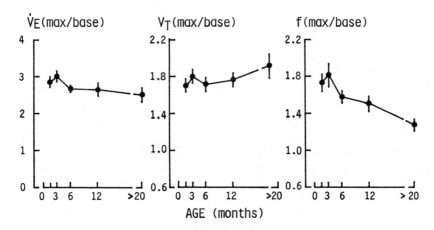

Fig. 5.   Magnitude of increase in ventilation during CO_2
inhalation. The ratio of the maximum values of $\dot{V}_E$,
V_T and f during CO_2 inhalation to those in baseline
condition before CO_2 inhalation is shown (mean ±
SE). Note reciprocal changes in the ratio between
V_T and f.

postnatal periods.(Bryan et al., 1986; Polgar and Weng, 1979; Rigatto, 1984; Woodrum et al., 1977). Deteriorations of respiratory functions in the aged human have been described (Begin et al., 1977; Cohn et al., 1963; Cotes, 1979; Muieson et al., 1971; Nunn, 1987). There have been, however, no systematic work on the regulation of respiratory function throughout entire life.

The present experiment is concerned with ventilation and metabolism during the breathing of air and their relationship to changes during respiratory stimulation by CO_2 breathing. Metabolic rates were the highest during a phase of rapid growth and thereafter decreased with increasing age. The age related reduction in metabolic rate, though partly due to an increase in accumulation of adipose tissue which has lower metabolic activity, suggests a general inhibition of metabolism after maturation. The $\dot{V}_E$ showed a similar parallel decay with metabolic rate. Therefore, ventilation is controlled in such a way that it matches with metabolic activity. Reductions in both V_T and f produced the decrease of $\dot{V}_E$. A slight increase in f at the age of 20-24 months was likely due to respiratory stimulation through peripheral chemoreceptor activation by hypoxemia. Slight hypercapnia and hypoxemia in the aged animal were considered due to increased dead apace, venous admixture or to impaired gas diffusion in the lung (Nunn, 1987).

The ventilatory responsiveness to CO_2 inhalation decreased also with increasing age. A clear limitation of f to increase was the main cause of reduction in $CO_2-\dot{V}_E$ response. This was also demonstrated when the ratio of maximum f during CO_2 inhalation to that in control condition was taken into account (Fig. 5). A slower f and smaller increase in f with relatively larger increase in V_T probably characterize the ventilatory pattern of all aged animals including humans. A limited increase in f was partly compensated by a relatively well maintained V_T-response during CO_2 breathing. These changes in ventilatory pattern may be due to alteration of mechanical properties of the lung and thorax such as loss of elasticity and stiffened or less compliant lung and thorax and to changes in Hering-Breuer inflation reflex which may follow structural change. Relationship between the mechanical properties of lung-thorax-airways and control function of breathing pattern should be examined.

REFERENCES

Begin, R., A.D. Renzetti,Jr, A.H. Bigler,and S. Watanabe (1977). Flow and age dependence of airway closure and dynamic compliance. J. Appl. Physiol., 38, 199-207.
Brody, J.S. and W.M. Thurlbeck (1986). Development, growth, and aging of the lung. In: Handbook of Physiology, Section 3, The respiratory system, Vol III, Mechanics of breathing (A.P. Fishman, P.T. Macklem, and J. Mead, Ed,), part 1, pp. 335-386.
Bryan, A.C., A.L. Mansell and H. Levison (1977) Development of the mechanical properties of the respiratory system. In: Development of the lung (W.A. Hodson Ed.), pp. 445-468.
Bryan, A.C., G.Bones and J.E.Moloney (1986) Control of breathing in the fetus and the newborn. In: Handbook of Physiology, Section 3, The respiratory system, Vol II, Control of Breathing (A.P. Fishman, N.S.Cherniack, and J.G.Widdicombe, Ed.), part 1, pp. 621-647.
Bryan, A.C. and M.E.B. Wohl (1986) Respiratory mechanics in children. In: Handbook of Physiology, Section 3, The respiratory system, Vol III, Mechanics of breathing (A.P. Fishman, P.T. Macklem, and J. Mead, Ed.), part 1, pp. 179-191.
Cohn, J.E. and H.D. Donosa (1963) Mechanical properties of lung in normal men over 60 years old. J. Clic. Invest., 42, 1406-1410.
Cotes, J.E. (1979) Lung function, 4th Ed., Blackwell Scientific Publication, Oxford, pp.329-387.
Fukuda, Y., W.R. See and Y. Honda (1982) Effect of halothane anesthesia on end-tidal Pco_2 and pattern of respiration in the rat. Pflügers Arch., 392, 244-250.
Muieson, G., C. Sorbini and V. Grassi (1971) Respiratory function in the aged.

Bull. Physio-pathol. Respir., _7_, 973–1009.

Nunn, J.F. (1987) Applied respiratory physiology, 3rd Ed., Butterworths, London.

Polgar, G. and T.R. Weng (1979) The functional development of the respiratory system. Am. Rev. Respir. Dis., _120_, 625–695.

Rigatto, H. (1984) Control of ventilation in the new born. Ann. Rev. Physiol., _46_, 661–674.

Woodrum, D.E., R.D. Guthrie and W.A. Hodson (1977) Development of respiratory control mechanisms in the fetus and newborn. In: Development of the lung (W.A. Hodson, Ed.), Marcel Dekker, New York & Basel, pp. 561–585.

Vulnerability of the Respiratory System: Disposition for Sudden Infant Death Syndrome?

T. Schaefer and M.E. Schlaefke

Department of Applied Physiology, Ruhr-University
Bochum, D-4630 Bochum 1, Germany

ABSTRACT

Impaired central respiratory control is suspected to be an important risk factor in the multifactorial genesis of Sudden Infant Death Syndrome. In order to study the development and disturbances of the respiratory system noninvasive whole night polysomnographies were performed in three groups: I) 181 healthy infants between 3 days and 18 months of age showed marked age dependent changes: Periodic and paradoxical breathing, number of breathing pauses and acute falls of $tcpO_2$ decreased, mean $tcpO_2$ increased with age. The respiratory response to CO_2 remained stable. II) 18 infants within the first month of life with cyanotic attacks ('apparent life threatening events') had a significant lower CO_2-response of tidal volume than group I. III) 70 formerly preterm infants aged 14 days to 18 months had significantly lower and more instable $tcpO_2$ values, less breathing pauses and increased respiratory frequencies than group I infants. We conclude that the respiratory system matures from a vulnerable state to a more stable and that infants at risk for SIDS may show impaired central respiratory control and hypoxic phases.

KEYWORDS

Development of respiration; CO_2-response; risk for Sudden Infant Death Syndrome; hypoxia.

INTRODUCTION

As infant mortality could drastically be reduced in industrial countries, the Sudden Infant Death Syndrome (SIDS) has become the most frequent death among infants between 2 and 52 weeks of life. Impaired central respiratory control is suspected to be causally involved in this phenomenon (Hunt and Brouillette, 1987). The data and conclusions in the literature, however, are controversial (Gaultier, 1985). The present study deals with two questions: 1) Are there developmental stages even in healthy infant with an increased 'vulnerability' of the respiratory system? 2) How do infants as members of risk groups for SIDS differ from healthy normal infants?

METHODS

In order to avoid disturbances of spontaneous night sleep as far as possible noninvasive techniques were used: respiratory inductive plethysmography (RIP) for measurement of breathing movements, transcutaneous electrodes for oxygen and carbon dioxide partial pressures, pulse oximetry, EEG, EOG, ECG. Being aware of the limitations given by these indirect methods, respiratory pattern, periodic and paradoxical breathing, transcutaneous blood gases and chemical drives of respiration were analysed. The CO_2-response was calculated as relative increase of breathing movements per Torr increased $tcpCO_2$ during a $FiCO_2$ of 0.02. The development of respiration was studied in 181 healthy, normal infants between 3 days and 18 months of life. These data were compared with those of two risk groups for SIDS: 16 infants within their first month of life with apparent life threatening (cyanotic) events and 70 formerly preterm infants aged 14 days to 18 months after discharge from hospital.

RESULTS

Data of 3 age groups of healthy infants are summarized in table 1. The Spearman's rank correlation coefficients of all infants (n=181) on age and on the ventilatory ratio of the CO_2-response was -0.02 (n.s.; T-test), on mean $tcpCO_2$ -0.01 (n.s.), on periodic breathing -0.46 (p<0.01), on paradoxical breathing -0.54 (p<0.01), on the number of acute falls of $tcpO_2$ per hour -0.39 (p<0.01), on the number of apneas (> 2 s) per hour -0.45 (p<0.01) and on mean $tcpO_2$ +0.21 (p<0.01).

One-month-old infants who suffered from a life threatening event had a significantly lower response of tidal volume to CO_2 (ratio per Torr increased $tcpCO_2$: 1.17 vs. 1.31, p<0.05) and a shorter maximal apnea duration (9 s vs. 10 s, p<0.05) compared to controls. The other parameters were not significantly different from controls (Table 1): Periodic breathing was found in 9 % (median; interquartile range 7-10 %) of total sleep time (TST), paradoxical breathing movements in 56 %TST (36-72 %). The number of apneas longer than 2 s was 50 /h (17-61 /h), mean $tcpO_2$ was 61.9 mmHg (58.6-66.4 mmHg). Table 2 shows median values of formerly preterm infants (gestational age 31-37 weeks) in comparison to controls. The numbers of infants per age group were (fullterm:preterm) 30:5, 31:17, 28:16, 25:10 and 25:20.

Table 1. Median values and interquartile ranges of
respiratory parameters during development

| | Age [months] | | |
	1	5+6	>9
CO_2-response (Ventilat. ratio)	1.28 (1.17-1.36)	1.20 (1.12-1.27)	1.32 (1.23-1.39)
Mean $tcpCO_2$ [mmHg]	40.3 (38.1-44.0)	40.3 (38.1-41.8)	40.3 (38.8-41.8)
Periodic breathing [% TST]	5 (2 - 10)	1 (0 - 2)	0 (0 - 1)
Paradoxical breathing [% TST]	49 (10 - 68)	21 (6 - 31)	0 (0 - 4)
Acute falls of $tcpO_2$ (>10mmHg in 1min)	3.17 (1.4 - 5.9)	1.65 (0.9 - 2.9)	1.29 (0.7 - 2.2)
Apneas (>2s) [1/h]	38.4 (29 - 47)	24.1 (17 - 34)	19.5 (16 - 25)
Mean $tcpO_2$ [mmHg]	65.4 (61 - 69)	70.1 (67 - 75)	68.4 (64 - 76)

Table 2. Comparison of healthy fullterm infants (F) and
preterm infants (P)

		Postnatal age [months]			
		2	3+4	5+6	7-9	>9
Minimal tcpO₂	F	45	51	52	50	52
[mmHg]	P	17 **	40 **	48	48	50
Mean tcpO₂	F	66	67	70	66	68
[mmHg]	P	45	63 **	64 *	66	71
Acute falls of	F	3.5	2.1	1.7	1.2	1.3
tcpO₂ [1/h]	P	1.7	4.1 *	1.8	1.3	1.0
Mean apnea duration	F	3.7	3.6	3.7	3.8	3.9
(>2s) [s]	P	3.8	3.5	3.4 *	3.4 *	3.6 **
Irregular breathing	F	59	54	48	43	46
[%TST]	P	73 **	62 **	53 *	49 *	42
Paradoxical	F	42	44	21	2	0
breathing [%TST]	P	33	43	34	40 **	3 *
Respiratory rate	F	34	33	27	26	21
[1/min]	P	41	40 *	39 **	30	25 *

$(*p<0.05; **p<0.01; U-Test)$

CONCLUSIONS

During human development several parameters of the respiratory system seem
to be stable: The CO_2-sensitivity as an important homeostatic mechanism of
respiration, carbon dioxide partial pressures during sleep, mean and
maximal duration of central apneas. Marked changes involve the respiratory
pattern: reduction of irregular breathing as a phenomenon of sleep stages,
decrease of respiratory rate, periodic and paradoxical breathing movements. These changes go along with an elevation of minimal and mean oxygen
partial pressures with increased stability indicating that the first six
months of life with the highest incidence of SIDS (about 75 - 90 % of all
cases) may be a phase of increased vulnerability due to developmental
processes.

The comparison of the data of healthy infants and infants at risk for SIDS
gives further evidence that 1. impaired central respiratory control may be
involved in SIDS and 2. that chronic hypoxia in some cases may lead to
SIDS, especially in preterm infants. Infants with cyanotic attacks had a
significantly reduced respiratory response to CO_2. The life threatening
effect of a reduced CO_2-sensitivity could be shown in humans as well as in
animal models (Schlaefke et al., 1990). The study of formerly preterm
infants revealed unknown hypoxic phases so that continued oxygen
monitoring (e.g. by pulse oximetry) is recommended.

REFERENCES

Gaultier, C. (1985). Review: Breathing and sleep during growth: Physiology
and pathology. Bull. Eur. Physiopathol. Respir., 21, 55-112.
Hunt, C.E. and R.T. Brouillette (1987). Sudden Infant Death Syndrome: 1987
perspective. J. Pediatrics, 110 (5), 669-678.
Schlaefke, M.E., T. Schaefer, D. Schaefer and C. Schaefer (1990). Development, disturbances, and training of respiratory regulation in infants.
In: Sleep and Health Risk (J.H. Peter, T. Podszus and P. von Wichert,
eds.). Springer, Heidelberg.

Effect of Halothane on Hypoxic and Hypercapnic Ventilatory Responses of Goats

Shin O. Koh and John W. Severinghaus

Department of Anesthesia and the Cardiovascular
Research Institute, University of California,
San Francisco, CA 94143-0542, USA

SUMMARY

In 4 chronically tracheostomized goats the effects of 0.5%, 1.0% and 1.25% end tidal halothane on the ventilatory responses to isocapnic hypoxia ($40 < P_{ET}O_2 < 45$ mmHg) were compared with the awake responses 11 times at 3 levels of $P_{ET}CO_2$. Hypoxia did not significantly increase the CO_2 response slope. At 1.25% halothane the CO_2 response slope fell to 36.3 ± 26.2 (s.d.) % of control, and the ventilatory increase (in L/min) produced by isocapnic hypoxia fell to 44.5 ± 18.6% of control. The mean ratio of hypoxic to normoxic ventilation increased from 1.71 ± 0.06 (s.e.) awake to 2.24 ± 0.20 at 1.25% halothane (N=33, P=0.025). It is concluded that, whereas previous studies have shown that halothane preferentially depresses hypoxic chemosensitivity in man, it depresses hypoxic and CO_2 chemosensitivity about equally in the goat.

Halogenated hydrocarbon anesthetics are known to decrease HCVR (hypercapnic ventilatory reponse) in a dose dependent manner [1,2]. They have been shown to more profoundly depress hypoxic ventilatory response in man even at low concentrations. Knill obtained evidence for a surprising fall in hypoxic response even at 0.1% halothane, and major depression at 1.1 MAC, even at increased PCO_2 [3]. This confirmed previous reports for dogs [4,5], although the degree of depression of hypoxic response was more severe in man. In decerebrate cats, Davies et al showed that halothane depressed neural output responses of the carotid body to hypoxia and hypercapnia about equally, but more profoundly to nicotine and cyanide [6]. In 1989 Ponte and Sadler [7] reported that in rabbits and cats peripheral chemoreceptor response to severe hypoxia ($P_{ET}O_2 \simeq 30$) was not depressed by anesthetics, although the response to more moderate hypoxia may have been attenuated.

METHODS

The following experiments were carried out on 4 healthy young castrated male goats that had been prepared for studies of the effect of high altitude on the pH of the brain ECF over central chemoreceptors. Logistic and technical problems with the electrodes had prevented that study. We had prepared carotid artery loops, but sampling proved impossible due to periarterial hemorrhage or clotting. Each goat had a chronic tracheostomy. We therefore decided to use the animals to compare the effects of halothane on the hypoxic and CO_2 chemosensitivities, since this could be accomplished by measuring end tidal concentrations of halothane, O_2 and CO_2.

For each study, a #7 French cuffed vinyl endotracheal tube was inserted after 4% lidocaine topical anesthesia of the trachea. The goats breathed through a #2 Fleisch pneumotachograph connected to a non-rebreathing valve. Sufficient gas was delivered to a 4 liter anesthesia inspired reservoir bag to keep it inflated.

Inspired minute ventilation was continuously recorded by electrically averaging the inspiratory flow with a 15 sec time constant. End tidal PO_2 and PCO_2 were continuously displayed and recorded using a Perkin Elmer 1100 mass spectrometer. End tidal halothane concentration was recorded using a Beckman LB2 infra-red halothane analyzer. Signals were recorded on strip chart recorders for later analysis. Pneumotachograph flow was calibrated over the range from zero to 60 L./min with a precision flow meter precalibrated with a Tissot spirometer.

Responses were tested awake and a 1.25, 1.0 and 0.5% end-tidal halothane concentration in that order because the lighter levels could not be studied first due to excitement. At each level of anesthesia, the first measurements were made without inspired CO_2, after 30 minutes of equilibration at that level of halothane to achieve a relatively constant brain halothane level [8]. At each anesthetic level, two levels of added CO_2 were obtained by adding 100% CO_2 to the inspired gas allowing at least 10 min for stabilization at each level. The hypoxic response was tested at each level of PCO_2 by changing the gas mixture delivered to the halothane by-pass type vaporizer from 100% O_2 to an air-N_2 mixture manually adjusted with flow meters to reduce end-tidal oxygen tension over several minutes to 40-45 torr and hold it constant for at least 2 minutes while holding $P_{ET}CO_2$ constant at its hyperoxic level. CO_2 slope was computed by linear regression. Hypoxic ventilatory response was measured in 3 ways:

1) increase in the CO2 response slope.
2) isocapnic increase in ventilation, L./min
3) hypoxic ventilatory ratio $F=V_{hypoxic}/V_{oxic}$.

Analysis of variance was used to assess difference, with p<0.05 taken as the threshold significance.

RESULTS

Eleven sets of data collected in the 4 goats, 2-4 in each animal over the course of 6 weeks, are presented in Table I. Hypoxia had no significant effect on the slope of the CO2 response either awake or at any level of halothane tested. As in man and other animals previously tested, both the CO2 response HCVR and the hypoxic response were decreased by halothane, but in these goats, the hypoxic response was not more depressed than the CO2 response. At 1.25% halothane the CO2 response slope fell to $36.3\pm26.2\%$ of control, and the ventilatory increase (in L.min-1) produced by isocapnic hypoxia fell to $44.5\pm18.6\%$ of control. These two depressant effects were not significantly different. The hypoxic ventilatory ration F was increased from 1.71 ± 0.06 awake to 2.24 ± 0.20 at 1.25% halothane (p=0.025).

DISCUSSION

The absence of arterial blood samples weakens the conclusions since end-tidal gas tensions may not reflect arterial values, especially with shallow breathing in deep anesthesia [9]. Placement of an cuffed tracheostomy tube in an awake goat might stimulate ventilation which could be interpreted as ventilatory depression with anesthesia. The animals usually coughed for a few seconds after intubation with topical anesthesia, but showed no subsequent evidence of discomfort or trachypnea. The anesthetic depressant effect on ventilatory response to CO_2 is in accord with previous studies [1,2] but in contrast to studies in man [3], the hypoxic response was not more depressed than CO2 response and the hypoxic ventilatory ratio F was increased at 1.25% halothane (p<0.05).

In other species, hypoxic drive mediated through carotid chemoreceptors is highly dependent on the level of PCO_2, and therefore is generally considered to operate by multiplying the central drive. Thus when central CO_2 drive is depressed by halothane, although total ventilation is less, one might attempt to compute the partial separate effect of hypoxia as a fractional change in ventilation or in CO_2 slope. In the goat, hypoxia increased ventilation proportionally more in deep halothane than awake.

These responses have not been previously studied in the goat, and may represent significant species differences. The hypoxic response was not significantly increased by hypercapnia at any level of halothane even though, via the Haldane effect, hypercapnia must have reduced arterial saturation at constant alveolar PO_2.

The effect of halothane on resting CO_2 level might be expected to vary widely between species because of the significant species differences in central and peripheral chemoreceptor physiologic and pharmacologic sensitivity [10]. Peripheral chemoreceptor hypoxic sensitivity is also variable depending on chronic hypoxic exposure [11]. Furthermore, the effect of halothane on resting PCO_2 may be far less than its effect on CO_2 response slope would lead one to expect [2,3]. At 1 MAC halothane in man [3] ventilation was decreased to 52% of the awake level while resting PCO_2 rose only to 43 torr, partly of course due to decreased CO_2 production. In dogs at 1 MAC, ventilation and resting PCO_2 did not change significantly [4].

The hypoxic responses were based on end tidal PO_2, which may differ considerably from arterial PO_2. Ideally we would have determined SaO_2 directly, but efforts to use several pulse oximeters on various locations in the goats failed. Two goats initially had carotid arterial loops, but both failed to provide blood samples and pulse oximeters failed to obtain dependable signals even when located to transilluminate the artery.

There are several ways to assess hypoxic ventilatory drive. Isocapnic minute ventilation during hypoxia rises linearly with arterial desaturation [12]. In this study, SaO_2 was not measured, but it would have been lower at constant $P_{ET}O_2$ as $P_{ET}CO_2$ rose both with halothane depth and with added CO_2. Halothane depressed the absolute ventilatory increase produced by hypoxia to 40-45 torr $P_{ET}O_2$, but did not depress the ratio of hypoxic to hyperoxic ventilation.

The CO_2 response slope showed no increase during hypoxia. Interaction in the ventilatory response between hypoxia and CO_2 has been shown to primarily orginate in the arterial chemoreceptors [13,14]. The mechanisms of carotid and aortic body stimulation are different for CO_2 and O_2 [15,16].

In 1989 Ponte and Sadler [7], recording carotid chemoreceptor nerve action potentials, showed persistently brisk responses to severe hypoxia (less than 35 torr (5.3KPa)) in the presence of several volatile anesthetics, inconsistent with previous findings [6]. They suggested that in severe hypoxia, peripheral chemoreceptor drive to the respiratory centers remains undepressed by anesthetics, although response at more moderate values of hypoxia may be attenuated.

REFERENCES

1. Dunbar BS, Ovassapian A, Smith TC: The effect of methoxyflurane on ventilation in man. ANESTHESIOLOGY 28:1020-1028, 1966
2. Munson ES, Larson CP JR, Babad AA, Regan MJ, Buechel DR, Eger EI: The effects of halothane, fluroxene, and cyclopropane on ventilation. A comparative study in man. ANESTHESIOLOGY 27 :716-728, 1966
3. Knill RL, Gelb AW: Ventilatory response to hypoxia and hypercapnia during halothane sedation and anesthesia in man. ANESTHESIOLOGY 49:244-251, 1978
4. Hirshman CA, McCullough, Cohen PJ, Weil JV: Depression of hypoxic ventilatory response by halothane, enflurane and

isoflurane in dogs. Br J Anaesth 49:957,1977

5. Weiskopf RB, Raymond LW, Severinghaus JW: Effects of halothane on canine respiratory response to hypoxia with and without hypercarbia. ANESTHESIOLOGY 41:350-360,1974

6. Davies RO, Edwards MW, Lahiri S : Halothane depresses the response of carotid body chemoreceptors to hypoxia and hypercapnia in the cat. ANESTHESIOLOGY 57: 153-159, 1982

7. Ponte J, Sadler CL : Effect of halothane, enflurane and isoflurane on carotid body chemoreceptor activity in the rabbit and the cat. Br J Aneaesth 62:33-39, 1989

8. Merkel G, Eger EI : A comparative study of halothane and halopropane anesthesia, including method for determining equipotency. ANESTHESIOLOGY 24:346-357, 1963

9. Eger EI, Bahlman SH: Is the end-tidal anesthetic partial pressure an accurate measure of arterial anesthetic partial pressure? ANESTHESIOLOGY 35:301-303,1971

10. Black AMS, Comroe JH, Jacobs L: Species difference in carotid body response of cat and dog to dopamine and serotonin. Am J Physiology 223:1097-1104,1972

11. Severinghaus JW, Bainton CR, Carcelen A: Respiratory insensitivity to hypoxia in chronically hypoxic man. Resp Physiol 1:308-334,1966

12. Rebuck AS, Campbell EJM: A clinical method for assessing the ventilatory response to hypoxia. Amer Rev Resp Dis 109:345-350,1974

13. Van Beek JHGM, Berkenbosch A, De Goede J, Olivier CN : Influence of peripheral O_2 tension on the ventilatory response to CO_2 in cats. Resp Physiol 51:379-388,1983

14. Lahiri S, Mokashi A, Delaney RG, Fishman AP: Arterial PO_2 and PCO_2 stimulus threshold for carotid chemoreceptors and breathing. Resp Physiol 34:359-375,1978

15. Fitzgerald RS, Dehghani GA: Neural response of the cat carotid and aortic bodies to hypercapnia and hypoxia J Appl Physiol 52:596-601,1982

16. Daristotle L, Berssenbrugge D, Bisgard GE: Hypoxic-hypercapnic ventilatory interaction at the carotid body of awake goats. Resp Physiol 70:63-77, 1987

Table 1.

%Halo(ET)	0(Awake)		0.5%		1.0%		1.25%	
	MEAN	SEM	MEAN	SEM	MEAN	SEM	MEAN	SEM
HCVR								
ox	1.23	0.14	0.67*	0.07	0.28*	0.03	0.39*	0.08
hy	1.33	0.14	0.90*	0.09	0.35*	0.06	0.32*	0.04
hy/ox	1.13	0.10	1.40	0.09	1.30	0.26	1.34	0.31
HVR, $P_ICO_2=0$								
$P_{ET}CO_2$	44.00	1.04	56.27	1.38	62.00	2.30	71.73	3.28
V_Iox	5.80	0.20	3.92*	0.32	2.72*	0.17	1.55*	0.15
V_Ihy	11.64	0.84	7.78*	1.09	5.09*	0.49	4.84*	0.86
$\dot{V}_I$	5.84	0.82	3.86	0.96	2.37*	0.44	3.29*	0.81
F	2.01	0.15	1.98	0.23	1.90	0.18	3.11*	0.44
P_ICO_2 step1								
$P_{ET}CO_2$	48.36	1.00	63.82	1.48	71.78	2.19	80.45	3.12
V_Iox	10.18	0.70	7.75*	0.58	4.64*	0.20	5.29*	1.13
V_Ihy	17.69	1.03	15.55	1.45	8.17*	0.76	8.25*	0.95
$\dot{V}_I$	7.51	0.68	7.80	1.18	3.54*	0.70	2.95*	0.53
F	1.76	0.08	2.02	0.14	1.77	0.17	2.07	0.31
P_ICO_2 step2								
$P_{ET}CO_2$	54.00	1.09	70.82	1.13	78.36	2.41	89.73	3.05
V_Iox	18.06	0.85	14.52*	0.93	7.47*	0.64	7.52*	1.04
V_Ihy	24.25	1.30	19.71	1.36	10.72*	0.81	10.00*	0.74
$\dot{V}_I$	6.20	0.81	5.19	0.64	3.25*	0.65	2.48*	0.58
F	1.35	0.04	1.36	0.04	1.48	0.12	1.53	0.18
MEAN F	1.71	0.07	1.79	0.12	1.71	0.13	2.24*	0.20

Data of 11 complete sets of studies in 4 goats in which ventilation was measured in hyperoxia and isocapnic hypoxia ($P_{ET}O_2=40-45$) awake and at 1.25, 1.0 and 0.5% end tidal halothane, at resting PCO_2 and at two elevated PCO_2 levels. * indicates a value significantly different from the awake value at p<0.05 by analysis of variance.

HCVR: Mean CO_2 response slopes at two elevated $P_{ET}CO_2$ levels, L./min/mmHg

HVR: Hypoxic ventilation response at constant $P_{ET}CO_2$

ox: hyperoxic. hy:hypoxic

V_I : ventilation, L./min

$\dot{V}_I$: VI (hy-ox), L./min

F:$V_{Ihypoxic}$ /V_{Ioxic}

*: significantly different from awake (p<0.05).

The Primary Analysis of Breathing Pattern in Elderly People

Ma Jiayong

1st Affiliated Hospital, Suzhou Medical College, Suzhou, China

ABSTRACT

To understand the significance of components of the breathing pattern in elderly people, we measured the breathing pattern of 21 normal elderly subjects and 24 elderly patients with COPD. In normal group, inspiratory time (Ti), mean inspiratory flow (Vt/Ti) and the fractional inspiratory time (Ti/Ttot) were 1.72 ± 0.59 sec, 400 ± 71ml/s and 0.407 ± 0.042, respectively. These values were not significantly different, comparing to those in a group of healthy middle-age. In patients with COPD, Ti and Ti/Ttot were 1.52 ± 0.43 sec and 0.402 ± 0.042, respectively, no differences to normal group, but Vt/Ti was 496 ± 88 ml/s, higher than normal elderly group ($p<0.01$). We conclude that (1)the mean values of the breathing pattern components in normal subjects were not affected by aging; (2)the increase in minute ventilation of patients with COPD is related to changes in the inspiratory drive.

KEYWORDS

Inspiratory drive; Breathing pattern.

It has been shown that the tidal volume divided by inspiratory time (mean inspiratory flow) could reflect respiratory center drive and in most COPD patients the respiratory drive was increasing, but the relationship between respiratory drive and aging was unknown. In this study , breathing pattern of normal elderly people and elderly people with COPD was recorded to provide a basis for understanding the effect of aging on respiratory center drive.

MATERIALS AND METHODS

The breathing pattern was recorded with a spirometer (FJD-80 model, Shanghai), 21 normal elderly subjects (≥60 years), FEV1%>75% and

without disorders of heart, lung and endocrine system; 24   elderly
patients with COPD (≥60 years), FEV1%<70%; 25 normal adults (52+6
years). All people were tested in standing position.
Baseline breathing was monitored for 10 minutes, at stable condition
5 respiratory waves were recorded with paper speed of 25 mm/s.   The
following parameters were calculated: minute ventilation (Vmin);tidal
volume (Vt); respiratory frequency (f); inspiratory time (Ti);
fractional inspiratory time (Ti/Ttot); mean inspiratory flow (Vt/Ti).
Student's unpaired t-test was used to test for significant difference
between mean values of breathing pattern , with $p < 0.05$ taken   as
significant.

RESULTS

In control group, there were no significant differences among   the
three waves (table 1).
The parameters in three groups were in table 2. Ti, Vt/Ti and Ti/Ttot
between normal elderly group and control group were no significant
difference. VC%pred in normal elderly group was higher than   COPD
group ($P < 0.05$). Vmin and Vt/Ti in COPD group was higher than normal
elderly group ($P < 0.01$), other indexes were no significant difference
between the two groups.

Table 1. Components of three waves in 25 normal
subjects (M±SD)

	First	Second	Third
Vt(ml)	696±167	718±249	721±222
Ti(s)	1.66±0.35	1.70±0.52	1.66±0.45
Te(s)	2.47±0.82	2.52±0.81	2.38±0.66
Vt/Ti(ml/s)	423±80	426±93	434±74
Ti/Ttot	0.411±0.053	0.405±0.045	0.414±0.045

P>0.1

DISCUSSION

Usually, minute ventilation was regarded as the product of mean
inspiratory flow (Vt/Ti) and fractional inspiratory time (Ti/Ttot).
Since neural impulses controlling inspiratory drive were independent
of reflex activity once inspiration has begun, Vt/Ti can reflected
respiratory center drive as it is the mechanical transformation   of

Table 2. Components of breathing pattern in three
groups (M±SD)

	Control	Normal elder	COPD elder
VC%pred	92.8±9.7	94.0±13.6	82.5±25.5*
FEV1/VC%	82.5±5.1	80.1±3.8	57.3±9.3**
Vmin(L/min)	10.30±1.66	9.72±1.80	11.72±1.96**
Vt(ml)	712±206	666±168	729±162
f	15±4	15±4	17±5
Ti(s)	1.67±0.41	1.72±0.59	1.52±0.43
Vt/Ti(ml/s)	427±75	400±71	496±88**
Ti/Ttot	0.409±0.042	0.407±0.042	0.402±0.042

*p<0.05; **p<0.01

phrenic nerve activity.(Milic-Emili et al.,1976, Tobin et al.,1983).
In this study, it was shown that there were no significant difference
in breathing pattern components between control and normal elderly,
indicating the respiratory center drive of normal elderly subject at
rest may be similar to the control group. Comparing to the normal
elder, in elderly patients with COPD Vt/Ti and Vmin increased. These
recordings revealed that increase of ventilation in COPD patients was
mainly due to the heightened respiratory center drive, which   may
relate to the reflex of vagal nerve (Savoy et al.,1981).

REFERENCES

Milic-Emili, J. and M.M. Grustein (1976). Drive and timing components
of ventilation. Chest, 70, 131-133.
Tobin, M.J., T.S.Chadha, G.Jenouri, S.J.Birch, H.B.Gazeroglu and
M.A.Sachner (1983). Breathing patterns. 1.Normal subjects. Chest,
84, 202-205.
Savoy, J., S.Dhingra and N.R.Anthonisen (1981). Role of vagal airway
reflexes in control of ventilation in pulmonary fibrosis.
Clin. Sci. Molecular. Med., 61, 781-784.

Respiratory-like Slow Wave Sympathetic Oscillations During Morphine-induced Central Apnea in Rabbits

N. Kimura, F. Kato, Y. Tsukamoto and
T. Hukuhara, Jr.

Department of Pharmacology II, The Jikei University
School of Medicine, Minato-ku, Tokyo 105, Japan

ABSTRACT

Sympathetic nerve rhythms during morphine-induced phrenic nerve quiescence were studied on vagotomized rabbits artificially ventilated. Slow sympathetic nerve rhythm having a period in the vicinity of the normal respiratory cycle (0.4 to 2 Hz) persisted after the phrenic respiratory discharge was ceased by morphine (6-14 mg/kg, iv). This slow sympathetic rhythm correlated with the EEG rhythm in the rabbits without baroreceptor inputs. After naloxone both the slow sympathetic and EEG rhythms correlated with the phrenic respiratory discharge.

KEYWORDS

Sympathetic nervous system; respiratory center; postganglionic autonomic fibers; phrenic nerve; electroencephalogram; morphine; naloxone; Fourier analysis.

INTRODUCTION

Respiratory rhythm in the sympathetic nerve discharge (SND) is generally assumed to be directly imposed on the brainstem sympathetic networks by simple intracentral propagation from the respiratory center. In contrast to this classical view, a central sympathetic oscillator hypothesis has explained the respiratory rhythm in SND as a result of entrainment of the respiratory and slow sympathetic oscillators (Gebber, 1980). This hypothesis is partly based on the observation that a slow sympathetic rhythm with a frequency around the normocapnic respiratory frequency often persisted during hyperventilation-induced phrenic nerve quiescence in cats (Barman and Gebber, 1976). However, Connelly and Wurster (1985) presented data not supportive of this hypothesis. The present study tested the hypothesis inducing the central apnea by morphine in the normocapnic rabbits.

METHODS

Twenty rabbits weighing between 2.0 and 3.1 kg were anesthetized with urethan (0.9-1.0 g/kg, ip), immobilized with gallamine triethiodide (3-5 mg/kg/hr, iv) and artificially ventilated. End-tidal CO_2 was kept at 4.4 ± 0.4 % and rectal temperature was maintained between 37 and 38°C. Bilateral vagus and depressor nerves were cut. Carotid sinus nerves were intact or cut. Efferent discharges of the renal sympathetic and phrenic nerves, frontal-occipital electroencephalogram (EEG) and arterial blood pressure (BP) were recorded simultaneously. Power spectra for SND, phrenic nerve discharge (PND), EEG and pump rhythm of the respirator and coherence spectra for these signals were calculated (frequency resolution, 0.03125 Hz; ensemble average of 20 raw spectra for 32-s data blocks) before and after administration of morphine (6-14 mg/kg, iv) or naloxone (0.1 mg/kg, iv). Statistical comparison between coherence values were made after adequate transformation with the Student's t-test. Values are expressed as means ± SD.

RESULTS

Slow sympathetic waves were locked in a 1:1 relation to the phrenic respiratory cycle before administration of morphine under the standard state (Fig. 1, IA). After the phrenic respiratory discharge was ceased by morphine, the slow rhythm having a period in the vicinity of the normal respiratory cycle (0.4 to 2 Hz) persisted in SND (Fig. 1, IB). In 7 of 14 rabbits with intact sinus nerves the slow sympathetic rhythm was related to the respirator-pump rhythm (0.75 Hz) during morphine-induced phrenic nerve quiescence. The mean BP was maintained at 101 ± 23 mmHg after morphine in these rabbits.

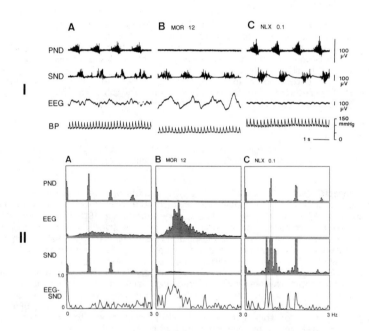

Fig. 1.   Slow sympathetic nerve rhythm during morphine-induced central apnea.   A, before morphine.   B, 5 min after morphine (12 mg/kg).   C, 5 min after naloxone (0.1 mg/kg).   Sinus nerves are intact.   I: original records.   II: autopower spectra for PND, SND and EEG and coherence spectra between EEG and SND (EEG-SND).   Data in I and II are from same rabbit.   Dotted line indicates the peak corresponding to the respiratory or slow sympathetic rhythm.

In the other 7 rabbits the mean BP decreased to less than 60 mmHg after morphine and the spectral peak corresponding to the cardiac-related rhythm disappeared in the coherence spectra between SND and BP. In these hypotensive rabbits after morphine, slow sympathetic waves were often related to the EEG activity and a broad spectral peak (0.4 to 2 Hz) was observed in the coherence spectrum between SND and EEG during morphine-induced phrenic nerve quiescence (Fig. 1, IB and IIB). The coherence value between SND and EEG in the 0.4- to 2-Hz band after morphine was significantly different from the control value (Table 1) and from the coherence value between random white noise and SND. In all the baroreceptor-denervated rabbits, the slow sympathetic rhythm correlated with the EEG rhythm during morphine-induced phrenic nerve quiescence (Table 1). After administration of naloxone the slow sympathetic rhythm synchronized with the PND in all the rabbits and often related to the EEG rhythm at the respiratory frequency (Fig. 1, IIC).

Table 1.   Coherence values between SND and EEG or PND
in the 0.4- to 2-Hz band.

	N	Control	Morphine	Naloxone
Hypotensive rabbits§				
PND-SND	7	0.95 ± 0.02	0.12 ± 0.07*	0.98 ± 0.004*
EEG-SND	7	0.30 ± 0.07	0.58 ± 0.14*	0.49 ± 0.26
Baroreceptor-denervated rabbits				
PND-SND	6	0.76 ± 0.30	0.22 ± 0.14*	0.91 ± 0.10*
EEG-SND	6	0.23 ± 0.05	0.43 ± 0.06*	0.43 ± 0.15

* Significantly (P<0.05) different from control.   § The mean BP decreased to less than 60 mmHg after morphine.

DISCUSSION

Persistence of the slow sympathetic rhythm during morphine-induced phrenic nerve quiescence would be supportive of the existence of the slow sympathetic oscillators. Correlation between slow sympathetic rhythm and EEG or pump rhythm after morphine suggests that the slow sympathetic oscillators in rabbits are capable of synchronizing with major periodic inputs from the respiratory oscillators, baroreceptors (Kimura, 1988) or higher center under a given condition. It still remains to be established whether the slow sympathetic rhythm during morphine-induced phrenic nerve quiescence persists after transection of the neuraxis between the brain stem and forebrain or not.

This study was partly supported by the Ministry of Education, Science, and Culture, Japan, Grant-in-Aid No. 62770157 and No. 01770144.

REFERENCES

Gebber, G.L. (1980). Central oscillators responsible for sympathetic nerve discharge. Am. J. Physiol. 239, H143-H155.
Barman, S.M. and G.L. Gebber (1976). Basis for synchronization of sympathetic and phrenic nerve discharges. Am. J. Physiol. 231, 1601-1607.
Connelly, C.A. and R.D. Wurster (1985). Sympathetic rhythms during hyperventilation-induced apnea. Am. J. Physiol. 249, R424-R431.
Kimura, N. (1988). Central rhythmic control of sympathetic nerve discharge. II. Sympathetic nerve rhythms during morphine-induced phrenic nerve quiescence. Jikeikai Med. J. 35, 535-548.

The Genesis of Gasps Provoked by Brain Ischemia in the Rabbit

S. Matsumoto, T. Shimizu, T. Kanno,
M. Yamasaki and T. Nagayama

Department of Physiology, Fukushima Medical College,
Fukushima 960-12, Japan

ABSTRACT

When the global brain ischemia was sustained for over 30 sec, the induction of gasps preceded by apnea was identified in the measurement of phrenic nerve activity (PNA). Gasping shifted to hyperpnea in the case with well maintenance of increased arterial pressure (AP), and the onset of gasping appeared again by reduction of AP due to nitroprusside administration. Under particular conditions in which the cerebral blood flow was perfused by the right common carotid blood flow (RCCBF) only, gasping following apnea was observed when the decrease of RCCBF was held at approximately 13 % of their control values. These results suggest that the genesis of gasping provoked by brain ischemia is probably due to a progressive change in the inherent rhythmicity of medullary inspiratory neurons.

KEYWORDS

Gasping; apnea; brain ischemia; common carotid blood flow; rabbit.

The global brain ischemia in the rabbit produces a characteristic effect in both respiration and circulation, for example, apnea, bradycardia and an increase in arterial pressure (Matsumoto, 1988; Shimizu and Miyakawa, 1970; Shimizu and Nomura, 1981; Shimizu et al., 1988). Concerning the bradycardia provoked by brain ischemia, this effect is greatly diminished or completely abolished by surgical denervation of the aortic nerves (Matsumoto, 1988; Shimizu and Nomura, 1981). Under these conditions, gasping preceded by apnea occasionally appears when brain ischemia is sustained for over 30 sec. To define the mechanism of the neurogenesis of gasping, we investigated the response of phrenic nerve activity (PNA) to brain ischemia sustained for over 30 sec in anesthetized rabbits with spontaneous breathing. Furthermore, we also examined the correlation between the onset of gasping and a decrease in the cerebral blood flow, by using the modified technique of brain ischemia.

Eleven rabbits weighing 2.5–3.5 kg were anesthetized with urethane (1 g/kg, i.p.). The trachea was cannulated and polyethylene catheters were inserted into a femoral artery and vein. AP and heart rate (HR) were measured by a pressure

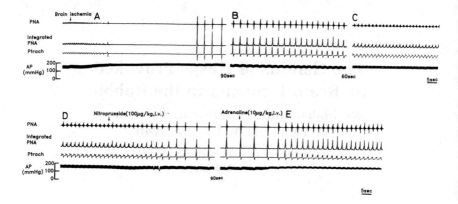

Fig. 1. Responses of phrenic nerve activity (PNA), tracheal
side-pressure (Ptrach) and arterial pressure (AP)
to brain ischemia before and after administration
of nitroprusside or adrenaline. (A): from apnea to
gasping, (B): gasping-like pattern, (C): from
gasping-like pattern to hyperpnea, (D): the onset
of gasping after administration of nitroprusside
and (E): the onset of hyperpnea after
administration of adrenaline.

transducer and a cardiotachometer, respectively. The tracheal side-pressure
(Ptrach), as an index of respiratory movement, was measured by a
pneumotachograph via a differential transducer. A phrenic root (C_5) on the
right side was exposed, sectioned and desheathed. Then, the central cut end of
phrenic nerve was placed on unipolar silver electrode and submerged under warm
liquid paraffin (37-38°C). To interrupt the vertebral blood flow, holes were
made on the ventral surface of the right and left transversal processes at C_3
and/or C_4. Then, a piece of a gause stick stiffened with bone wax was
forcefully inserted into each hole. After interrupting the vertebral blood
flow, the global brain ischemia was performed by clamping both common carotid
arteries at C_3 level. In some animals, after the interruption of blood flow of
the vertebral arteries, the blood flow of the right common carotid artery was
measured by connecting a probe (cannula type) of the electromagnetic flowmeter
to a polyethylene catheter inserted into the artery, while clamping the left
common carotid artery. A decrease in the cerebral blood flow was performed by
occluding the catheter connecting to the probe.

The sequence of changes on PNA and AP in the time course of sustained brain
ischemia is shown in Fig. 1A-D. When the magnitude of the increased AP was well
maintained during brain ischemia, gasping shifted to hyperpnea. In the same
preparation, under the particular condition of brain ischemia, the onset of
gasping was produced by administration of nitroprusside (see Fig. 1D) whereas
adrenaline counteracted this specific respiratory effect (Fig. 1E). Fig. 2
shows the typical responses of Ptrach and AP to progressive decrease of the
RCCBF in a rabbit without intact aortic nerve. Note that the induction of
gasping occurs when RCCBF is reduced remarkably. The values of RCCBF in control
condition were 20.5±2.0 ml/min (means±S.E., n=5). When progressive occlusion of
the right common carotid artery elicited the onset of gasping, the values of
RCCBF were 3.5±2.5 ml/min.

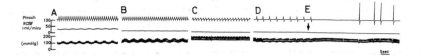

Fig. 2.   Responses of tracheal side-pressure (Ptrach),
right common carotid blood flow (RCCBF) and
arterial pressure (AP) to progressive occlusion
of the right common carotid artery. (A) before
occlusion (RCCBF=25 ml/min), (B) during occlusion
(10 ml/min), (C) during occlusion (5 ml/min), (D)
during occlusion (6 ml/min) and (E) during
occlusion (↓) (3 ml/min).

It is well known that the onset of gasping preceded by apnea is observed in a
characteristic course during either progressive asphyxiation or hypoxemia
(Guntheroth et al., 1975; Hukuhara et al., 1959; Lawson and Thach, 1977).
Lawson and Thach (1977) suggested that gasping due to sustained airway occlusion
occurs as a result of the progressive changes in respiratory patterns observed
before the onset of primary apnea. In this study, the onset and the
disappearance of gasps during brain ischemia were provoked by the change in AP
to influence the cerebral blood flow and the responses were usually associated
with the hyperpneic phase. Furthermore, marked reduction of the cerebral blood
flow elicited gasping preceded by apnea as well as hyperpnea. The results
suggest that the onset of gasping during brain ischemia probably reflects the
level of the cerebral blood flow and is part of a progression of changes in the
inherent rhythmicity of medullary inspiratory neurons.

REFERENCES

Guntheroth, W. G., I. Kawabori, D. Breazeale and G. McGough (1975). Hypoxic
    apnea and gasping. J. Clin. Invest., 56, 1371-1377.
Hukuhara, T., S. Nakayama and M. Yamagami (1959). On the behavior of the
    respiratory muscles in gasping. Jpn. J. Physiol., 9, 125-129.
Lawson, E. E. and B. T. Thach (1977). Respiratory patterns during progressive
    asphyxia in newborn rabbits. J. Appl. Physiol., 43, 468-474.
Matsumoto, S. (1988). The abilities of myelinated and non-myelinated aortic
    fibers on the brain ischemia-mediated reflex bradycardia in the rabbit.
    Fukushima J. Med. Sci., 34, 95-108.
Shimizu, T. and K. Miyakawa (1970). Cardiac output and stroke volume during
    complete interruption of blood supply to the brain in rabbit. Med. J. Shinshu
    Univ., 15, 47-70.
Shimizu, T., T. Nagayama, T. Kanno, S. Matsumoto and M. Yamasaki (1988).
    Effects of acute global brain ischemia on cardiovascular functions and
    reversibility of these brain ischemic responses in rabbits. In: High-altitude
    Medical Science (G. Ueda et al., ed.), pp. 56-60. Shinshu Univ., Matsumoto.
Shimizu, T. and H. Nomura (1981). The functional and anatomical differences of
    the left and right aortic nerves on the brain ischemia-mediated reflex
    bradycardia in the rabbit. Med. J. Fujitagakuen, 5, 111-115. (in Japanese).

Carotid Chemoreceptor Discharge in the Rat

R. Maruyama and Y. Fukuda

Department of Physiology, School of Medicine, Chiba
University, 1-8-1 Inohana, Chiba 280, Japan

ABSTRACT

Carotid chemoreceptor discharge response to various chemical stimuli were studied
in the urethane-anesthetized, vagotomized, artificially ventilated rat. The mean
carotid sinus nerve (CSN) discharge and amplitude of oscillation synchronized
with the phase of artificial respiration increased gradually as end-tidal P_{O2} was
decreased from a hyperoxic to hypoxic level at a maintained end-tidal P_{CO2}.
Hypercapnia, however, did not increase the CSN discharge in both background hyperoxic and hypoxic conditions indicating no CO_2-hypoxia interaction at the
chemoreceptor site. Intra-carotid artery injections solution containing H^+, K^+ or
Acetylcoline (ACh) induced chemoreceptor activation. The results indicated that
the rat carotid chemoreceptor responses to hypoxia or hypercapnia and their
interaction differ significantly from those reported on the cat.

KEYWORDS

Rat carotid chemoreceptor discharge; Hypoxia; Hypercapnia.

INTRODUCTION

Recently, the rat has been widely used in cardiovascular, respiratory researches.
However, there have been only a few studies on the characteristic of afferent
discharge response of the rat carotid chemoreceptors to various chemical stimuli
(Brokaw et al. 1985. Fukuda et al. 1987). In the present experiments we have investigated the effect of hypoxic, hypercapnic and other chemical stimuli on the
discharge pattern of afferent mass activity in the rat carotid sinus nerve.

MATERIAL and METHODS

Male Wistar rats weighing 300 - 400g were anesthetized with urethane (0.8g/kg).
The animal was trachectomized, bilaterally vagotomized and artificially ventilated. Afferent mass discharges from the carotid chemoreceptors were recorded
from the cut central end of the carotid sinus nerve with bipolar platinum electo-
rodes during systemic hypoxia and/or hypercapnia. Also external carotid artery
was catetherized to stimulate the carotid body locally with solutions containing

© 1991 Pergamon Press plc.
Printed in Great Britain.

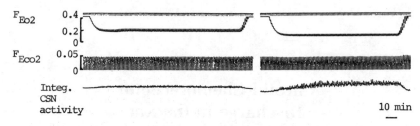

Fig. 1. Carotid sinus nerve discharge response normoxia
(left) and hypoxia (right) at a maintained end-tidal
F_{ECO2}. F_{EO2} and F_{ECO2}, fractional concentration of O_2
and CO_2 tracheal gas; integ. CSN activity, Integrated
carotid sinus nerve mass discharges.

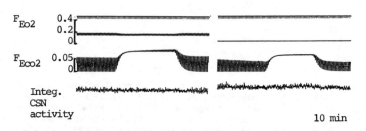

Fig. 2. Effect of hypercapnia on the afferent carotid sinus
nerve discharge in background normoxia(left) and
hypoxia(right). F_{EO2} and F_{ECO2} , O_2 and CO_2 fractional concentration of tracheal gas; integ. CSN
activity, integrated carotid sinus nerve mass
discharges.

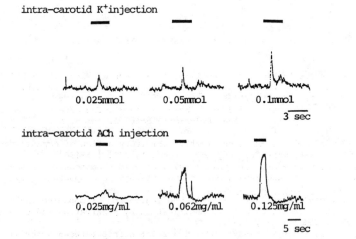

Fig. 3. Effect of intra-carotid injection of K^+ (upper) and
Acetylcoline (lower).

H$^+$, K$^+$ or ACh (0.1ml/vol).

RESULTS

The afferent mass discharges of the rat CSN consisted mostly of chemoreceptor activities, and this enebled us to estimate discharge response semi-quantitatively. Figure 1 shows an example of CSN mass discharge response to hypoxic stimulation at a maintained end-tidal Pco2. The integrated CSN discharges increased, and the amplitude of discharge oscillation synchronized with ventilatory cvcle due to artificial respiration were augmented. Figure 2 illustrates typical examples of CSN activities during hypercapnia (end-tidal CO2 up to about 70 mmHg) in background hyperoxic and hypoxic conditions. Hypercapnia did not increase the CSN discharges and suppressed the magnitude of discharge oscillation. Figure 3 shows the effect of intra-carotid injections of solution containing K$^+$ and ACh. Both and H$^+$ injection induced an increase in discharge in dose dependent manner.

DISCUSSION

Many previous studies on the response of carotid body chemoreceptor to chemical stimulation performed mostly in the cat (Band et al., 1978, Linton and Band, 1988) An interesting observation is that though the chemoreceptor is stimulated by both the hypoxic and hypercapnic stimuli, but is sensitive to small rapid change in arterial Pco2. This result in CO2 related discharge oscillation being synchronized with instantaneous cyclic Paco2 (or pH) variation due to ventilatory phasing. Our results indicated that carotid chemoreceptor responses differ significantly from those reported for the cat. First, the rat carotid chemoreceptor showed neglibly small response to CO2. Secondly, the CSN discharge oscillation in the rat could be increased by hypoxic stimulation and suppressed by hypercapnia. These particular differences especially the lack of response to CO2 in the rat, may represent some structual or biochemical differences in the chemosensing mechanism between two species. A differrent contribution of dopaminergic mechanism within the carotid body has been known (Hanbauer and Hellström, 1978, Brokoaw et al., 1985). Dopamine which is related from Type 1 cell by hypoxia facillitates the chemoreceptor response in rats (Mishra et al., 1979). Whereas in cats, dopamine has an inhibitory effect (Docherty and MaQueen, 1978). These findings, can not totally explain the different chemorecptor response between two species, and more extensive stidies on the chemosensing mechanism in rat are required.

REFERENCES

Band, D.M., M. Mcclelland, D.L. Phillips, K.B. Saunders and C.B. Wolff (1978). Sensitivity of the carotid body to within-breath changes in arterial Pco2. J. Appl. Physiol., 45, 768-777.

Brokoaw, J.J., J.T. Hansen and D.S. Christie (1978). The effects of hypoxia on catecholamine dynamics in the rat carotid body. J. Auton. Nerv. Syst., 13, 35-47.

Docherty, R.J. and D.S. MaQueen (1978). Inhibitory action of dopamine on the cat carotid chemoreceptors. J. Physiol. (London), 279, 425-436.

Fukuda, Y. A. Sato and A. Trzebski (1987). Carotid chemoreceptor discharge response to hypoxia and hypercapnia on normotensive and spontaneously hypertensive rats. J. Auton. Nerv. Syst., 19, 1-11.

Haubauer, I. and S. Hellström (1978). The regulation of dopamine and noradrenalin in the rat carotid body and its modification by denervation and by hypoxia. J. Physiol. (london), 282, 21-34.

Linton, R.A.F. and D.M. Band (1988). The relationship between arterial pH and chemoreceptor firing in anesthetized cats. Respir. Physiol., 74, 218-229.

Mishra, J. H.N. Sapru and A. Hess (1979). Physiolgical effects of dopamine agonist and antagonist on the rat carotid body. Fed. Proc. Exp. Biol., 38, 1143.

Effect of Sudden Withdrawal of Respiratory CO_2 Oscillation on the Phrenic Nerve Activity

E. Takahashi, I. Tateishi and T. Mikami

Division of Biomedical Systems Engineering, Faculty of
Engineering, Hokkaido University, Sapporo 060, Japan

ABSTRACT

The effect of sudden withdrawal of respiratory oscillations of arterial P_{CO_2} (CO_2 oscillations) was examined in anesthetized vagotomized dogs. Reciprocally ventilating the right and left lungs resulted in complete abolition of CO_2 oscillations while the mean level of arterial blood gases were unaffected. We found negligible change in the respiratory center output as a result of the withdrawal of CO_2 oscillations. Thus, we conclude that CO_2 oscillations do not play an important role in the control of respiration at a resting metabolic rate.

KEYWORDS

CO_2 oscillations; control of respiration; pH electrode; anesthetized dog.

INTRODUCTION

Yamamoto and Edwards Jr. (1960) were the first to suggest that CO_2 oscillations play an important role in the control of respiration. Reducing CO_2 oscillations may be a way to examine the significance of CO_2 oscillations in maintaining respiratory rhythmicity in the normal resting condition. The effect might be demonstrated by unloading CO_2 from the venous circulation using a membrane lung (Phillipson et al., 1981), a use of a mixing chamber in the carotid artery (Linton et al., 1977), or in patients in which CO_2 oscillations are considerably dampened due to lung diseases (Cochrane et al., 1981). In the present paper, we propose a new technique which could completely abolish respiratory CO_2 oscillations without affecting the mean level of arterial blood gases in anesthetized animals. Our results suggest that CO_2 oscillations do not exert an important effect on the respiratory center output at rest.

METHODS

Eleven dogs weighing 8–19.5 kg were used. The dog was anesthetized with ketamine hydrochloride (10 mg/kg, i.m.) followed by intravenous injection of a mixture of urethane and chloralose (400 mg/kg and 40 mg/kg, respectively). Arterial and venous catheterizations were conducted. The phrenic neurogram was recorded from a branch of the C_5 root by a standard technique, which was then moving time averaged to assess the activity of the respiratory center. We inserted a 35 Fr. double lumen endotracheal tube through a tracheostomy, which was connected to a newly devised pressure type ventilator providing 2 independent gas outlets. The device delivered   room air or mixed gas at arbitrary flow rate to the right and left lungs (through tracheal and bronchial ports of the endotracheal tube, respectively) alternatively or simultaneously at arbitrary inspiratory and expiratory durations. The dog was paralyzed by gallamine triethiodide (1 mg/kg, i.v.) and vagotomized.

Respiratory CO_2 oscillations were assessed by a rapidly responding intra-arterial pH electrode (Kuraray, PH-1035) where the amplitude of respiratory oscillations of pH were converted to that of $Paco_2$ using a pH-log Pco_2 buffer line determined in vitro (Takahashi and Ashe, 1989). Alveolar gas was sampled and analyzed by a mass spectrometer (SRI, MS-8).

The effect of sudden withdrawal of CO_2 oscillations on the phrenic nerve activity was examined as follows. Firstly, the dog was ventilated with both lungs inflated/deflated simultaneously for 3 minutes (first control). Then, the operating mode of the ventilator was suddenly switched so that the right and left lungs were alternatively ventilated for 3 minutes (withdrawal of CO_2 oscillations). Lastly, we bracketed the withdrawal of CO_2 oscillations with another control where the lungs were simultaneously ventilated for 3 minutes. Arterial blood was sampled at the end of each phase and analyzed by standard electrodes (Radiometer, BMS3Mk2 and PHM71Mk2). We also conducted CO_2 inhalations to confirm that the dog was sensitive to steady-state changes in the chemical stimuli.

RESULTS

Experiments were conducted in normoxic normocapnia (mean Pao_2 and $Paco_2$ were 83.9 mmHg and 41.0 mmHg, respectively). We accepted 50 complete runs for further analysis in which changes in the minute phrenic activity (peak height of the phrenic neurogram x numbers of burst per minute) from the first to the second control was less than 30 % of the first control. Mean levels of $Paco_2$ in the first and second controls did not differ significantly (41.2+2.6 mmHg and 40.8+2.3 mmHg, respectively; mean+SD). Also, the amplitude of CO_2 oscillations were identical in the first and second controls (2.33+0.87 mmHg and 2.33+0.90 mmHg, respectively). The respiratory center output in the second control was 100.9+10.8 % of the first control and hence the base line drift was minimal.

By reciprocally ventilating the right and left lungs, we could completely abolish the respiratory CO_2 oscillations (Fig.1) without affecting the mean level of $Paco_2$ (40.9+2.5 mmHg). The difference of the minute phrenic activity from the base line was -0.02+6.11 % of the control (N.S.). Thus, the effect of changing CO_2 oscillations on the phrenic nerve activity was negligible.

DISCUSSION

The importance of the CO_2 oscillations in maintaining regular respiratory movement in a resting animal was most successfully but indirectly demonstrated by Phillipson et al. (1981). They showed in unanesthetized sheep that the removal of metabolicaly produced CO_2 from the venous circulation resulted in apnea without a decrease in $Paco_2$. Since CO_2 oscillations must have been considerably dampened or abolished during venous CO_2 unloadings, it might be claimed that almost all respiratory drive in the sheep depended exclusively on the oscillatory component of arterial Pco_2 if one postulates that CO_2 oscillations were responsible for this isocapnic hypopnea/apnea. However, recent CO_2 unloading studies conducted in unanesthetized dogs substantially contradict this speculation. Bennett et al. (1984) and Tallman et al. (1986) demonstrated CO_2 unloading resulted in hypocapnic hypopnea which could be extrapolated from the hypercapnic ventilatory response to inhaled CO_2. The present experiment in anesthetized and vagotomized dog in which arterial CO_2 oscillations were selectively altered suggests negligible involvement of CO_2 oscillations in the control of respiration at rest.

If CO_2 oscillations are involved in the control of respiration at rest, the respiratory controller should be sensitive enough to recognize the CO_2 oscillations as small as 2 mmHg in the amplitude (which is also a function of a respiratory frequency). With such a high sensitivity, the respiratory controller would confront the disturbances elicited by various spontaneous activities such as sigh, phonation and so on, and the stability of the respiratory control might be impaired. The possible role of the CO_2 oscillations in the control of respiration, if any, might become detectable when the oscillations are considerably augmented.

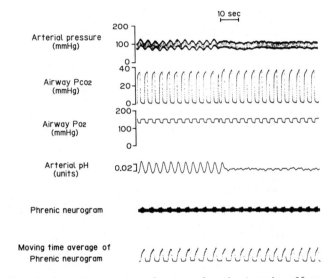

Fig. 1. Recorder tracings from one dog showing the effect of sudden withdrawal of respiratory CO_2 oscillations on the phrenic nerve activity.

REFERENCES

Bennett, F.M., R.D. Tallman, Jr. and F.S. Grodins (1984). Role of V̇co₂ in control of breathing of awake exercising dogs. J. Appl. Physiol., 56, 1335-1337.
Cochrane, G.M., J.G. Prior and C.B. Wolff (1981). Respiratory arterial pH and Pco₂ oscillations in patients with chronic obstructive airways disease. Clin. Sci., 61, 693-702.
Linton, R.A.F., R. Miller and I.R. Cameron (1977). Role of Pco₂ oscillations and chemoreceptors in ventilatory response to inhaled and infused CO₂. Respir. Physiol., 29, 201-210.
Phillipson, E.A., J. Duffin and J.D. Cooper (1981). Critical dependence of respiratory rhythmicity on metabolic CO₂ load. J. Appl. Physiol., 50, 45-54.
Takahashi, E. and K.A. Ashe (1989). Role of carbon dioxide oscillation in the control of respiration in the anesthetized dog. Jpn. J. Physiol., 39, 267-281.
Tallman, R.D., Jr., R. Marcolin, M. Howie, J.S. McDonald and T. Stafford (1986). Cardiopulmonary response to extracorporeal venous CO₂ removal in awake spontaneously breathing dogs. J. Appl. Physiol., 61, 516-522.
Yamamoto, W.S. and M.W. Edwards, Jr. (1960). Homeostasis of carbon dioxide during intravenous infusion of carbon dioxide. J. Appl. Physiol., 15, 807-818.

Effect of Vagal Nerve Cooling on Hypercapnic and Hypoxic Ventilatory Responses in Anesthetized Dogs

Y. Sagara, K. Koike, T. Nakada and
S. Fujimura

Department of Surgery, The Research Institute for Chest
Disease and Cancer, Tohoku University, 4-1, Aobaku,
Sendai, Japan

ABSTRACT

We studied ventilatory responses using a vagal nerve cooling technique and found
that the effect of the vagus nerve on respiratory regulation was different between
hypercapnic and hypoxic gas inhalation.

KEYWORD

vagal cooling;hypercapnia; hypoxia; J-receptor.

Phillipson *et al.* (1973) utilized a vagal cooling technique in dogs and found
that reduction of the increment of the respiratory frequency response to hypercapnia was related to the cessation of the Hering-Breuer inflation reflex. They
concluded that the increase in respiratory frequency during hypercapnia was due
to the irritant receptor. However, Russell *et al.* (1984) concluded that respiratory frequency with hypercapnic gas inhalation increased due to stimuli from the
C-fiber receptor. It has not been clarified how the Hering-Breuer inflation
reflex and other vagally mediated stimuli affect the hypoxic respiratory response.
    The purpose of this study is to elucidate how the Hering-Breuer inflation
reflex and other vagally mediated stimuli affect hypercapnic and hypoxic respiratory responses.

MATERIALS AND METHODS

Surgical preparation
    We anesthetized 18 dogs (8-15kg), inserted an endotracheal tube. and main-
teined anesthesia by continuous intravenous infusion of chloralose and urethane.
The right cervical vagosympathetic trunk was cut at the level of the 4th cervical
vertebra. We made a vertical incision on the left side of the cervix and dissected the left cervical vagosympathetic trunk for about 5 cm long at about 8 cm
peripheral to the distal vagal ganglion.

Vagus nerve cooling
A copper cooling probe was attached to the left cervical vagosympathetic trunk.
The cooling probe was perfused with water having a temperature of 37°C in the
control experiment and with water a temperature of 7°C in the vagus nerve cooling
experiment.

Experimental protocol
We divided the animals into two groups; hypercapnic (n=9) and hypoxic (n=9)
groups.
    In the control experiment of the hypercapnic group. the nerve cooler was

TABLE 1. Vantilatory responses in control, vagal nerve cooling and vagotomy

Condition	n	f (breath/min)	V_T (ml)	$\dot{V}_E$ (liter/min)
Room air	9			
Control		14.4±3.6	279±67	4.1±1.6
Vagal nerve cooling		14.4±4.9	361±126*	5.1±2.5*
Vagotomy		14.3±4.7	346±125*	4.7±1.8
7% CO_2	9			
Control		22.7±5.2	503±191	11.8±6.4
Vagal nerve cooling		23.7±7.1	742±247*	18.1±9.4*
Vagotomy		17.9±5.0†	850±390*	15.7±10.0*
5% CO_2+20% O_2 in N_2	9			
Control		18.2±7.0	404±129	6.7±1.3
Vagal nerve cooling		18.3±10.9	578±232*	8.8±2.1*
Vagotomy		15.2±10.8†	704±273†	8.7±2.6*
5% CO_2+10% O_2 in N_2	9			
Control		25.6±9.7	452±127	10.9±4.0
Vagal nerve cooling		25.7±12.6	702±254*	15.8±5.0*
Vagotomy		23.2±12.3	818±314†	16.4±4.5*

Results are given as mean±S.D. *$p<0.05$ against corresponding control values (paired t-test). †$p<0.05$ against corresponding values during vagus nerve cooling (paired t-test). n. numbers of dogs; f. respiratory frequency; V_T, tidal volume; $\dot{V}_E$,expired minute ventilation.

perfused with 37℃ water. Then we clamped the endotracheal tube and inflated the lungs by the rapid injection of about 400 ml air into the tube untill the airway pressure rose to 20-30 mmHg. Animals exhibiting apnea for 30 sec were determined as having the inflation reflex. The animals were the subjected to hypercapnic test, rebreathing 7% CO_2+20% O_2 in N_2 for 5 min, and all variables were measured. In the vagus nerve cooling experiment, we perfused the nerve cooling probe with water at 37℃ .We inflated the lung as described above and found that the inflation reflex had ceased. The animals were placed in room air and all variables were measured. Then the animals subjected to hypercapnic test and all variables were again measured. In the vagotomy experiment, we measure all variables under room air and hypercapnic trials after severing the left cervical vagosympathetic trunk. These experiments were conducted by using the same animals.

In the hypoxic group, we confirmed the presence of the inflation reflex at the beginning of the control experiments. In the control, vagus nerve cooling and vagotomy experiments, we measured all variables by the same protocol as employed in the experiments with the hypercapnic groups. We used 5% CO_2+20% O_2 in N_2 and 5% CO_2+10% O_2 in N_2 gas instead of room air and 7% CO_2+20% O_2 in N_2 gas.

Measurement

We continuosly measured the respiratory frequency (f). the tidal volume (V_T) and the expired minute ventilation ($\dot{V}_E$) by pneumotachogragh (47303A. Hurett-Pakkard. Waltham. MA. USA). We collected heparinized arterial blood samples at the end of each test period to measure the blood gases and pH by blood gas analyzer (ABL2. Radiometer, Copenhagen. Denmark). We measured the fractions of O_2 and CO_2 in inhalation gas by the Scholander method.

Data analysis

We averaged the ventilatory responses for 30 sec at the end of 5-min gas inhalation. This value was assumed to indicate the response to this gas inhalation.

Statistical analysis was done by Student's t-test for paried variables, and $p<0.05$ was considered to be significant.

RESULTS

During the experiments, the ciliary reflex of the animals existed. The summarized data of the ventilatory responses and arterial blood gases are shown in Table 1. The composition of gas used for the hypercapnic experiments were 7% CO_2 and 20% O_2 in N_2 . Vagus nerve cooling and vagotomy did not affect the respiratory frequencies under normocapnic conditions. In the hypercapnic experiments.vagus nerve cooling did not affect the respiratory frequency. but vagotomy caused respiratory frequency to decrease in 8 of 9 dogs. Comparing vagus nerve cooling and vagotomy, respiratory frequency was significantly less in vagotomy. Vagus nerve cooling and vagotomy caused tidal volume to increase significantly under both normo⁻and hypercapnic conditions.

Under normocapnic conditions, vagus nerve cooling caused expired minute ventilation to increase, but vagotomy did not. Under hypercapnic conditions, both
vagus nerve cooling and vagotomy caused expired minute ventilation to increase.
There was no defference in $PaCO_2$ among the three conditions in hypercapnic gas
inhalation experiments.

The composition of gas used for the normoxic experiments were 20% O_2 + 5% CO_2
in N_2, and for hypoxic experiments were 10% O_2 + 5% CO_2 in N_2.

Vagus nerve cooling and vagotomy did not affect the respiratory frequency under
normo⁻and hypoxic conditions. But the respiratory frequency was significantly
less in vagotomy compared to the vagus nerve cooling under nomoxic conditions.
Vagus nerve cooling and vagotomy caused expired minutes ventilation to increased
signifficantly under normo⁻and hypoxic conditions. There was no difference in
SaO_2 among the three conditions in normo⁻ and hypoxic gas inhalation experiments.

DISCUSSION

Our results show thatthe cervical vagosympathetic trunks regulate respiratory
frequency under hypercapnic conditions, and do not contribute to the control of
respiration under hypoxic conditions. In hypercapnic gas inhalation experiments,
vagus verve cooling did not influence respiratory frequency. not vagotomy caused
frequency to decrease. These results suggest that the cervical vagosympathetic
trunks regulate the increment of the respiratory frequency due to hypercapnic
conditions. It has been known that there were three peripheral receptors in
lungs· the pulmonary stretch receptors, irritant receptors and J-receptors (Sant'
Ambrogio 1982). We decided on a cooling temperature of 7℃, as it was the highest
temperature at which the Hering-Breuer inflation reflex was assumed to be ceased
in all dogs in our experiments. The non-myelinated fibers. which is not blocked
by a temperature of 7℃, conduct the stimuli from J-receptors (Coleridge and
Coleridge 1984). We found that vagus nerve cooling did not affect respiratory
frequency and that vagotomy caused a reduction in the increment of the respiratory frequency under hypercapnic; this suggests that non-myelinated fibers, which
conduct the stimuli from the J-receptors, increase respiratory frequency under
conditions of hypercapnic gas inhalation.

In hypoxic experiment, respiratory frequency and tidal volume were affected
to 5%CO_2 gas mixture. We concluded that the vagus nerve did not increase respiratory frequency during hypoxic loading. The effect of the vagus nerve seemed to be
less under hypoxic conditions than under hypercapnic conditions. The expired
minute ventilation was greater under conditions of vagus nerve cooling and vagotomy than under control conditions before and during hypoxic gas inhalation. But
there was no difference in the expired miniute ventilation among the three conditions. We concluded that the expired minute ventilation during hypoxic gas
inhalation was also reflected by the effects of 5% CO_2 gas mixture and that
strength of the output from the respiratory centers overcame the input from the
vagus nerve during hypoxic gas inhalation.

REFERENCES

Colerige. J.C.G. & Colerige. H.M.(1984) Afferent vagal C-fiber innervation of the
    lungs and airways and its functional significance. *Rev. Physiol. Phalmaco.*, *99*,
    1-100.
Phillipson. E.A.. Fishman. N.H.. & Nadal. J.A.(1973) Effect of differential vagal
    blockade on ventilation responses to CO_2 in awake dog. *J. Apple. Physiol.*, *34*,
    759-763.
Russell. N.J.W.. Raybould. H.E. & Trenchard. D. (1984) Role of vagal C-fiber
    afferents in respiratory response to hypercapnia. *J. Apple. Physiol.*, *56*,
    1550-1558.
Sant' Ambrogio. G. (1982) Information arising from the tracheobronchial tree
    mammals. *Physiol Rev.*, *62*, 531-569.

Abnormalities of Vagal Reflexes in Asthmatic Rabbits

M. Sibuya, A. Kanamaru, M.B. Sibuya and
I. Homma

Department of Physiology, Showa University, School of
Medicine, 1-5-8 Hatanodai, Shinagawa-ku, Tokyo 142,
Japan

ABSTRACT

The effects of airway mechanoreceptor afferents on the respiratory pattern were
studied by vagal cooling block and airway mechanical stimulation in normal and
Alternaria-sensitized rabbits. The results of these applications suggested that
the vagal reflex induced by slowly adapting receptors (SAR) is less apparent and
that induced by rapidly adapting receptors (RAR) is more apparent in sensitized
rabbits.

KEYWORDS

SAR; RAR; Vagal cooling; High-frequency inflation (HFI)

INTRODUCTION

It has been suggested that reflex bronchoconstriction mediated by the vagal
nerve plays a role in the pathophysiology of asthma (Mills et al., 1969; Koller,
1969; Koller and Ferrer, 1970; Gold et al., 1972). It is also known that vagal
afferents modify central respiratory motor output. In this study, the change in
phrenic efferent activity induced by alteration of vagal afferents in normal and
allergic rabbits was compared under no antigen exposure. Vagal afferents were
altered by vagal cooling block and high frequency inflation (HFI, Homma et al.,
1987) applied to the airway.

METHOD

The 9 normal and 13 asthmatic rabbits, sensitized according to the method of
Shampain et al. (1982), were anesthetized with urethane and chloralose, and
breathed spontaneously through a tracheal cannula.   The phrenic efferent activity was recorded.   Respiratory pattern parameters, such as total respiratory
time (Ttot) inspiratory time (TI), expiratory time (TE) and amplitude of integrated phrenic activity (IPA), were measured breath by breath. Integration time
constant was always 30 ms.

Unilateral vagotomy was carried out and the contralateral vagal nerve was attached to a cooling plate. The temperature of the vagal nerve (Tvag) was monitored. HFI was applied to the airway from an arm of the tracheal cannula for
15 to 20 s. 100 Hz HFI was generated with a moving coil transducer driven by
triangular-shaped pulses (6 ms in width). The peak airway inflation pressure
was about 7 cmH_2O.

Hypersensitivity of the sensitized rabbits as measured by homologous passive
cutaneous anaphylaxis method as described by Shampain et al. (1982), was
positive in all sensitized rabbits and ranged from x2-x256.

RESULTS and DISCUSSION

In normal rabbits progressive vagal cooling block induced IPA augmentation and
Ttot prolongation. Ttot prolongation was caused mainly by TI prolongation to
approximately 12 °C, and below this, TI was constant. On the other hand, IPA
and TI remained almost constant during the cooling in allergic rabbits. This
was seen in 7 of 12 allergic rabbits (Fig. 1A).

The IPA augmentation and TI prolongation in normal rabbits was probably due to
inhibition of vagal reflex induced by SAR afferents, which is known to "off-
switch" inspiratory activity. In 7 out of 12 allergic rabbits, neither IPA augmentation nor TI prolongation was observed during vagal cooling. This suggested
that the reflex induced by SAR afferents was weak or disappeared in allergic
rabbits.

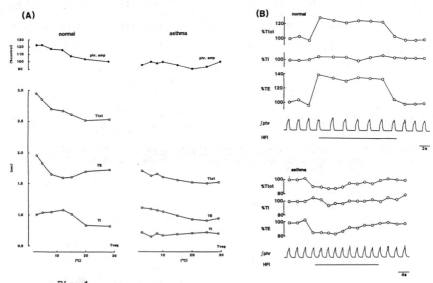

Fig. 1.
(A) Effect of vagal cooling on respiratory pattern of
normal (left) and allergic (right) rabbits. Horizontal
axis:Tvag, Vertical axis: upper:IPA, lower:Ttot, TI, TE.
(B) Effect of HFI on respiratory time of normal (upper),
allergic (lower) rabbits. From upper to downward, percent
control of Ttot, TI, TE, integral phrenic activity curve,
and HFI application.

In all normal rabbits, HFI application prolonged Ttot, which was caused by TE prolongation (Fig. 1B). In 7 of 13 allergic rabbits, HFI shortened TE. HFI had almost no effect on TI in both normal and allergic rabbits.

Homma et al. have reported that 100 Hz HFI stimulates both SAR and RAR (1987). Thus the effect of HFI depends on the balance between the reflex induced by SAR afferents and that induced by RAR afferents. HFI prolonged TE in all 9 normal rabbits. This indicates that SAR reflex is dominant in normal rabbits. In allergic rabbits, TE was shortened, indicating dominance of RAR reflex.

The SAR reflex and RAR reflex have reciprocal effects from many view points (Widdicombe, 1974) including airway smooth muscle tone. Thus the shift in dominance from SAR reflex to RAR reflex in allergic rabbits may be one of the critical pathophysiological characteristics in the present allergic rabbit model.

ACKNOWLEDGMENT

This work was supported by Grants-in-Aid for Scientific Research from the Ministry of Education, Science and Culture, Japan.

REFERENCES

Gold , W. M., G. F. Kessler, D. Y. C. Yu (1972). Role of vagus nerves in experimental asthma in allergic dogs. J. Appl. Physiol., 33, 719-725.
Homma, I., A. Isobe, M. Iwase, H. Onimaru, M. Sibuya (1987). Cross-correlation between vagal afferent impulses from pulmonary mechanoreceptors and high-frequency inflation (HFI) and deflation (HFD) in rabbits. Neurosci. Lett.,75, 299-302.
Koller, E. A. (1969). Respiratory reflexes during anaphylactic bronchial asthma in guinea-pigs. Experientia, 25, 368-369.
Koller, E. A., P. Ferrer (1970). Studies on the role of the lung deflation reflex. Resp. Physiol., 10, 172-183.
Mills, J., H. Sellick, J. G. Widdicombe (1969). The role of lung irritant receptors in the respiratory responses to multiple pulmonary embolism, anaphylaxis and histamine-induced bronchoconstriction. J. Physiol. (London), 200, 79P-80P.
Shampain, M. P., L. Behrens, G. L. Larsen, P. M. Henson, (1982). An animal model of late pulmonary responses to alternaria challenge. Am. Rev. Respir. Dis., 126, 493-498.
Widdicombe, J. G. (1974). In: Respiratory Physiology (J. G. Widdicombe, ed.), Vol. 2, Chap. 10, pp. 273-296. University Park Press, Baltimore.

Vagal Afferents Augmented Respiratory Reflex Facilitation Induced by Muscle Nociceptive Inputs

D.G. Simbulan, Jr., E.T. Tadaki, Y. Kozaki, K. Eguchi and T. Kumazawa

Department of Nervous and Sensory Functions, Research Institute of Environmental Medicine, Nagoya University, Nagoya 464-01, Japan

ABSTRACT

The vagal influence on respiratory reflex facilitation induced by muscle nerve stimulation was examined in the anesthetized, glomectomized, paralyzed and artificially ventilated cats. Facilitation was much greater during the intact state than after vagotomy. "Evoked post-inspiratory phrenic activity" (or EPIPA), induced during expiratory phase-locked muscle nerve electrical stimulation in the intact state, was attenuated or almost completely abolished by vagotomy. The EPIPA was restored by inspiratory phase-locked vagal conditioning stimulation combined with expiratory phase-locked muscle nerve stimulation. The results suggest that vagal facilitatory reflexes augment the respiratory reflex facilitation during muscle nociceptive stimulation.

KEYWORDS

Phrenic activity, muscle nerve stimulation, phase-locked stimulation, muscle nociceptive reflex facilitation, vagal afferent facilitation, vagotomy

INTRODUCTION

Thin-fiber muscular afferents' activation facilitates respiration (Senapati, 1966). Polymodal receptors, signalling nociceptive information, mediate this respiratory reflex facilitation (Kumazawa and Mizumura, 1976). The facilitation was greater when muscle nerve stimulation was applied during the inspiratory phase than during the expiratory phase (Simbulan et al., 1987). To investigate the vagal influence on the respiratory reflex facilitation during these respiratory phase-locked muscle nociceptive stimulations, the following experiment was carried out. Respiratory activity from the right phrenic nerve preparation was recorded in anesthetized, glomectomized, paralyzed and artificially ventilated cats ($N= 14$). The medial and lateral branches of the left gastrocnemius muscle nerve were prepared and electrically stimulated to obtain the muscle twitch threshold (T) before neuro-muscular block. The central cut ends of the muscle nerves were electrically stimulated at 400-600 T (13 pulses per breath, at 12.5 Hz) during the inspiratory (T_I-locked) or expiratory (T_E-locked) phases in the intact and vagotomized states. Vagal conditioning stimulation was also done to simulate responses during T_E-locked muscle nerve stimulation in the intact state. The following changes in integrated phrenic nerve activity were measured by microcomputer: the peak amplitude (PK); inspiratory phase duration (T_I); maximum rate of rise $(SLOPE)$ and average rate of rise (PK/T_I) of integrated phrenic nerve activity and $AREA (A)$ of the integrated phrenic neurograms to express the "evoked post-inspiratory phrenic activity" (EPIPA) during T_E-locked muscle nerve stimulation such as that shown in Fig. 1.

Table 1. Parameters of respiratory reflex facilitation during muscle nerve stimulations during five consecutive breaths, before and after vagotomy (average ± S.E.M., % pre-stimulus).

	TI-LOCKED MUSCLE NERVE ES			TE-LOCKED MUSCLE NERVE ES			
	VAGI-INTACT	VAGI-CUT		VAGI-INTACT	VAGI-CUT		
PK	177.4 ± 30 +++	115.3 ± 3.4 ++	(**)	121.1 ± 4.5 +++	106.4 ± 1.4	++	(**)
A	NA	NA		157.8 ± 19.1 +	110.1 ± 5.8	NS	(**)
S	287.6 ± 80.5 +	136.5 ± 9.0 ++	(***)	148.8 ± 16.2 +	111.8 ± 3.6	++	(**)
PK/TI	224.6 ± 50.2 +	130.0 ± 7.2 ++	(***)	143.1 ± 12.5 ++	112.8± 3.0	++	(**)

+ p <0.05, ++ p <0.01, +++ p <0.001, NS = not significant (compared to pre-stimulus); (**) p <0.01, (***) p<0.001 (intact vs. cut state). PK = peak amplitude; A = area of integrated phrenic neurogram to express "evoked post-inspiratory phrenic activity" (or EPIPA); S = slope or maximum rate of rise of integrated phrenic activity; PK/TI = average rate of rise of integrated phrenic activity. NA = not applicable; area is only used to measure EPIPA during TE-locked muscle nerve stimulation.

VAGOTOMY ATTENUATED OR ABOLISHED NOCICEPTIVE RESPIRATORY REFLEX FACILITATION

In the vagi-intact state, *PK*, *SLOPE*, and *PK/T$_I$* increased sharply during five-consecutive breath T$_I$-locked muscle nerve stimulation (Table 1). During T$_E$-locked muscle nerve stimulation, the *PK*, *SLOPE, and PK/TI* also increased (Table 1), but less than that of T$_I$-locked stimulation. "Evoked post-inspiratory phrenic activity" (EPIPA) during T$_E$-locked muscle nerve stimulation appeared as a hump on the declining slope of the integrated phrenic neurogram as shown in the typical example from one cat in Fig. 1A (thick line). This EPIPA is expressed as a significant increase in the mean *AREA* (p< 0.05) of the neurograms during T$_E$-locked muscle nerve stimulation from 14 cats as shown in Table 1 and the bargraph in Fig. 1D (vagi intact, ME). After vagotomy, there were smaller increases in *PK*, *SLOPE*, and *PK/T$_I$* during T$_I$-locked muscle nerve stimulation compared to those in the intact state; this was also the case for T$_E$-locked muscle nerve stimulation (Table 1). EPIPA was almost completely abolished in most cases after vagotomy. In some cases, EPIPA was attenuated as shown by the smaller hump in the example in Fig. 1B (thick line). On the average, this EPIPA is expressed as an insignificant change in *AREA* of the integrated phrenic neurogram during T$_E$-locked muscle nerve stimulation as shown in Table 1 (vagi cut) and the bargraph in Fig. 1D (vagi cut, ME).

EPIPA RESTORED BY VAGAL CONDITIONING STIMULATION

T$_I$-locked vagal nerve conditioning stimulation (100 uA, 100 Hz) alone produced a sharp rise in *SLOPE* and T$_I$-shortening, which is shown by the thin-lined neurogram in an example from one cat in Fig. 1C. The EPIPA was restored after T$_I$-locked vagal conditioning stimulation (VI) followed by T$_E$-locked muscle nerve stimulation (ME) as shown by the thick-lined neurogram in Fig. 1C. This restored EPIPA is expressed as a significant increase in the mean *AREA* (p<0.05) of the integrated phrenic neurogram from 14 cats as shown in the bargraph in Fig. 1D (VI + ME).

While these results implicate the vagal afferents contributing to the augmentation of muscle nociceptive respiratory reflex facilitation, no direct evidence from this study implicates which sensory system of the vagus is specifically involved. While pulmonary stretch receptors (PSRs) generally mediate the characteristic inspiratory inhibitory Hering-Breuer reflex (Younes and Polacheck, 1985), other investigators have also implicated a positive feedback facilitation from PSRs (Dimarco et al., 1981; Cohen et al., 1986). In addition, rapidly adapting receptors may also mediate augmentation of phrenic neural activity during rapid, large inflation in the dog (Pack et al., 1981). It is also of interest to investigate the possible relation of EPIPA, which appears during the early expiratory phase in response to nociceptive inputs in the presence of vagal influence, to that of "post-inspiratory inspiratory activity" (PIIA) of "early expiratory phase I" (Richter, 1982). Further studies need to be carried out to elucidate the sensory characteristics of this vagal augmentation of muscle nociceptive reflex facilitation.

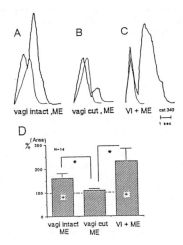

Fig. 1　EPIPA during TE-locked muscle nerve stimulation (ME) before and after vagotomy, and during combined TI-locked vagal conditioning stimulation (VI) and ME in the vagotomized state. Neurograms in A,B,C come from the same cat; averaged neurogram of 2nd-5th breath responses during ME (thick-lined) superimposed on averaged neurogram of 5 pre-stimulus control breaths (thin-lined) in A and B; the thin-lined neurogram in C is average of 2nd-5th breath responses during VI alone superimposed by the ave rage of 2nd-5th breath responses during VI + ME (thick-lined). The *PK* of the control neurograms (thin-lined) in A, B, and C have been normalized to be able to show the relative changes before and during test stimulations. D shows the change in mean total *AREA* (± S.E.M.) of the 2nd-5th breaths, to represent EPIPA during ME, before and after vagotomy which is expressed as percent change of pre-stimulus mean value (% pre-ES); mean total *AREA* during VI+ ME is expressed as percent change of *AREA* during VI (N= 14).

REFERENCES

Cohen, M. I., W.R. See, A.L. Sica and I.R. Moss (1986). Influence of central nervous system state on inspiratory facilitation by pulmonary afferents. In: *Neurobiology of the Control of Breathing*, ed. by Euler, C. von and Lagercrantz, H., Raven Press, New York, pp. 251-256.

Dimarco, A.F., C. von Euler, J.R. Romaniuk and Y. Yamamato (1981). Positive feedback facilitation of external intercostal and phrenic inspiratory activity by pulmonary stretch receptors. *Acta Physiol. Scand.*, 113: 375-386.

Kumazawa, T. and K. Mizumura (1976). The polymodal C-fiber receptor in the muscle of the dog. *Brain Res.*, 101: 589-593.

Pack, A.I., R.G. DeLaney and A.P. Fishman (1981). Augmentation of phrenic neural activity by increased rates of lung inflation. *J. Appl. Physiol.*, 50: 149-161.

Senapati, J.M.(1966). Effect of stimulation of muscle afferents on ventilation of dogs. *J. Appl. Physiol.*, 21: 242-246.

Simbulan, D., E. Tadaki, Y. Kozaki, K. Eguchi and T. Kumazawa (1987). Phrenic responses to muscle afferent nerve stimulation applied to different respiratory phases. *Environ. Med.*, 31: 61-67.

Younes, M. and J. Polacheck (1985). Central adaptation to inspiratory-inhibiting expiratory-prolonging vagal input. *J. Appl. Physiol.*, 59: 1072-1084.

Endogenous Opioid-mediated Respiratory Modulations Induced by Nociceptive Muscular Afferents

T. Kumazawa, E. Tadaki, Y. Kozaki,
D. Simbulan, K. Eguchi and T. Hirano

Department of Nervous & Sensory Functions, Research
Institute of Environmental Medicine, Nagoya University,
Nagoya 464-01, Japan

ABSTRACT

Following intensity-dependent respiratory facilitation, long lasting respiratory changes were induced by muscular nociceptive afferent (polymodal receptor) stimulation in anesthetized, paralyzed and artificially ventilated dogs and cats. The post-stimulus suppression was induced by strong stimulus and was reversed by an opioid antagonist, naloxone. Involvement of N. parabrachialis in the opioid-mediated respiratory suppression is highly suggested.

KEYWORDS

Endogenous opioid; respiratory suppression; nociceptive reflex; muscular afferents; polymodal receptor; N. parabrachialis; naloxone;

Respiratory facilitation induced by muscular polymodal receptor inputs. The great majority of the thin-fiber muscular afferents are of the polymodal receptor type, signalling nociceptive informations (Kumazawa and Mizumura, 1977). Arterial injection of various algesic substances into the gastrocnemius muscle of anesthetized, spontaneously ventilated dogs caused an increase in minute respiratory volume similar to the increase in discharge rates of muscular polymodal receptors in response to the same stimulus, suggesting implication of the muscular polymodal receptors in the respiratory response (Mizumura and Kumazawa, 1976). After the end of stimulation, however, the reflexive respiratory responses declined faster than the discharge-responses, presumably due secondary to hyperventilation.

Respiratory responses induced by polymodal receptor inputs under constant end-tidal CO_2 and O_2. To avoid the secondary effects of hyperventilation, a similar experiment was performed in anesthetized dogs which were artificially ventilated with the end-tidal CO_2 and O_2 kept constant. The product of the peak amplitude and the instantaneous respiratory rate of the integrated phrenic nerve activity averaged for a 30- or 60-sec period was used as the neural respiratory output. As shown in Fig.1.A, intra-arterial injection of hypertonic saline, which is a consistent stimulant of the polymodal receptor, into the gastrocnemius muscle caused concentration-dependent increases in the respiratory outputs. Few minutes after washing the solution (FO), the respiratory outputs decreased below the pre-stimulus level (post-stimulus suppression) with the 3.6 and 4.5% solutions, while with the 1.8% solution,

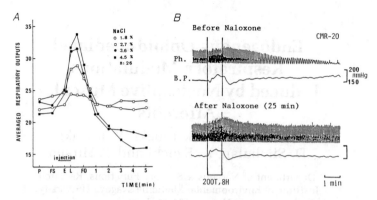

Fig. 1. Averaged changes in the phrenic outputs induced by intra-arterial injection of 4 concentrations of hypertonic saline into the gastrocnemius muscle in dogs (A) and the effect of naloxone (0.1mg/kg, iv) on the post-stimulus respiratory suppression induced by stimulation of the muscle nerve in a cat (B). Ph.: integrated phrenic discharges, B.P.: mean arterial pressure.

they remained high in the following several minutes (post-stimulus facilitation) (Kumazawa et al., 1983). Similar post-stimulus suppression effects were observed by electrical stimulation above the C fiber threshold of the muscle nerve in dogs and also in cats (Kumazawa and Tadaki, 1983). These results indicate an involvement of a certain inhibitory mechanism triggered by the polymodal receptor inputs. The degree and duration of the post-stimulus suppression varied among animals; in some cases it took more than 1 hour to return to the pre-stimulus level. Repeated stimulation generally caused less prominent suppression.

Involvement of endogenous opioids in the post-stimulus respiratory suppression. The long lasting suppression suggests an intervention of neuro-humoral factors such as endogenous opioids, since nociceptive stimulation induces opioid release (Yaksh and Elde, 1981). As shown in Fig.1,B, the post-stimulus suppression was abolished by pretreatment of naloxone (0.1-0.5mg/kg, i.v.) in dogs as well as cats (Kumazawa, et al., 1980, Kumazawa and Tadaki, 1983). On the other hand, perfusion of the IVth ventricle with peptidase-inhibitors (thiorphan and bestatin, 10µg/ml each) enhanced the post-stimulus suppression. Marked attenuation of the post-stimulus suppression by repeated stimulations with an interval of 15 min. was reversed by low dose of proglumide, a cholecystokinin (CCK) antagonist, (continuous i.v. injection, 0.08mg/kg/hr) (Tadaki et al., 1986). This result is similar to the effect of the CCK antagonist on the shock-induced opioidergic analgesia (Watkins et al., 1984).

Possible implication of N. parabrachialis in opioid-mediated respiratory suppression. This opioid-mediated respiratory suppression was still obtained after intercollicular decerebration, but abolished by a slightly caudal transection (Kumazawa et al., 1985). Micro-stimulation of the parabrachial region in 20 successive expiratory phases (0.3ms, 100µA, 5 pulses at 1kHz) as well as micro-injection of morphine (2.7nmol in 0.1µl) into the nucleus (Fig.2,A & B) caused respiratory suppressions similar to that induced by the muscular afferent stimulation and these respiratory suppressions were abolished by naloxone (Eguchi et al., 1987). Evoked discharges recorded in this region revealed nociceptive inputs from the calf-muscle to the nucleus. These results suggest implication of N. parabrachialis in the post-stimulus respiratory suppression induced by nociceptive muscular afferents.

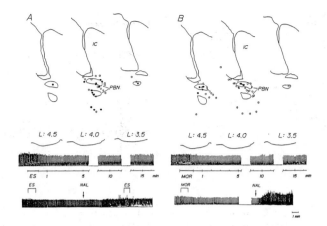

Fig. 2. Respiratory suppression induced by microstimulation (ES) of the parabrachial region (A) as well as microinjection of morphine (MOR) into the nucleus (B). Upper traces: location of effective (●) and non-effective (○) sites shown in sagittal planes of the rostral pons. IC: inferior colliculus, PBN: nucleus parabrachialis. Lower traces: responses induced by both types of stimulation. NAL: naloxone, 0.1mg/kg, iv.

REFERENCES

Eguchi,K., E.Tadaki, D.Simbulan Jr. and T.Kumazawa (1987). Respiratory depression caused by either morphine microinjection or repetitive electrical stimulation in the region of the nucleus parabrachialis of cats. Pflügers Arch., 409, 367-373.

Kumazawa,T., K.Eguchi and E.Tadaki (1985). Naloxone-reversible respiratory inhibition induced by muscular thin-fiber afferents in decerebrated cats. Neurosci. Lett., 53, 81-85.

Kumazawa,T. and K.Mizumura (1977). Thin-fibre receptors responding to mechanical, chemical, and thermal stimulation in the skeletal muscle of the dog. J. Physiol., 273, 179-194.

Kumazawa,T. and E.Tadaki (1983). Two different inhibitory effects on respiration by thin-fiber muscular afferents in cats. Brain Res., 272, 364-367.

Kumazawa,T., E.Tadaki and K.Kim (1980). A possible participation of endogenous opiates in respiratory reflexes induced by thin-fiber muscular afferents. Brain Res., 199, 244-248.

Kumazawa,T., E.Tadaki, K.Mizumura and K.Kim (1983). Post-stimulus facilitatory and inhibitory effects on respiration induced by chemical and electrical stimulation of thin-fiber muscular afferents in dogs. Neurosci. Lett., 35, 283-287.

Mizumura,K. and T.Kumazawa (1976). Reflex respiratory response induced by chemical stimulation of muscle afferents. Brain Res., 109, 402-406.

Tadaki,E., D.Simbulan, K.Eguchi, H.Yasui and T.Kumazawa (1986). Effects of proglumide, a cholecystokinin antagonist, on opiate-mediated respiratory suppression induced by thin-fiber muscular afferent. Environ. Med., 30, 47-53.

Watkins,L.R., I.B.Kinscheck and D.J.Mayer (1984). Potentiation of opiate analgesia and apparent reversal of morphine tolerance by proglumide. Science, 224, 395-396.

Yaksh,T.L. and R.P.Elde (1981). Factors governing release of methionine enkephalin-like immunoreactivity from mesencephalon and spinal cord of the cat in vivo. J. Neurophysiol., 46, 1056-1075.

Positive Pressure Ventilation Reverses Phasic Respiratory Glottis Narrowing in Anesthetized Dogs

S. Sakurai, H. Toga, J. Huang, Y. Nagasaka
and N. Ohya

Division of Respiratory Diseases, Department of Internal
Medicine, Kanazawa Medical University School of
Medicine, 920-02 Ishikawa, Japan

ABSTRACT

We made a hypothesis that phasic respiratory glottic motion will reflect lower
airway pressure (Plaw) rather than lung volume and we studied the relationship
between Plaw and glottic motion as changes of glottic resistance to air flow
(Rglott) in anesthetized dogs. The reverse relationship between Rglott and
lung volume was observed in this experimental condition. But when the
relationship between Plaw and Rglott was concerned, there was parallel shift.
We conclude that control of respiratory glottic motion is dependent on Plaw,
not lung volume in this experimental condition.

KEYWORDS

respiratory glottic motion;positive pressure ventilation;resistance.

INTRODUCTION

Since Baier et al.(1977) reported that lung volume affected glottic aperture
size only when there was extreme change of it, it has been commonly thought
that lung volume is not a major determinant of respiratory glottic motion.
However, There is still no conclusive evidence concerning the regulatory
factors other than the lung volume. In the present study, the following
experiments were performed using anesthetized dogs mainly to clarify the
degree of involvement of changes in the airway pressure and the lung volume in
glottic movement is a phenomenon based more on changes in airway pressure than
on the lung volume. Studies were performed (1) the effects of increases in
lower airway pressure on changes in the glottic resistance to airflow, and (2)
effects of changes in lung volume on glottic resistance.

MATERIALS AND METHODS

Thirteen anesthetized mongrel dogs (average weight:10.8Kg) were used. Cannulae
were individually inserted into the opening of the trachea on rostral and
the condition of continued spontaneous respiration. Mouth pressure (Pmouth),

upper airway pressure (Puaw), upper airway flow ($\dot{V}$uaw), lower airway pressure (Plaw) or esophageal pressure (Peso) were serially recorded in the constant airflow at 1 L/sec using an electric blower protruding from the cannula on rostral side toward the oral cavity (Fig.1). Glottic resistance (Rglott) was calculated from the Puaw and $\dot{V}$uaw records using the fomula (I):

$$\text{Rglott} = \text{Puaw} / \dot{V}\text{uaw} \text{ ---- (I)}$$

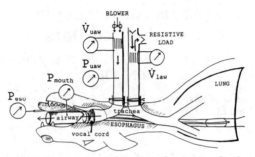

Fig.1 Diagram of experimental setup. Resistive load or ventilator was attached at lower airway cannula.

Protocol for Study 1:Constant resistive load was applied in 6 dogs at only expiration during spontaneous respiration. The effect of an increase in Plaw due to the expiratory resistive loading on changes in Rglott was studied.

Protocol for Study 2 :The relationship between change in Plaw (or Peso) and change in lung volume (Vlung) was reversed to that during spontaneous respiration by positive pressure ventilation in 7 dogs. The change in Rglott seen in these reversed condition was compared with the change in Rglott at spontaneous respiration.

RESULTS

Result of Study 1: Puaw and Vuaw changed slightly with a change in respiratory phase. The Rglott at expiration was always greater ($p < 0.05$) than that at inspiration (Fig.2), and the mean Rglott at expiration with expiratory resistive loading was 156.7% in contrast to 100%, the Rglott at inspiration.

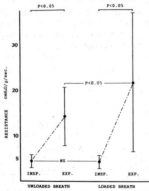

Fig.2   Changes in glottic resistance during loaded, unloaded breathing.

Results of Study 2: Changes in Rglott were determined according to changes in Vlung. Rglott was increased with an increase in Plaw both during spontaneous respiration and it was decreased with a decrease in Plaw (Table 1).

| | | MODE OF VENTILATION | | |
| | | SPONTANE. | | VENTILATOR. | |
V_{lung}		MAX.	MIN.	MAX.	MIN.
RESISTANCE *	①	2.0	13.3	11.2	7.3
	②	4.0	8.6	20.0	7.5
	③	0.5	20.0	13.3	3.3
	④	3.5	40.0	40.0	3.5
	⑤	6.5	20.0	20.0	8.0
	⑥	6.5	20.0	10.0	14.0
	⑦	8.0	12.5	24.0	12.5
mean ± SD		4.42 ± 2.49	19.2 ± 9.46	19.78 ± 9.54	8.01 ± 3.76

* cmH₂O/L/sec

$*cmH_2O/L/sec$

Table 1. Compalisons of changes in glottic resistance during spontaneous respiration (spontane.) versus positive pressure ventilation (ventilator).

DISCUSSION

Stanescu et al.(1972) reported a significant positive relationship between the glottic aperture and lung volume during panting at a flow 1.0 L/sec. However, Since Baier et al(1977) reported that lung volume affected glottic aperture size only when there was extreme change of it, it has been commonly thought that lung volume is not a major determinant of respiratory glottic motion. The present report is the first study of changes in glottic resistance during positive pressure ventilation. It discussed which factor is the main reguratory factor of changes in glottic resistance, lower airway pressure or changes in lung volume, by utilizing property showing that the relationship between lower airway pressure and lung volume during spontaneous respiration. Glottic movement controls upper airway resistance and regulation of expiration time in cat presumably by volume related feedback control (Bartlett,D.et al.1973). However, this presumption is not confirmed yet and the possibility of regulation by pressure related feed back cannot be excluded. In the present study, phasic respiratory change in glottic resistance were found increase lung volume independently (study 2). Thus these results suggest the possibility that lower airway pressure is the main regulatory factor in phasic respiratory changes in glottic resistance.

REFERENCES

Baier, H., Wanner, A., Zarzecki, S. and Sackner,M.A. (1977). Relationships among glottis opening , respiratory flow, and upper airway resistance in humans. Respirat Environ Exercise Physiol, 43, 603-611.
Gautier, H., Remmers, J.E., and Bartlett, Jr.,D. (1973). Control of the duration of expiration. Respir. Physiol. 54, 1726-1735.
Stanescu, D.C., Pattijin, J., Clement, J., and Van de Woestijine, K.P.(1972) Glottic opening and airway resistance.J. Appl. Physiol. 32, 460-466

The Long-term Follow-up of Respiratory Chemosensitivity in COPD Families

M. Yamamoto, M. Nishimura,
A. Yoshioka, Y. Akiyama, F. Kishi and
Y. Kawakami

First Department of Medicine, Hokkaido University
School of Medicine, N-15, W-7, Kitaku, Sapporo 060,
Japan

ABSTRACT

In 22 healthy sons of patients with chronic obstructive pulmonary disease,
ventilatory responses to hypoxia and hypercapnia were examined twice at
intervals of 7 to 10 years. The individual values of both tests obtained in the
initial study had a weak but a significant correlation with those of the present
study, suggesting that the wide inter-individual variability in respiratory
chemosensitivity remains relatively unchanged over the years in healthy
subjects.

KEYWORDS

ventilatory response; hypoxia; hypercapnia; sons of COPD patient; follow-up
study

INTRODUCTION

We have previously shown that respiratory chemosensitivity is at least partly
determined by genetic factors (Kawakami et al., 1982a, 1984) and that
respiratory chemosensitivity to hypoxia may modulate the clinical course of COPD
because low hypoxic ventilatory responses are more frequently detected in
families of COPD patients with abnormal arterial blood gases (Kawakami et al.,
1982b) . However there have been, to our knowledge, no longitudinal studies
concerning the individual constancy in such chemosensitivity over a number of
years. We therefore conducted a long term follow-up study in sons of COPD
patients who participated in our original study 7 to 10 years ago.

SUBJECTS AND METHODS

Twenty-two healthy sons of 18 families of COPD patients participated in the
present study. After the standard spirographic data were obtained, the
ventilatory responses to isocapnic progressive hypoxia and to normoxic
progressive hypercapnia were measured in the same manner as in the initial study
(Kawakami et al., 1981, 1982b,) . Hypoxic ventilatory response was evaluated by
the slope factor (A) for the PO_2 response hyperbola of the PO_2-ventilation
relation, and hypercapnic ventilatory response by the slope factor (S) for the
PCO_2-ventilation response line. Both "A" and "S" were standardized by body
surface area (BSA). In addition, we examined both ventilatory responses 3 times

Table1.

Anthropometric Data	Initial Study	Present Study	p-value
Age (y.o.)	33.0 ± 8.4	41.8 ± 8.3	
Height (cm)	167.4 ± 5.3	167.8 ± 5.4	NS
Body Weight (kg)	64.2 ± 8.8	64.7 ± 9.4	NS

Respiratory Function			
VC (cc)	4638 ± 623	4462 ± 515	<0.05
%VC (%)	115.6 ± 13.0	115.8 ± 11.1	NS
$FEV_{1.0}$ (cc)	3867 ± 535	3512 ± 547	<0.01
$FEV_{1.0}$% (%)	83.7 ± 5.0	78.6 ± 6.6	<0.01
MVV (ℓ/min)	143.5 ± 25.8	132.3 ± 27.8	<0.05

Ventilatory Response			
A/BSA (ℓ/min·Torr/m²)	54.2 ± 43.1	46.6 ± 35.0	NS
S/BSA (ℓ/min/Torr/m²)	0.88 ± 0.33	1.11 ± 0.41	<0.05

mean ± S.D.
NS : not significant

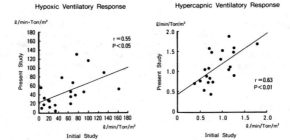

Hypoxic Ventilatory Response   Hypercapnic Ventilatory Response

Fig. 1.

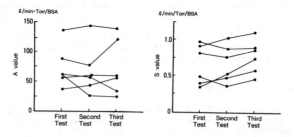

Fig. 2.

at one week intervals in a different group of normal volunteers in order to
evaluate the reproducibility of these tests after a short interval.

RESULTS

A summary of the data from the initial and the present studies is shown in Table
1. Although there were no significant changes in physical characteristics after
an interval of 7-10 years, pulmonary function tests revealed an age-dependent
decline in vital capacity (VC) , forced expiratory volume in 1sec (FEV$_1$) and
maximum voluntary ventilation (MVV). Although there was no significant
difference in the average value of A/BSA in the two studies, the S/BSA in the
present study was significantly higher than that in initial study. In both
ventilatory responses, the individual values showed a weak but significant
correlation in the two studies (Fig.1) , suggesting that the wide inter-
individual variability in respiratory chemosensitivity remained unchanged
over the years in these subjects. Figure2 shows the reproducibility of
ventilatory responses examined at one week intervals in our laboratory. The
coefficient of variance for A was 22.4% and that for S is 17.9%, which are
comparable to the values reported from aoother laboratory (Sullvian et al.,
1984). The variance between the two test values after a long interval was
significantly larger than that obtained after a short interval.

DISCUSSION

It is well-known that ventilatory responses to hypoxia and hypercapnia are quite
variable among healthy subjects as well as in patients with cardiopulmonary
disease (Sahn et al., 1977). Such a wide variation in respiratory
chemosensitivity, particularly in hypoxia, has been reported to possibly
influence the clinical courses of some diseases including COPD (Kawakami et al.,
1981, Fleetham et al., 1984, Oren et al., 1987). However, to our knowledge,
there have been no longitudinal data concerning whether the individual values in
respiratory chemosensitivity really remain unchanged over the years. This study
provides firm evidence that inter-individual variability in the ventilatory
response to hypoxia and hypercapnia is maintained after an interval of 7-10
years in healthy subjects.

However, it must be noted that the reproducibility of ventilatory responses
tested after a long interval was not as good as that exmined after a short
interval. This suggests that the inherent individual value in respiratory
chemosensitivity is not strictly fixed but is influenced by some environmental
factors, including changes in physical characteristics, pulmonary function data
and behavioral aspects associated with aging. Smoking habits should also be
considered (Kawakami et al., 1982c, Yamamoto et al.,1985).
Nevertheless, the significant relation between the ventilatory response values
obtained after such a long interval seems to indicate a strong genetic influence
on respiratory chemosensitivity.

The reason why the S values, but not the A values, significantly increased over
the years in this study is unknown.

REFERENCES

Kawakami Y, Irie T, Kishi F, Asanuma Y, Shida A, Yoshikawa T, Kamishima K,
Hasagawa H, Murao M. (1981) Familial aggregation of abnormal ventilatory control
and pulmonary function in chronic obstructive pulmnary disease. Eur J Respir Dis
62:56-64
Kawakami Y, Yoshikawa T, Shida A, Asanuma Y, Murao M. (1982a)
Control of breathing in young twins. J Appl Physiol 52:537-42
Kawakami Y, Irie T, Shida A, Yoshikawa T. (1982b) Familial factors affecting
arterial blood gas values and respiratory chemosensitivity in chronic
obstructive pulmonary disease. Am Rev Respir Dis 125:420-425
Kawakami Y, Yamamoto H, Yoshikawa T, Shida A. (1982c) Respiratory

chemosensitivity in smokers. Am Rev Respir Dis 126:986-990
Kawakami Y, Yamamoto H, Yoshikawa T, Shida A. (1984) Chemical and behavioral
control of breathing in adult twins. Am Rev Respir Dis 129:703-707
Fleetham JA, Arnup ME, Anthonisen NR (1984) Familial aspects of ventilatory
control in patients with chronic obstructive pulmonary disease. Am Rev Respir
Dis 129:3-7
Oren J, Kelly DH, Shannon DC. (1987) Long-term follow-up of children with
congenital central hypoventilation syndrome. Pediatrics 80:375-80
Sahn SA, Zwillich W, Nathan D, McCullough RE, Lakshminarayan S, Weil JV (1977)
Variability of ventilatory responses to hypoxia and hypercapnia J Appl Physiol
43:1019-25
Sullivan TY, Yu P. (1984) Reproducibility of CO_2 response curve with ten minutes
separating each rebreathing test. Am Rev Respir Dis 129:23-26
Yamamoto H, Inaba S, Nishiura Y, Kishi F, Kawakami Y. (1985) Acute inhalation of
cigarette smoke augments hypoxic chemosensitivity in humans. J Appl Physiol
58:717-23

Breathing of Hyperventilation Syndrome Patients at Rest, the Hyperventilation Stage and the Posthyperventilation Stage

K. Chin, M. Ohi and K. Kuno

Department of Clinical Pulmonary Physiology, Chest
Disease Research Institute, Kyoto University, Kyoto,
Japan

ABSTRACT

We investigated the breathing patterns of three hyperventilation
syndrome (HVS) patients in the resting (non attack) stage, in the
involuntary hyperventilation (HV) stage and in the posthyperventilation (PHV) stage, with non-invasive monitoring systems, used
commonly in polysomnography (inductive plethysmography, ear
oximeter, transcutaneous PCO ($PtcCO_2$) and so on). During the PHV
state two of three HVS patients had several episodes of hypoxemia
($SaO_2 \leq 90\%$) without any respiratory disease except for HVS. Lowest
SaO_2 was 81% in patient No.1 and 60% in patient No.3. In the
involuntary HV stage, changes of ventilation from the resting level
were caused by central inspiratory activity, respiratory timing,
or both. Using the inductive plethysmography and $PtcCO_2$ to teach
the proper breathing pattern (slow and shallow) helps the some HVS
patients in their early attack stage. We conclude that physicians
who treat HVS patients must know about the possibility of hypoxemia
during the recovering period from hypocapnia, and it is important
to know the prevalence of the PHV hypoxemia in HVS patients.

KEYWORDS

Hyperventilation syndrome; breathing of hyperventilation syndrome
patients; post hyperventilation hypoxemia; involuntary hyperventilation

INTRODUCTION

Hyperventilation syndrome (HVS) is said to occur in about 6-11% of
the general patients' population (Brashear, 1983, Waites, 1978).
There are few reports concerning the breathing patterns and
physiology of the HVS patients. PHV breathing, from hypocapnia to
normocapnia, is always accompanied by hypoventilation (including
apnea) during the recovery stage, so HVS patients may show
hypoxemia during their PHV stage. We monitored the breathing
patterns of HVS patients at rest, in the involuntary HV state, in
the PHV state, and in the recovery state, using non-invasive

monitoring systems, commonly applied in polysomnography, such as
inductance plethysmography, oximeter, and transcutaneous PO_2 and
PCO_2 measurements.

METHODS

Patients

Three HVS patients were investigated. Patient No.1 was 28 year old
male. Patient No.2 was 38 year old male. Patient No.3 was 75 year
old female. Their pulmonary functions and arterial blood gas
analysis at rest (non attack state) were almost normal. Diagnosis
of HVS depends on the blood gas analysis at an attack and clinical
features.

Monitoring

Surface electrodes for an electroencephalogram (EEG),electromyogram
(EMG) of the chin, electrocardiogram (ECG) and an electrooculogram
(EOG), were applied, using standard techniques, to know whether the
subjects were awake or sleeping. Ventilation was monitored non-
invasively with an inductive plethysmography (Respitrace).
Calibration   factors were obtained by multiple linear regression
methods (Loveridge *et al.*, 1983). Arterial O_2 saturation (SaO_2) was
monitored continuously with an ear oximeter (Hewlett Packard model
47201A). Transcutaneous PCO_2 ($PtcCO_2$) and PO_2 ($PtcO_2$) were continuously monitored with transcutaneous electrodes (Hoffman La Roche
630) heated to 45° C.

Experimental Protocol

Respiratory measurements were conducted in the supine position,
during the daytime, after fasting for at least 3h. The supine
subjects (HVS patients in the non attack state) breathed naturally
for about 30 min. After the ventilation of subjects became stable,
the consecutive 4 min of ventilation in the stable state was
collected as resting ventilation (non attack ventilation). After we
measured the resting ventilation, we requested the HVS patients to
think of the situation which caused them to enter the HV state.
Using this procedure we were able to get data of the HV state for
two (patients No.1 and No.2) of three patients. We could not get
the data of the HV state from patient No.3 on the same day when we
measured her resting ventilation. Some weeks later however, she
came to our hospital because she was in the HV state with symptoms.
After we measured the patients' breathing parameters in the
involuntary HV state for the 4 min, we ordered the patients to
breath slowly and shallowly, while observing their breathing with
Respitrace. Patients No.1 and No.2 could keep their breathing slow
and shallow, their $PtcCO_2$ rose to almost the normal range and their
symptoms disappeared. Patient No.3 could not make her breathing
slow and shallow.

DATA ANALYSIS

The parameters were quoted as means±sd. We applied the Student's t
test, and $p < 0.05$ was considered to be significant.

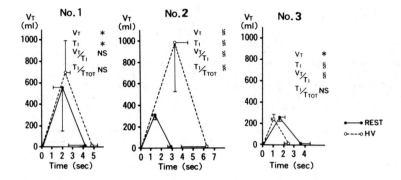

Fig. 1. Average respiratory cycles in patients
No. 1, 2 and 3 at rest (closed circle)
and in a involuntary hyperventilation
state (open circle). Mean inspiratory
flow (V_T/T_I) is represented by the slope
of the ascending limb of the schematic
spirogram. Bars indicate 1 SD. *p<0.05,
§p<0.001 compared to breathing at rest.
NS, not significant.

RESULTS

Values of Breathing Pattern Components in the Involuntary HV State

The changes of breathing components between the resting state and
the involuntary HV state are shown in Fig. 1. The changes of
breathing components between the resting state and the involuntary
HV state were caused by central inspiratory activity, respiratory
timing, or both.

Recovery Stage after the Involuntary HV State

After almost ten minutes of involuntary HV PtcCO$_2$ of patient No.2
decreased from 38 Torr to 27 Torr, and we asked him to breathe
slowly and shallowly, looking at his breathing with Respitrace. His
breathing was irregular, but he could control it and keep it
shallow as we advised and his symptoms began to disappear as the
value of his PtcCO$_2$ increased. Patient No.1 also improved his
symptoms and his HV by following our advice.

After we recorded the involuntary HV breathing of Patient No.3, she
began to sleep. She showed periodic breathing with central apnea.
Her lowest SaO$_2$ was almost 60%. Patient No.1 also showed 81% SaO$_2$
while recovering from the HV state.

DISCUSSION

PHV hypoxemia, due to PHV apnea and hypoventilation, was also reported in a few papers (Saltzman et al., 1963, Bates et al., 1966, Macdonnell et al., 1976). PHV apnea is apt to occur in relaxed conditions (Bainton and Mitchell., 1966). It is reported that HVS is usually chronic (Waites, 1978), and involuntary, so HVS patients may be accustomed to frequent shift between hypocapnia and normocapnia. For this reason, HVS patients may have many episodes of hypoxemia due to apnea and hypoventilation during their PHV state. So we think that the physicians who treat HVS patients must know about the possibility of hypoxemia.

In our study, patients No.1 and No.2 could breathe slowly and shallowly, as advised, by observing Respitrace. These two patients could almost control their breathing in the early stage of a HV attack, and since the day of our experiment they have had few severe HV attacks. Our explanations were not effective, however, for patient No.3 who was already in a severe HV attack. Investigation of HVS patients with non-invasive respiratory monitors such as used in our experiments is useful for the treatment of HVS, and may enable patients to control their abnormal breathing (HV breathing) in the early stages of an attack.

REFERENCES

Bainton, C.R. and R.A. Mitchell (1966). Posthyperventilation apnea in awake man. J. Appl. Physiol., 21, 411-415.
Bates, J.H., J.S. Adamson and J.A. Pierge (1966). Death after voluntary hyperventilation. N. ENG. J. MED., 274, 1371-1372.
Brashear, R.E.(1983). Hyperventilation syndrome. Lung, 161, 257-273
Loveridge, B., P. West, N.R. Anthonisen and M.H. Kryger (1983). Single-position calibration of the respiratory inductance plethysmograph. J. Appl. Physiol., 55, 1031-1034.
Macdonnell, K.F., J.T. Bower and R.E. Flynn (1976). Poshyperventilation apnea associated with severe hypoxemia. Chest, 70, 554-557.
Saltzman, H.A., A. Heyman and H.O. Sieker (1963). Correlation of clinical and physiologic manifestations of sustained hyperventilation. N. ENG. J. MED., 268, 1431-1436.
Waites, T.F. (1978). Hyperventilation-chronic and acute. Arch. Intern. Med., 138, 1700-1701.

Effect of Theophylline on Brain Tissue Oxygenation and Acid-base Status in Patients with COPD

M. Nishimura, A. Suzuki, T. Hiraga,
A. Yoshioka, F. Kishi and Y. Kawakami

First Department of Medicine, School of Medicine,
Hokkaido University, Sapporo 060, Japan

ABSTRACT

To assess the possible adverse effect of theophylline on brain tissue oxygenation due to decreased cerebral blood flow (CBF), we measured internal jugular venous PO_2 (PjO_2) simultaneously with arterial and mixed venous blood PO_2 (PaO_2 and $P\bar{v}O_2$) during right heart catheterization in 10 patients with chronic obstructive pulmonary disease (COPD) before and after theophylline infusion. Additionally we examined the hypothesis that the ventilation-stimulating effect of theophylline is due to the change of the acid-base status in the brain as a result of reduced CBF. PaO_2 stayed at the same level, but PjO_2 decreased markedly after theophylline infusion. Both jugular venous PCO_2 ($PjCO_2$) and pH (pHj) were kept constant, despite significant changes in arterial PCO_2 ($PaCO_2$) and pH (pHa), which suggested increased ventilation. These changes seemed specific to the brain circulation, because mixed venous blood gases behaved similarly to arterial blood gases. These data suggest that a clinical dose of theophylline substantially reduces brain tissue PO_2 in patients with COPD. In addition, theophylline seems to stimulate ventilation without changing the brain acid-base status.

KEY WORDS

theophylline; brain; tissue hypoxia; acid-base status; cerebral blood flow; chronic obstructive pulmonary disease.

INTRODUCTION

Theophylline is widely used in the treatment of patients with COPD as well as asthmatic patients. However, it is well known that theophylline, an adenosine receptor antagonist, substantially reduces cerebral blood flow (CBF). We, therefore, addressed two questions in this study. First, is there any possibility that theophylline selectively decreases the brain tissue PO_2, leading to significant brain hypoxia, particularly when the drug is administered to hypoxemic patients with COPD. Second, is there any possibility that the ventilation-stimulating effect of theophylline is due to the change of the acid-base status in the brain as a result of reduced CBF? Partial gas pressures in jugular venous blood were considered to reflect those of the brain tissue in this study.

SUBJECTS AND METHODS

Ten male patients who were clinically diagnosed as having COPD participated in this study with informed consent. Anthropometric and pulmonary function data are as follows: age, 62±12SD years; height, 162±6 cm; body weight, 51±7 kg; %vital capacity(VC), 70±17%; forced expiratory volume in 1 sec(FEV1), 1.22±0.39 L; FEV1/FVC, 57±9%. Before the study, right heart catheterization was done and catheters were placed into the left bracheal artery and the right internal jugular vein. Blood gases and pH were analyzed soon after sampling with a pH/blood gas analyzer (type 1303, Instrumentation Laboratory). Oxygen hemoglobin saturation (SO$_2$) was determined by a co-Oximeter (Model 282, Instrumentation Laboratory). Cardiac output (CO) was measured by means of the computerized thermodilution technique. Mixed venous samples were obtained from the main pulmonary artery.

Experimental Protocol

Subjects were instructed to refrain from coffee, tea, or caffeinated beverages on the day of the study and all medications were restricted from the day before. They were all in a clinically stable condition. The subjects were placed in the supine position with their eyes closed and were allowed to breathe spontaneously in room air throughout the experiment. After the subject showed stable heart rate and arterial pressure for at least 10 min, hemodynamic parameters were obtained and then blood samples were collected at the same time from the three lines (systemic artery, internal jugular vein and main pulmonary artery). Following this, a clinical loading dose of theophylline (6mg/kg body weight) was intravenously infused over 10 min. Fifteen min after this, hemodynamic parameters and blood samples were obtained again for comparison.

RESULTS

The most striking results were marked drops in PjO$_2$ and SjO$_2$ after theophylline infusion, whereas PaO$_2$ and SaO$_2$ remained constant and PvO$_2$ and SvO$_2$ showed only a small decrease (Table 1). An expected decrease in PaCO$_2$ by 2.7 torr and an associated increase in arterial pH by 0.02 which occured reflected ventilation augmented by theophylline. However, neither PjCO$_2$ nor pHj changed. There were no significant changes in either mean systemic arterial pressure or cardiac output.

Table 1. Effect of theophylline on blood gases and pH

	Control	Theophylline		Control	Theophylline
PaO$_2$, torr	72.9±3.2	73.2±3.2	SaO$_2$, %	93.9±0.7	94.3±0.7
PjO$_2$, torr	34.7±2.2	29.1±1.8*	SjO$_2$, %	60.6±4.1	49.5±4.1*
PvO$_2$, torr	36.7±0.9	35.2±0.9*	SvO$_2$, %	67.7±1.4	65.8±1.6**
PaCO$_2$, torr	40.5±1.4	37.8±1.2*	pHa	7.42±0.01	7.44±0.01*
PjCO$_2$, torr	47.8±1.6	48.8±1.3	pHj	7.37±0.01	7.38±0.01
PvCO$_2$, torr	45.0±1.4	43.3±1.2*	pHv	7.40±0.01	7.41±0.01*

Values are expressed as mean±SE (n=10).
a: arterial, j: jugular venous, v: mixed venous
*: p<0.01, **: p<0.05 compared to control data

DISCUSSION

The present study demonstrates that, in patients with COPD, a clinical dose of theophylline markedly decreases PjO_2 and SjO_2 in the presence of unchanged arterial oxygenation and that ventilation seems to be stimulated without changing the acid-base status in the brain. In addition, these findings seem specific to the brain circulation, because mixed venous blood gases and pH behave quite differently from those of jugular venous blood.

Theophylline, which is now known as an adenosine receptor antagonist, has been repeatedly shown to reduce CBF in humans as well as in some other animal species. A recent study (Bowton et al., 1987) showed that a clinical dose of theophylline caused a decrease in CBF by as much as 26% in patients with COPD. Such a considerable decrease in CBF, combined with the possible increase in local brain metabolism due to theophylline, may induce substantial brain tissue hypoxia, which is of potential clinical importance, particularly when the drug is administered to hypoxemic subjects. In this study, we have demonstrated that PjO_2, which is considered to reflect the average brain tissue PO_2, decreases by as much as 5.6 torr after theophylline infusion. Although no definite conclusion can be drawn concerning the clinical relevance of this finding, it might be possible that brain tissue hypoxia induced by theophylline has an adverse effect on brain higher integrative functions in a chronic term. Chronic hypoxia has been cited as one of the important variables accounting for neuropsychological impairment reported in patients with COPD (Grant et al., 1987).

In this study we did not measure ventilation, because we wanted to avoid any effects on ventilation from an apparatus such as a mouthpiece or a facemask. However, the significant decrease in $PaCO_2$ after theophylline infusion indicates that ventilation was actually stimulated, assuming that the metabolic rate remained unchanged. If theophylline causes a reduction in CBF without a change in the cerebral metabolic rate, it should increase cerebral tissue PCO_2. The change in ventral medullary extracellular fluid acid-base variables might mediate the stimulatory effect of theophylline on ventilation. However, neither $PjCO_2$ nor pHj changed in this study, suggesting that this hypothesis is unlikely. This is in good agreement with a recent animal study (Javaheri et al., 1989), which demonstrated that in spontaneously breathing, peripherally chemodenervated cats, PCO_2 and H^+ in the ventral medullary extracellular fluid did not change with theophylline. Recent studies (Hedner et al., 1982, Eldridge et al., 1985) indicate that adenosine and its analogues exert an inhibitory action on respiratory activity in the brain. Therefore, the stimulatory effect of theophylline on ventilation may be mediated through competitive inhibition of theophylline for an adenosine receptor.

REFERENCES

Bowton, D.L., P.T. Alford, B.D. McLees, D.S. Prough and D.A. Stump (1987). The effect of aminophylline on cerebral blood flow in patients with chronic obstructive pulmonary disease. Chest, 91, 847-877.
Grant, I., G.P. Prigatano, R.K. Heaton, A.J. McSweeny, E.C. Wright and K.M. Adams (1987). Progressive neuropsychological impairment in relation to hypoxemia in chronic obstructive pulmonary disease. Arch. Gen. Psychiatry, 44, 999-1006.
Javaheri, S., J.A.M. Evers and L.J. Teppema (1989). Increase in ventilation caused by aminophylline in the absence of changes in ventral medullary extracellular fluid pH and carbon dioxide tension. Thorax, 44, 121-125.
Hedner, T., J. Hedner, P. Wessberg and J. Jonason (1982). Regulation of breathing in the rat: indications for a role of central adenosine mechanisms. Neuroscience Letters, 33, 147-151.
Eldridge, F.L., D.E. Millhorn and J.P. Kiley (1985). Antagonism by theophylline of respiratory inhibition induced by adenosine. J. Appl. Physiol., 59, 1428-1433.

Factors Responsible for a Wide Variation in PaCO$_2$ in Patients with Chronic Obstructive Pulmonary Disease

Y. Akiyama, M. Nishimura,
M. Yamamoto, F. Kishi and
Y. Kawakami

First Department of Medicine, Hokkaido University
School of Medicine, N-15, W-7, Kita-ku, Sapporo 060,
Japan

ABSTRACT

To examine factors responsible for inter-individual variation in resting PaCO$_2$, we studied 55 clinically stable patients with chronic obstructive pulmonary disease by physical characteristics, pulmonary function tests, resting breathing patterns, and chemosensitivity to hypoxia and hypercapnia. We concluded that body weight is an independent determinant for PaCO$_2$ when pulmonary mechanics are severely impaired, and that dead-space ventilation is important when airflow limitation is moderate.

KEYWORDS

Chronic obstructive pulmonary disease; PaCO$_2$; Chemosensitivity; Hypoxia; Hypercapnia; Nutrition.

INTRODUCTION

In patients with chronic obstructive pulmonary disease (COPD), even in a clinically stable period, resting PaCO$_2$ varies quite markedly among individuals. Several factors have been implicated in this variability, although they may be interrelated to some degree. For example, mechanical respiratory limitation, reduced chemosensitivity to hypoxia or hypercapnia (either as an inherent characteristic or as a phenomenon secondary to the disease itself), changes in breathing pattern, and respiratory muscle weakness have been considered to have undesirable effects on PaCO$_2$ levels (Weinberger et al., 1989, West, 1971). However, few studies have extensively investigated these factors in a large number of patients. We studied the physical characteristics, pulmonary function tests, resting breathing patterns, and chemosensitivity to hypoxia and hypercapnia of 55 clinically stable patients with COPD.

METHODS

Fifty-five patients who were clinically diagnosed as having COPD were studied. Their anthropometric and pulmonary function data are shown in Table 1. Averaged arterial blood gas values of several measurements during clinically

Table 1. Patient characteristics.

Subjects, n (M:F)	55 (50:5)	Brinkman index	960±636
(emphysematous:bronchitic)		%VC, %	74±18
	(35:20)	%FEV$_1$, %	47±18
Age, yr	62±11	FEV$_1$/FVC, %	52±11
Height, cm	160.4±7.3	pH	7.39±0.03
Weight, kg	54.2±9.9	PaCO$_2$, Torr	41.5±3.8
BSA, m^2	1.55±0.15	PaO$_2$, Torr	77.4±9.6

Values are means±SD.

stable periods prior to the ventilatory response tests are also listed in
Table 1.

Ventilatory and $P_{0.1}$ responses were measured, while subjects were supine,
using a servo-control system of arterial blood gases (Kawakami et al., 1981).
First, the resting breathing pattern was measured. Ventilatory and $P_{0.1}$
responses to isocapnic progressive hypoxia and hyperoxic progressive
hypercapnia were examined in this order with a 30-min interval. The
chemosensitivity to hypoxia was assessed by $\Delta\dot{V}_E/\Delta SaO_2$ and $\Delta P_{0.1}/\Delta SaO_2$. The
chemosensitivity to hypercapnia was evaluated by $\Delta\dot{V}_E/\Delta P_{ET}CO_2$ and $\Delta P_{0.1}/\Delta P_{ET}CO_2$.

Statistical analyses used were linear regressions and unpaired t-tests. P
values of less than 0.05 were accepted as significant.

RESULTS

For the whole group, PaCO$_2$ weakly correlated with %VC ($r=-0.30$, $p<0.05$), %FEV$_1$
($r=-0.28$, $p<0.05$), and ventilatory responses to hypercapnia ($r=-0.27$, $p<0.05$).
$P_{0.1}$ responses to hypercapnia as well as ventilatory and $P_{0.1}$ responses to
hypoxia were unrelated to PaCO$_2$. We compared 2 sub-groups with similar, low
%FEV$_1$ levels (29±5 and 28±4%) and different PaCO$_2$ levels (47.8±2.6 and 40.5±1.9
Torr)(Fig. 1., vertical comparison). There were no differences in $P_{0.1}$
responses to hypoxia and hypercapnia, and resting breathing pattern. However,
the high PaCO$_2$ group (n=6) had heavier body weight than the low PaCO$_2$ group
(n=6)(58.4±6.5 and 48.7±4.4 kg, $p<0.02$). Further, by comparison of 2 sub-
groups with similar, high PaCO$_2$ levels (44.0±2.2 and 44.6±2.3 Torr) and
different %FEV$_1$ (57±7 and 26±6%)(Fig. 1., horizontal comparison), the high
%FEV$_1$ group (n=6) showed higher resting ventilation standardized by body
surface area than the low %FEV$_1$ group (n=6)(5.2±0.5 and 4.1±0.8 L/min/m^2,
$p<0.05$). The resting $P_{ET}CO_2$ in the high %FEV$_1$ group was lower than that in
the low %FEV$_1$ group (33.5±2.1 and 43.0±7.3 Torr, $p<0.05$).

DISCUSSION

Although the PaCO$_2$ level at rest had a weak but significant correlation with
the lung mechanical disturbance assessed by %FEV$_1$, there was a large variation
for a given level of %FEV$_1$. This suggests that factors other than the
mechanical disturbance are involved as determinants of PaCO$_2$ in patients with
COPD.

To search for such factors, we compared 2 sub-groups whose pulmonary mechanics
were severely impaired to the same degree, but whose PaCO$_2$ was different.
We found the difference in body weight alone could explain the difference
in PaCO$_2$. Malnourished COPD patients are shown to have increased resting
energy expenditure, and malnutrition may result in reduced respiratory and

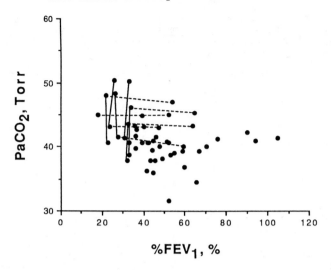

Fig. 1.   We paired 12 patients so that each pair had
similar, low %FEV_1 and different $PaCO_2$ levels
(solid lines), and so that similar high $PaCO_2$
levels and different %FEV_1 (broken lines),
without prior knowledge of other factors.

limb muscle strength, increased muscle fatigability and breathlessness, as
well as reduced performance (Efthimiou et al., 1988, Hunter et al., 1981).
However, the present study suggests that that there is another view concerning
the nutritional status in COPD.   Patients with greater body weight may have
greater CO_2 production, and this may be associated with an increase in $PaCO_2$
if airflow limitation is severe enough to prevent CO_2 elimination.

Comparing 2 sub-goups with the same high $PaCO_2$ levels and different %FEV_1,
the high %FEV_1 group showed larger resting ventilation and lower resting
$P_{ET}CO_2$.   These findings imply that there are patients with only moderate
airflow limitation and large dead-space ventilation.   The increase in dead-
space ventialtion may derive from rapid shallow breathing (Javaheri et al.,
1981) or a considerable ventilation-perfusion mismatch (West, 1971), although
we could not confirm these possibilities in the present study.

We conclude that body weight is an independent determinant for $PaCO_2$ in
patients with COPD when pulmonary mechanics are severely impaired, and that
dead-space ventilation is important when airflow limitation is moderate.

REFERENCES

Efthimiou, J., J. Fleming, C. Gomes, and S.G. Spiro (1988).   The effect of
    supplementary oral nutrition in poorly nourished patients with chronic
    obstructive pulmonary disease.   Am. Rev. Respir. Dis., 137, 1075-1082.
Hunter, A.M.B., M.A. Carey, and H.W. Larsh (1981).   The nutritional status
    of patients with chronic obstructive pulmonary disease.   Am. Rev. Respir.
    Dis., 124, 376-381.
Javaheri, S., J. Blum, and H. Kazemi (1981).   Pattern of breathing and carbon
    dioxide retention in chronic obstructive lung disease.   Am. J. Med., 71,
    228-234.

Kawakami, Y., T. Yoshikawa, Y. Asanuma, and M. Murao (1981). A control system
  for arterial blood gases. J. Appl. Physiol., 50, 1362-1366.
Weinberger, S.E., R.M. Schwartzstein, and J. Woodrow Weiss (1989).
  Hypercapnia. N. Engl. J. Med., 321, 1223-1231.
West, J.B. (1971). Causes of carbon dioxide retention in lung disease.
  N. Engl. J. Med., 284, 1232-1236.

New Disease with Ankyloglossia, Dislocation of the Epiglottis and of the Larynx — Dyspnea of Newborn and Suckling Infants

Susumu Mukai and Chikako Mukai

Kaseikai Mukai Clinic, Mukai Research Institute of
Microbiology, Yamatominami 2-8-9, Yamato,
Kanagawa, 242 Japan

ABSTRACT

A new congenital disease with ankyloglossia and associated dislocation of the
epiglottis and of the larynx is described. Newborn and suckling babies with this
anomaly had dyspnea, and showed typical skin and hair signs. In addition, the
following symptoms were observed : suckling difficulties, they cried hard and
frequently, their extremities were cold and had a low muscle tone, their forehead
appeared dark and frown, they snored, their development was either too fast or
slow, weak and dependent and were rather inactive.
After the operation dyspnea disappeared and the other symptoms and signs
improved dramatically.

KEYWORDS

Dyspnea, Ankyloglossia, Larynx, Epiglottis, Anomaly, SIDS.

PRESENTATION OF THE CASES

The patients were 51 babies, 3-59 weeks old, who were brought to Mukai Clinic
from May to October, 1989, with chief complaints of feeding difficulties, nasal
obstruction and snore. Although these babies had been diagnosed as having no
particular abnormalities by their pediatricians, on examination, dislocation of the
epiglottis and of the larynx associated with ankyloglossia was found.

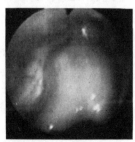

Fig.-1. Larynx, fiberscopic view via nose
The Larynx raised and curved ventrally.

The epiglottis leaned towards the radix linguae
and some cases it was impossible to see it all from
epipharynx by fiberscope via nose; the larynx
raised and curved ventrally (Fig.-1). The vocal
cord did not open widely during inspiration.
Moreover the following symptoms were observed
: suckling difficulties, they cried hard and
frequently, their extremities were cold and had a
low muscle tone, their forehead appeared dark
and frown, they snored, their development was
either too fast or slow, they had difficulties in
following an object with their eyes, they looked
pale, weak and dependent and were rather
inactive. Their sleeps were shallow and they
awaked easily.

Frenoplasty involving the anteriorgenioglossal muscles was carried out to correct the dislocation of the tongue, the epiglottis and the larynx. Before and after the operation variations in their blood oxygen saturation rate, as well as skin and hair signs were recorded. Patients were divided into three groups according to their age : newborn (3,4 weeks), 6 patients ; suckling (5-14 weeks), 24 patients ; and, post-suckling (15-59 weeks), 21 patients

1) *Blood   oxygen saturation   rate   (SpO2)* was measured during sleeping, while awaken and while sucking with a pulse oximeter (CSI 502: Tokyo). In this oximeter between 99 and 96 was considered within normal range and when below 95 it was hypoxemia. Patients were classified in two groups: A) in normal range and B) when below 95, according to measurements.

Table-1. Relationship between patients' age and SpO2

Weeks	Cases	Sleep A	B	Awake A	B	Suckling A	B
3,4	6	0	6	2	4	1	5
5-14	24	2	22	13	11	10	14
15-59	21	10	11	13	8	13	8
Total	51	12	39	28	23	24	27

(A; 99-96, B; presented below 95)

SpO2 during   sleep; As shown in table 1, there were 12cases (24%) in group A and 39 (76%) in group B. That is, among the newborn babies there was none in A group and 6 (100%) were in B group. Of the suckling babies, 2 (8.3%) were in group A and 22 (91.7%) were in group B. And of the post-suckling infants, 10 (47.6%) were group A and 11(52.4%) were in group B. Inter-group statistical analysis revealed that SpO2 during sleep varied significantly according to patients' age (p<0.005).
SpO2 while   awaken; 28 patients (55%) had normal SpO2 and 23 cases (45%) showed below 95 (Table-1). That is, among the newborn babies 2 (33.3%) were in group A and 4 (66.7%) were in group B. Of the suckling babies, 13 (54.2%) were in group A and 11 (45.8%) were in group B.And of post-sukling infants, 13 (61.9%) were in group A and 8 (38.1%) were in group B. There was no significant difference between these groups. SpO2 were unstable under 14 weeks of age.
SpO2 while   sucking; 24 (47%) were allocated to group A and 27 (53%) to group B (Table-1). That is, among the newborn babies, 1 (16.7%) was in group A and 5 (83.3%) were in group B. Of the suckling babies, 10 (41.7%) were in group A and 14 (58.3%) were in group B. And in the post-suckling infants, 13 (61.9%) were in group A and 8 (38.1%) were in group B.
However, three kinds of suckling difficulties were noted in all cases: **a)** When the patients started sucking, their pulse rate increased but suddenly it decreased the SpO2 decreased below 95 and they could not continue feeding. They stopped their sucking and sometimes cried out loudly. After breathing several times they recommenced sucking. **b)** Their pulse rate increased to 170 or more and while their pulse rate was high they stopped sucking to start again when their pulse rate went back to normal or they finished their sucking. While feeding their SpO2 was at the maximum value of 99. **c)** They continued sucking, but it was difficult for their mothers to tell whether they had stopped sucking or not.

2) *SKIN* ; Regarding the color of their skin before operation, patients were allocated to three different groups: to group A those who had normal color (9 patients, 18%), to group B when their skin was marmorated (32 patients, 63%) and to group C when their skin showed signs of cyanosis (10 patients, 20%) (Table-2). The number of newborn babies in groups A, B and C was 1,3 and 2 respectively: among the suckling babies, it was 0, 20 and 4; and of the post-suckling infants there was 8,9 and 4. The inter-group statistical analysis revealed significant differences with regard to skin signs between these groups (P<0.01).

3) HAIR ; Before the operation some patients had normal hair [group A-8 cases (16%)], others had very scanty hair [group B- 19 cases (37%)] and others showed piloerection [group C-24 cases(47%)]. When both signs were observed in one patients he was allocated to either B or C according to predominant sign. The number of newborn babies in group A, B and C, was 1,4 and 1 respectively; among suckling babies, it was 2,10 and 12; and of the post-suckling infants there were 5,5 and 11. There was no significant relationship between the patients' hair characteristics and the SpO2 either.

RESULTS

After the operation, the SpO2 was 98-99 in all the patients. Their skin acquired a normal color. Their hair stopped falling and, in those patients who had piloerection before the operation, this tended to disappear. They were able to follow an object with their eyes and their eyes looked more vivid. Their cheeks got color and their features became soft. Snoring also disappeared. According to the observations of their mothers, the babies stopped crying hard, they slept well and could play alone. Mothers even reported that they were more fond of their babies after the operation than before.

DISCUSSION

Phylogenetically, in babies, the epiglottis conjugate with the epipharynx during feeding and as a result they can breath while sucking [1]. But in this anomaly the epiglottis and the larynx are in a ventral position ; consequently, a complete conjugation between epipharynx and the epiglottis can not be obtained. This results in an increased respiratory resistance; and, since newborn and suckling infants have weak respiratory muscles, babies with this anomaly probably fall into dyspnea readily. After the operation all symptoms of respiratory distress as well as other clinical signs disappeared. The data presented here strongly suggest that the symptoms and signs observed in these patients are due to the patients' dyspneic state.

Moreover, it is important to note that the symptoms and signs present in patients with ankyloglossia and associated dislocation of the epiglottis and larynx as described here, are surprisingly similar to those reported in the literature for sudden infant death syndrome (SIDS) [2]. Full awareness of pediatricians in this respect would prevent these infants falling victims to SIDS.

REFERENCES

1) Negus, V. (1929). The mechanism of the larynx. W.H.Heinemann Ltd. , Paris.
2) Naeye, R.L. (1989). Underlying disorders associated with recognized risk factors for sudden infant death syndrome. XXVth congress of the Japan Society of Neonatology. Tokyo.

The authors are grateful to Mrs. P. Lopetegui, DDS,
Tokyo Tanabe Pharmaceutical Ltd.,Tokyo,
for assistance in preparing the English language manuscript.

Analysis of Dyspnea Episodes in Children with Obstructive Sleep Dyspnea

K. Togawa*, S. Miyazaki*, K. Yamakawa*,
H. Tada*, Y. Itasaka* and M. Okawa†

*Department of Otolaryngology;
†Department of Neuropsychiatry, Akita University
Hospital, 1-1-1, Hondo, Akita 010, Japan

ABSTRACT

The main cause of obstructive sleep dyspnea in children is adenotonsillar hypertrophy. On such patients polysomnography was carried out. The severity of sleep
dyspnea was classified into three groups depending on the amplitude of intraesophageal pressure ; slight (15-19 cmH$_2$0), moderate (20-39 cmH$_2$0), and severe
(40 cmH$_2$0 and over). Up to the moderate obstruction, the polysomnograms showed
normal pattern in sleep-stage changes. Those who with severe obstruction could
not reach in deep-sleep stage. When the sleep stage changed from non-REM to REM-
sleep stage, tcPO$_2$ and SaO$_2$ decreased abruptly. Definite increase in tcPCO$_2$ and
bradycardia were observed. Some of these cases fell in cyanosis. Such evidence
in severe sleep dyspnea may cause sudden infant death.

KEYWORDS

Obstructive sleep dyspnea; REM sleep; polysomnography; intraesophageal pressure;
adenotonsillar hypertrophy; SIDS

INTRODUCTION

Influence of obstructive sleep dyspnea on children has been investigated with
multifactorial interests among otolaryngologists and pediatricians. The main
cause of this clinico-pathological conditions is adenotonsillar hypertrophy
(89.5 %). Polysomnographic studies on these cases revealed certain evidences
which may cause sudden infant death (SID). In this paper the analysis of our
polysomnographic data is introduced.

MATERIAL AND METHOD

Seventeen children of less than 7 years of age who had sleep dyspnea and snoring
underwent all night polysomnography under natural sleep pre and postoperatively.
Polygraphic recordings included EEG (C3-A2, C4-A1, O1-A2 and O2-A1), EMG of the
chin muscles, eyemovements (EOG-vertical and horizontal), ECG, airflows at the
nares and mouth with thermistors, abdominal and thoracic movements with strain-
gauges, the intraesophageal pressure (Pes.) with balloon method, transcutaneous

PO_2 and PCO_2 ($tcPO_2$, $tcPCO_2$), oxygen saturation ratio (SaO_2), expiratory gas
contents (FO_2 & FCO_2), respiratory rate and heart rate. All the parameters were
stored in a datarecorder, and analysed later on demands. Based on the amplitude
of Pes., the severity of sleep dyspnea was classified into 3 groups ; slight (15
-19 cmH_2O), moderate (20-39 cmH_2O) and severe (40 cmH_2O and over).

RESULTS

The influence of respiratory disturbance during sleep was slight up to moderately
obstructed group. In the severely obstructed group, the influences on sleep and
cardiorespiratory functions were remarkable. In severely obstructed cases,
respiratory pattern was irregular with apnea and hyperpnea during the light-
sleep period. Blood gas levels fluctuated correspondingly. Hypoxia and hypercapnia, caused by apnea, enforced the respiratory effort reflexibly. When the
intraesophageal pressure reached more than -50 cmH_2O and prevailed over the
stenosis, ventilation started accompanied with loud snoring. Deviated blood gas
levels returned to normal. Then, the intraesophageal pressure was reduced
reflexibly, which resulted in the onset of apnea again (Fig. 1, A). Extremely
obstructed cases could not obtain a deep-sleep level because of frequent arousal
responses. But, if the patient tolerated such disturbed respiratory condition
and fell into the deep-sleep level, the breathing pattern turned to constant.
Ventilation was kept by the respiratory force of 40-60 cmH_2O intraesophageal
pressure-change (Fig. 1, B). In REM-sleep stage, ventilatory insufficiency was
more evident than that in non-REM-sleep stage, in which the intraesophageal
pressure fluctuated between 30-50 cmH_2O, with unstable, low $tcPO_2$ and high
$tcPCO_2$ correspondingly (Fig. 1, C). In slightly or moderately obstructed cases
also, such phenomena in relation to the sleep stage were found, but minimal or
slight.

After adenotonsillectomy such phenomena as marked increase in the intraesophageal
pressure and the change in blood gases returned in normal level. Breathings were
regular and quiet (Fig. 1, D). The ratio of decrease in $tcPO_2$ in severely
obstructed group was significantly greater than those in other groups. The ratio
of increase in $tcPCO_2$ showed the same tendency. However, statistical analysis
did not show significant difference, due to wide distribution of data (Fig. 2).

The influence of obstruction on EEG-staging was slight up to the moderately
obstructed group. In the severely obstructed group, EEG revealed a disturbed
sleep condition with definite increase in the ratio of the sleep stage 1 and
decrease in those of the sleep stages 3, 4 and REM stage.

DISCUSSION

Monitoring of the intraesophageal pressure and blood gas levels is useful in
evaluating the severity of respiratory effort and in determining apneic patterns
(obstructive, central or mixed type). Our data showed that the infant with
severe airway obstruction has been suffered from cardio-respiratory dysfunction
during sleep. Especially, in REM sleep stage characterized with excessive
muscular hypotonia, autonomic dysfunction and less sensitivity of respiratory
center to hypercapnia and hypoxia, such influence of the upper airway obstruction was much more severe than presumed. In a few extreme cases, sudden
infant death may happen. Careful observation and proper treatment would save the
suffering infants from such risk.

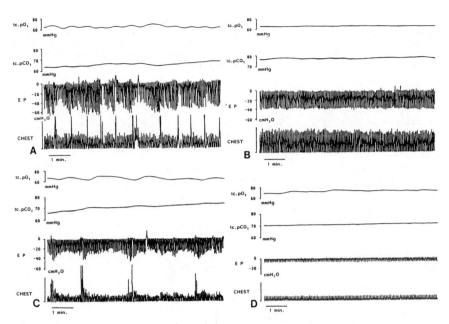

Fig. 1. Typical preoperative respiratory patterns in the
light (A), deep (B), and REM (C) sleep stages in a
case of severe obstruction, and postoperative
respiratory pattern during light sleep (D).

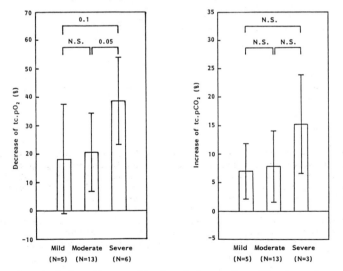

Fig. 2. Left : Mean amplitude of change in $tcPO_2$ when sleep
stage changed from non-REM to REM stage.
Right : Mean amplitude of change in $tcPCO_2$ in
similar transitional stage.

Sleep Disturbance and Decreased Vagal Tone in Respiratory and Cardiovascular Disorders

M. Adachi, Y. Ichimaru, Y. Sato and
T. Yanaga

Medical Institute of Bioregulation, Kyusyu University,
Tsurumibaru 874, Beppu, Japan

ABSTRACT

With the purpose of clarifying the roles of sleep and of autonomic disturbances in respiratory and cardiovascular disorders,ambulatory polygraphic monitoring was performed in 9 patients and 5 normal controls. Patients with ischemic heart disease (IHD)showed decreased sleep efficiency compared with the controls (59.0% vs 89.1%), and patients with the sequel of cerebral bleeding (CB), sleep apnea syndrome (SAS), or IHD also showed decreased heart rate variability (HRV) both at awakening and during sleeping. Especially, HRV at sleep stage 4 showed decreases from 14.6 ± 2.2/min for control to 0.96 ± 2.2/min for CB, 0.98 ± 1.2/min for IHD, and 1.59 ± 1.8/min for SAS. Thus, although the influence of aging and the small number of cases are involved, patients with respiratory and cardiovascular diseases were shown to present with decreased vagal tone while sleeping.

KEYWORDS

heart rate variability ; vagal tone ; sleep apnea syndrome ; ambulatory polygraphic monitoring

Heart rate variability (HRV)

HRV, which is regarded as the estimative index for autonomic nerve function, has variously been reported and especially plays an important role in predicting severe arrhythmia and sudden cardiac death in sleep. In the present study, assessing cardiac parasympathetic activity using 24 hour electrocardiogram according to Ewing and his associate , we comparatively examined HR(Heart Rate), RR(Respiratory Rate), and HRV of each sleep stage between patients with respiratory and cardiovascular diseases and control subjects.

M. Adachi *et al.*

Table 1.   Clnical Chaeactristics of Patients

Pt.No.	Age	Sex	Clinical diagnosis	Ht/Wt (cm) (kg)	BMI*	Apnea episodea
1	49	M	SAS	164.5/92.0	34.0	+
2	56	M	CB	153.0/53.0	22.6	+
3	64	F	SAS	146.0/47.0	22.0	+
4	59	F	Af	145.0/46.5	22.1	−
5	62	F	Angina	152.5/65.0	27.9	−
6	41	M	HL	163.0/67.0	25.2	−
7	74	M	OMI	166.0/67.0	24.3	+
8	61	M	Af	152.2/48.0	20.6	−
9	45	M	SAS	162.0/77.0	29.3	−

SAS : Sleep apnea syndrome
Af : atrial fibrillation
OMI : old myocardial infarction
CB : cerebral bleeding
HL : Hyperlipidemia

$$*BMI(Body\ mass\ index) = \frac{Wt(Kg)}{Ht(m)^2}$$

Methods

As shown in Table 1, 9 patients (6 males, 3 females, mean 56 ± 9.7 years) and 5 healthy, normal controls (3 males, 2 females, mean 23.0 ± 5.3 years) were studied. EEG, ECG, Respitogram, EOG and EMG were recorded by Oxford Medilog 9000(Oxford), and the sleep stage and RR were read by the doctor from real time regeneration records over a total of 8 hours from 10:00 p.m. to 6:00 a.m. HR and HRV were determined by digitalization of the successive   RR interval according to sixtyfold high-speed play back. Accordingly, HR and HRV could not be determined for patient 1, 4, 7, 8, and 9 because of the erroneous records involved. For the remaining 4 patients, HR, RR, and HRV, by sleep stage, were expressed in values every minute and were entered into the paired-T test to determine any significant difference from the controls.

Results

sleep efficiency (actual sleeping time / recording time) was 96.7, 91.5, 89.1, and 59.0% for CB, SAS, control, and IHD, respectively, being lowest for the latter . HR, RR, and HRV at wakening, sleeping stages 2 and 4, and REM sleep are shown in Table 2. HR and RR tended to decrease for the patient group compared with the control group, but not to a significant extent. Patients 2 and 3 presented with apnea at recording and with remarkable hypopnea and sinus bradycardia at sleeping. HRV was lowest (2.12 ± 2.91/min) for IHD at wakening, while at sleeping it was lowest for CB (stage 2; 0.93 ± 2.4/min, stage 4; 0.96 ± 2.2/min) . In REM sleep, CB, IHD, SAS, and HL(Hyperlipidemia) patients showed 1.00, 1.06, 2.50, and 5.48, respectively. In terms of the mean values for 4 patients, significant decrease was noted at each sleep stage compared with the controls.

Table 2   Comparison of HR, HRV, and RR for control group and patients
               in each sleep stages.*

	awakening			stage 2			stage 4			REM		
	HR	HRV	RR	HR	HRV	RR	HR	HRV	RR	HR	HRV	RR
control	71.4	16.2	16.0	61.8	13.4	20.8	66.2	14.6	16.2	63.6	12.6	21.0
(n=5)	±9.2	±1.4	±8.4	±5.9	±1.4	±6.7	±13.5	±2.2	±10.4	±6.0	±2.2	±8.1
P t.	59.7	3.48‡	15.8	56.7	2.80‡	14.7	55.6	3.04‡	14.8	57.3	2.51‡	16.1
(n=4)	±5.4	±1.6	±1.8	±5.4	±2.0	±1.5	±4.4	±3.2	±1.5	±5.1	±1.8	±1.9

HR : Heart rate
HRV: Heart rate variability
RR : Respiratory rate
* Values are means±SD
‡ P<0.001

Discussion

Many reports are available in which HRV in normal subjects has been
determined at each sleep stage. In the control group of the present
study, however, HRV at REM sleep tended to decrease, but not to a
remarkable extent. For such young, normal subjects, supposed to be
free from autonomic functional disturbance, HRV itself had a great
change, but a small standard deviation, reflecting a respiratory
variation. On the other hand, for the patient group, HR and RR also
tended to decrease, and to a remarkable extent for patients
presenting with sleep apnea syndrome(patients 2 and 3), and that
was presumed to be ascribable to bradycardia due to apnea. The
decrement in HRV for the patient group seemed to show the reduction
of vagal tone and was strongest for central nervous system
and cardiovascular diseases , reflecting a response
approximate to that for normal control in hyperlipidemic
patients. For patients with sleep apnea syndrome , whose apnea
type and apnea index have not been determined , the
possibility was suggested that , or indistinct organic
impairment , the reduction of vagal tone was facilitated to a
stronger extent by sleep.

References

Ewing , D.J.,J.M. Neilson and P. Travis , P(1984).New method for
    assessing cardiac parasympathetic activity using 24 hour
    electrocardiograms. Br. Heart. J.,52,396-402.
Bond , W.C., C. Bohs and J.J. Ebey (1973). Rhythmic heart rate
    variability(sinus arrhythmia related to stages of sleep).
    Conditional Reflex,8,98.
Baust , W. and B. Bohnert (1969). The regulation of heart rate
    during sleep. Exp. Brain. Res.,7,169.
Guilleminault , C. and W. C. Dement (1978).Sleep Apnea Syndrome .
    Alan R . Liss, Inc., New York.
Zwillich , C. , T. Devlin , D. White , N. Douglas , J. Weil and
    R. Martin (1982). Bradycardia during sleep apnea . J.
    Clin. Invest. , 69, 1286-1292.

Changes of Respiratory Variables in Sleep Apnea Syndrome

Y. Inoue, K. Ueda, T. Tamura and
H. Hazama

Department of Neuropysychiatry, Tottori University
School of Medicine, Nishimachi 86, Yonago, Japan

ABSTRACT

We examined the relationship between respiratory variables and pathogenesis of
sleep apnea syndrome (SAS) in patients with or without conditions of upper airway
obstruction (UAO).
In mild SAS cases without UAO, the coefficient of variation of tidal volume (VT-
CV) increased significantly through all sleep stages compared with healthy
subjects , and periodic breathings were frequently observed even in apnea-free
periods. In mild SAS cases with UAO, the total compartmental displacement per
tidal volume (TCD/VT) increased through all sleep stages compared with healthy
subjects, whereas VT-CV did not show any definite difference. In severe SAS cases
of both groups with and without UAO, high incidence of periodic breathing was observed, but frequent hypoxic events were observed only in severe SAS cases with UAO.
From these results, obstruction of upper airway manifested as the increase of TCD
/VT was thought to play a pathogenetic role of sleep apnea in patients with UAO,
and periodic breathings triggered with hypoxia might contribute to an aggravating
process. On the other hand in patients without UAO, periodic breathing was thought
to be the primary feature of SAS originating from dysfuction of respiratory control system.

KEY WORDS

sleep apnea,respiratory inductive plethysmography,periodic breathing, desaturation.

INTRODUCTION

In order to clarify the difference of pathogenesis and progression process of sleep
apnea syndrome (SAS) between two groups of patients with and without conditions of
upper airway obstruction (UAO), the relationship between respiratory variables and
appearance mode of apneic episodes on polysomnogram was examined.

SUBJECTS AND METHOD

Polysomnographic recordings and measurements of respiratory variables were carried
out on 7 healthy subjects with mean age of 46.7 ± 9.4 years and 24 SAS patients. SAS

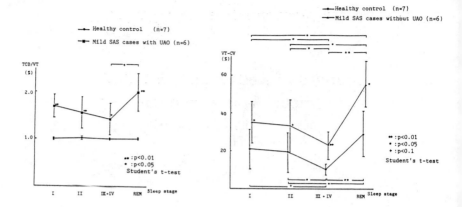

Fig. 1. Comparison of respiratory variables during each sleep
stage between healthy subjects and mild SAS cases
Left : Comparison of VT-CV between healthy subjects and mild
SAS cases without UAO
Right: Comparison of TCD/VT between healthy subjects and mild
SAS cases with UAO

patients with or without UAO were judged from the fiberscopic findings of the upper
airways. SAS patients were divided into four groups with 6 subjects each; mild
SAS cases with UAO (mean age 55.1±5.0 yrs: apnea index 8.1±1.6), mild SAS cases
without UAO (mean age 56.2±6.1 yrs: apnea index 7.4±3.2), severe SAS cases with
UAO (mean age 42.1±3.3 yrs: apnea index 36.6±3.7), and severe SAS cases without
UAO (mean age 53.5±10.3 yrs: apnea index 37.9±5.8).
Respiratory variables such as coefficient of variation (CV) of respiratory frequency, CV of tidal volume (VT-CV), and total compartmental displacement per tidal
volume (TCD/VT) were measured by use of a respiratory inductive plethysmograph (
RIP) calibrated with isovolume maneuver. In patient groups, these variables were
measured only during periods free from apnea. Then, comparison of these respiratory variables was made between SAS patient groups and healthy control
subjects in each sleep stage.

RESULTS

CV of respiratory frequency showed the lowest value during sleep stage III-IV and
the highest value during sleep stage REM in all subject groups. But statistical
difference of this variable was not observed between healthy control subjects and
SAS groups with or without UAO. Regarding VT-CV, sleep stage related change of
the value showed almost the same tendency as CV of respiratory frequency in both
SAS groups and healthy subjects, but mild SAS cases without UAO showed significantly higher value during each sleep compared with healthy subjects (Fig.1). In
mild SAS cases with UAO, values of TCD/VT during each sleep stage were significantly higher compared with healthy subjects (Fig.1), whereas VT-CV did not show
statistically higher value.
In mild SAS cases without UAO, the periodic breathing, a pattern of alternating
hyperpnea and hypopnea, was frequently observed during light sleep as well as REM
sleep, and apnea occured only at the nadir of such periodic breathing. In mild
SAS cases with UAO, however, the appearance of apneic episode was not likely to
relate to periodic breathing. Percent time appearance of periodic breathing
during sleep was 14.7±6.1% in mild SAS cases with UAO and 56.9±19.3% in mild SAS cases
without UAO, and there existed significant difference between two group (P<0.01
). On the other hand in both severe SAS cases with and without UAO, periodic
breathing were observed in more than 80% of total sleep time, and there lacked

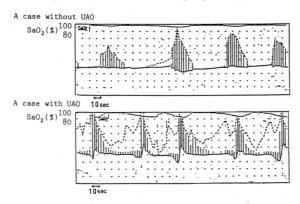

A case without UAO

$SaO_2(\%)$ $^{100}_{80}$

A case with UAO 10 sec

$SaO_2(\%)$ $^{100}_{80}$

10 sec

Fig. 2. Respiratory inductive plethysmogram demonstrations
of severe SAS cases with or without UAO. Real vertical lines indicate VT and broken lines indicate TCD.

significant difference between the two groups. Concerning with SaO_2, 221.1 ± 43.8
times of desaturation events during sleep when SaO_2 fell over 4% from the awake
value in severe SAS cases with UAO were significantly more frequent than 70.4±26.3
times in severe SAS cases without UAO (P<0.01). Though apneic episodes were
frequently observed at the nadir of the periodic breathing in both severe SAS
cases with and without UAO, remarkable increase of TCD/VT was only observed in the
cases with UAO (Fig.2).

DISCUSSION

From these results, obstruction of the upper airway manifesting as the increase
of TCD/VT during sleep was though to play a pathogenetic role of SAS, and instability of respiration due to narrowing of the upper airway seemed to lead to apneic
episodes. Also in severe SAS cases with UAO, the periodic breathing triggered
with hypoxia occuring during apneic episodes were thought to act as one of the
essential aggravating factors of SAS (Önal et al., 1986).
On the other hand, respiratory dysrhythmia manifesting as increase of VT-CV was
considered as the primary cause of sleep apnea in patients without UAO. As Webb
(1974) reported, the periodic breathing was observed frequently even during apnea-
free periods and was thought to be the primary feature of SAS in patients without
UAO. Increase of frequency and amplitude of the periodic breathing might lead to
aggravation of sleep apnea in both severe cases with and without UAO. However,
desaturation events in severe cases without UAO showed less frequency than in cases
with UAO, and actually hypoxia did not seem to be related with aggravating process
of SAS so much as in cases with UAO. Many reports indicated that respiratory
dysrhythmia is the main cause of SAS in elderly subjects without any particular
background conditions. Pathogenesis of SAS in patients without UAO in our study
is most likely coincided with that of elderly subjects.

REFERENCE

Önal, E. and Burrows, D.L.(1986). Induction of periodic breathing during sleep
cases upper airway obstruction in humans. J. Appl. Physiol., 61, 1438-1443.
Webb, P.(1974). Periodic breathing during sleep. J. Appl. Physiol., 37, 899-903.

Measurement of the Pharyngeal Area in Patients with Obstructive Sleep Apnea (OSA) During Sleep Using Acoustic Reflection Technique

H. Shen, J. Huang, S. Kitagawa,
K. Yamanouchi, S. Sakurai, H. Toga,
T. Fukunaga, Y. Nagasaka and N. Ohya

Division of Respiratory Diseases, Department of Internal
Medicine, Kanazawa Medical University,
Ishikawa 920-02, Japan

ABSTRACT

We measured the pharyngeal area of patients with OSA during sleep by the
acoustic reflection technique(ART) and found that their pharyngeal area which
is smaller than normal subjects decreased even further while they were asleep.
This is the first report of successful measurement of the pharyngeal area by
ART while breathing room-air(Air) in sleeping OSA patients.

KEYWORDS

Acoustic reflection technique; Airway area; Upper airway; OSA.

Although the factors producing closure of the upper airway(UAW) in patients
with OSA are still poorly understood, it is apparent that UAW in patients with
OSA is narrow even in the sitting position. Moreover, it is thought that OSA
patients are predisposed to the development of UAW occlusion during sleep
because of a decreased neural drive to the UAW muscles. However, there are few
reports on the morphology of UAW in sleeping OSA patients due to the lack of
suitable technique. Jackson et al.(1977) have invented a new technique permitting measurement of the airway area referred to as ART. Although there have
been many reports on UAW in awake OSA patients using ART, there have been none
concerning the UAW of sleeping patients using this technique. We measured the
pharyngeal area in OSA patients using ART in both the sitting and supine positions while they were awake and while asleep. This is a preliminary report.

SUBJECTS and METHODS

First, eight normal subjects were studied when breathing Air and when
breathing $80\%He-20\%O_2(He-O_2)$ to clarify if measurement of the airway area differs when using these two methods. Then, four OSA patients were studied while
they were awake and asleep during normal tidal breathing of Air following an
inspiration to total lung capacity in the sitting and supine positions. The
pharyngeal areas were measured every 0.3s; 50 area-distance functions were
determined during a single run spanning 4 to 5 tidal breaths. Then the patients fell asleep, after which measurements were made during tidal breathing
and apnea. Neither electroencephalogram nor electromyogram was recorded.

Advances in the Biosciences Vol. 79

207

ART is based on the analysis of acoustic pulse response measurement described
by Jackson et al.(1977) and Fredberg et al.(1980,1984). The apparatus consisted of a 4-m wave-tube, a horn driver centrally located on the tube, a pressure
transducer, and a minicomputer. A spirometer was attached to the tube at the
distal end to measure air-flow. A 33-cm curved tube was connected to the
other end of the wave-tube permitting measurement in the supine position.

RESULTS

Area-distance functions of each subject were arbitrarily divided into 9
divisions in order to compare the areas determined by the two methods(Fig.1).
The areas determined by breathing Air were identical to those determined by
breathing He-O$_2$ from P3 to P1; namely in the area of the pharynx(Fig.2).

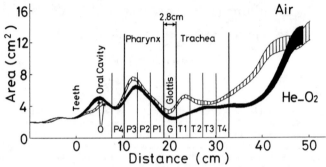

Fig.1. Typical area-distance functions obtained by breathing
He-O$_2$ and Air during quiet tidal breathing in the
same subject. The anatomic landmarks are indicated.
O:the largest area of the oral cavity, G:glottal segment, P:a part of the pharyngeal segment, T:a part of
the tracheal segment, He-O$_2$:80%He-20%O$_2$, Air:room-air.

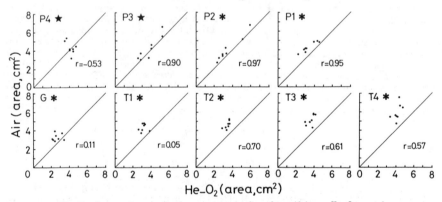

Fig.2. Comparison of airway areas by breathing He-O$_2$ and
breathing Air in all subjects. Solid line is line of
identity. r:correlation coefficient. ★:Not significant difference(P>0.05) in the average airway areas
of 8 normal subjects between the Air and the He-O$_2$.
✱:Significant difference(P<0.05). See Fig.2 for
definitions of abbreviations.

Pharyngeal cross-sectional areas of the 4 OSA patients were smaller than those of normal controls even in the sitting position. They became smaller in the supine position. While the patients were asleep, acoustic pulses were launched without interrupting their sleep, and we could obtain data except for a few instances in which the responses to the acoustic pulses passed through the open velum. Measurements were performed during apnea in one patient(Fig.3), during hypopnea in two, and during near normopnea in the remaining one. In all the patients, the pharyngeal areas were the narrowest while asleep.

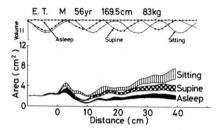

Fig.3. Pharyngeal areas in an OSA patient while awake in the
sitting and supine positions, and while asleep(apnea).

DISCUSSION

Details of the ART have been described by Jackson et al.(1977). Fredberg and his coworkers(1980;1984) modified it further and reported that by using He-O_2, the tracheal area determined by ART is highly accurate and reproducible. Although there have been many reports on UAW of awake OSA patients using ART both in the sitting and the supine positions(Hoffstein et al.,1984), there has been none on UAW of sleeping patients. It is thought to be difficult to measure UAW in sleeping patients using ART(He-O_2) because of difficulty in maintaining the concentration of He-O_2 within the airway and the system. There was small or no significant difference between the airway areas measured by both ART(He-O_2) and ART(Air) within the pharynx. These results are similar to those reported by Fredberg et al.(1980). When using Air, there was no problem of the gas concentration like He-O_2. When measureing the pharyngeal area particularly during asleep, breathing Air instead of the He-O_2 mixture is practical and adequate.

We preliminarily measured the pharyngeal area in 4 sleeping OSA patients. In all 4 patients the upper airway was narrower during sleep than while awake in the sitting or supine positions. We plan to study further how the stage of sleep affects the upper airway area.

REFERENCES

Brooks, L.J., R.G. Castile, G.M. Glass, N.T. Griscon, M.E.B. Wohl, and J.J. Fredberg(1984). Reproducibility and accuracy of airway areaby acoustic reflection. J. Appl. Physil., 57:777-787.
Fredberg, J.J., M.E.B. Wohl, G.M. Glass, and H.L. Dorkin(1980). Airway area by acoustic reflections measured at the mouth. J. Appl. Physiol., 48:749-758.
Hoffstein, V., N. Zamel, E.A. Phillipson(1984). Lung volume dependance of pharygeal cross-sectional area in patients with obstructive sleep apnea. Am. Rev. Respir. Dis., 130:175-178.
Jackson, A.C., J.P. Butler, E.J. Millet, F.G.Jr. Hoppin, and S.V. Dawson(1977). Airway geometry by analysis of acoustic pulse response measurements. J. Appl. Physiol., 43:523-536.

Load Compensation to Postural Change in Patients with Obstructive Sleep Apnea

M. Satoh, T. Chonan, W. Hida, S. Okabe,
H. Miki, O. Taguchi, Y. Kikuchi, N. Iwase,
C. Miura and T. Takishima

First Department of Internal Medicine, Tohoku
University School of Medicine, Sendai 980, Japan

ABSTRACT

We examined the effects of postural change on CO_2 responsiveness and breathing efficiency in 18 patients with obstructive sleep apnea (OSA). We measured responses of minute ventilation ($\dot{V}E$) and $P_{0.1}$ (mouth pressure 0.1 sec after the onset of occluded inspiration) to hypercapnia ($\Delta \dot{V}E/\Delta PCO_2$, $\Delta P_{0.1}/\Delta PCO_2$) produced by rebreathing. The ratio of the two ($\Delta \dot{V}E/\Delta P_{0.1}$) was taken as an index of breathing efficiency both in sitting and supine positions. There were no systematic changes in the resting values of end-tidal PCO_2, $P_{0.1}$, tidal volume, respiratory rate or $\dot{V}E$ between the two positions in all subjects, although functional residual capacity decreased significantly in the supine position as compared to the sitting position (mean decrease 0.55 L, $P<0.001$). The ratio of forced expiratory flow to forced inspiratory flow at mid-vital capacity (FEF_{50}/FIF_{50}) obtained from the maximal expiratory-inspiratory flow volume curve was significantly greater in the supine than in the sitting position (supine, 0.96 ± 0.05, mean $\pm$ SE; sitting, 0.90 ± 0.05, $P<0.01$). During CO_2 rebreathing, $\Delta \dot{V}E/\Delta P_{0.1}$ decreased significantly from the sitting to the supine position (sitting, 4.6 ± 0.5 L/min/cmH2O; supine, 3.9 ± 0.4, $P<0.01$), but $\Delta P_{0.1}/\Delta PCO_2$ was significantly greater in the supine than in the sitting position (supine, 0.67 ± 0.08 cmH2O/torr; sitting, 0.56 ± 0.09, $P<0.05$) and $\Delta \dot{V}E/\Delta PCO_2$ did not differ between the two positions. In 6 patients who underwent uvulopalatopharyngoplasty (UPPP) for treatment of OSA, breathing efficiency improved significantly in the supine, but did not change in the sitting position compared to the pre-UPPP state. These results suggest that in patients with OSA the postural change from the sitting to the supine position increases upper airway resistance and decreases breathing efficiency, but the inspiratory drive increases compensately to maintain the same level of ventilation. Load compensation mechanisms in OSA patients for increase in upper airway resistance appear to be operating during wakefulness.

KEYWORD

Breathing efficiency; control of breathing; hypercapnic ventilatory response; obstructive sleep apnea; position.

INTRODUCTION

Upper airway resistance in patients with obstructive sleep apnea (OSA) increases

TABLE 1 CO_2 responsiveness and breathing efficiency
in sitting and supine positions

	Sitting	Supine
$\Delta\dot{V}E/\Delta PCO_2$ (L/min/torr)	2.1 ± 0.2	2.1 ± 0.2
$\Delta Po.1/\Delta PCO_2$ (cmH2O/torr)	0.56 ± 0.09	0.67 ± 0.08*
$\Delta\dot{V}E/\Delta Po.1$ (L/min/cmH2O)	4.6 ± 0.5	3.9 ± 0.4**

Values are means ± SE.   *, **; Significantly different
from the vale in sitting position (* p<0.05, ** p<0.01)

significantly in the supine position (Anch et al., 1982), but the compensatory
capacity for an externally added load to breathing has been reported to be
impaired in patients with OSA (Rajagopal et al., 1984). However, the ability of
patients with OSA to compensate for internal increase in ventilatory load has
not been examined.   To assess the respiratory response of patients with OSA to
the increase in upper airway resistance induced by postural change, we measured
ventilatory and occlusion pressure responses to progressive hypercapnia in the
sitting and supine positions.

METHODS

The study was carried out in eighteen patients (17 males, 1 female) with OSA
previously diagnosed by polysomnography.   The age of the group was 45 ± 10 yr
(mean ± SD) and the weight was 76 ± 13 kg.   The subjects' apnea indices ranged
from 23.8 to 82.3 episodes/hour.   All were in a clinically stable condition and
free of complications such as lung disease or heart failure.   Written informed
consent was obtained from each subject before starting of this study.

Ventilatory response was measured with a circuit similar to that reported previously (Hida et al., 1987, Chonan et al., 1988).   After measurement of resting
values of respiratory frequency (f), tidal volume (VT), minute ventilation ($\dot{V}E$),
Po.1 (mouth pressure 0.1 sec after the onset of occluded inspiration) and end-
tidal PCO_2, ventilatory response to hypercapnia was measured by the rebreathing
method both in the sitting and supine positions.   Responses of $\dot{V}E$ and Po.1 to
the increase in PCO_2 were analyzed by linear regression.   The slope of ventilatory response to hypercapnia ($\Delta\dot{V}E/\Delta PCO_2$) divided by the slope of occlusion
pressure response to hypercapnia ($\Delta Po.1/\Delta PCO_2$) is $\Delta\dot{V}E/\Delta Po.1$, i.e., the increase
in ventilation obtained by a given rise in neuromuscular output.   This charac-
teristic index was defined as the breathing efficiency during hyperventilation
(Chonan et al., 1988).   In the supine position, the subjects laid on a height-
adjustable bed, the head supported by a pillow, and the neck contour was adjusted to be similar to that in the sitting position.   For each study, the rebreathing circuit was positioned to allow the subject to breathe through a mouthpiece
(rotated 90 for supine studies) with minimal effort.   All subjects remained
awake throughout the study.   The order of posture was randomized.   The change in
functional residual capacity (FRC) from the sitting to the supine position was
measured using a spirometer or by the helium dilution method.   Forced inspiratory and expiratory flow-volume curves were measured with a spirometer using a
direct pen-writing system (Takishima et al., 1972).   Three reproducible flow-
volume curves were obtained and the highest values of the forced inspiratory and
expiratory flows at mid-vital capacity (FIF50, FEF50) were calculated.   Upper
airway function was estimated by the ratio of the two, FEF50/FIF50 (Kryger et
al., 1976, Nishimaki et al., 1988).   Six patients who underwent uvulopalatopha-

ryngoplasty (UPPP) for treatment of OSA were retested 2-6 months after the operation. Statistical analysis were performed with the paired t-test and the values of $p<0.05$ were accepted as significant.

RESULTS

There were no systematic changes in the resting values of end-tidal PCO_2 (sitting vs supine, 36.5 ± 0.9 torr; 37.3 ± 0.9), $P_{O.1}$ (2.3 ± 0.2 cmH2O; 2.5 ± 0.1), tidal volume (0.65 ± 0.03 L; 0.62 ± 0.03), respiratory rate (15.5 ± 0.7 /min; 15.4 ± 0.7) or $\dot{V}_E$ (10.0 ± 0.5 L/min; 9.3 ± 0.5) between sitting and supine positions in all subjects. Functional residual capacity decreased significantly in the supine as compared to sitting position (mean decrease 0.55 L, $P<0.001$). The ratio of forced expiratory flow to forced inspiratory flow at mid-vital capacity (FEF_{50}/FIF_{50}) was significantly greater in the supine than in the sitting position (supine, 0.96 ± 0.05, mean $\pm$ SE; sitting, 0.90 ± 0.05, $P<0.01$). During CO_2 rebreathing, $\Delta\dot{V}_E/\Delta PCO_2$ did not differ between the two positions (supine, 2.1 ± 0.2 L/min/torr; sitting, 2.1 ± 0.2), but $\Delta P_{O.1}/\Delta PCO_2$ was significantly higher in the supine than in the sitting position (supine, 0.67 ± 0.08 cmH2O/torr; sitting, 0.56 ± 0.09, $P<0.05$). Breathing efficiency ($\Delta\dot{V}_E/\Delta P_{O.1}$) decreased significantly from the sitting to the supine position (sitting, 4.6 ± 0.5 L/min/cmH2O; supine, 3.9 ± 0.4, $P<0.01$). In 6 patients who underwent uvulopalatopharyngoplasty (UPPP), breathing efficiency improved significantly in the supine (before 3.8 ± 0.5; after 4.8 ± 0.5), but did not change in the sitting position (before 4.6 ± 0.7; after 4.7 ± 0.7), in comparison to the pre-UPPP state.

CONCLUSION

These results suggest that in patients with OSA, the postural change from the sitting to the supine position increases upper airway resistance and decreases breathing efficiency, but at a given level of CO_2 the inspiratory drive increases to maintain the same level of ventilation. Load compensation mechanisms in patients with OSA for increase in upper airway resistance appear to be operating during wakefulness.

REFERENCES

Anch AM, Remmers JE, Bunce H (1982). Supraglottic airway resistance in normal subjects and patients with occlusive sleep apnea. *J. Appl. Physiol.*, <u>53</u>, 1158-1163.

Chonan T, Hida W, Kikuchi Y, Shindoh C, Takishima T (1988). Role of CO2 responsiveness and breathing efficiency in determining exercise capacity of patients with chronic airway obstruction. *Am. Rev. Respir. Dis.*, <u>138</u>, 1488-1493.

Hida W, Suzuki R, kikuchi Y, Shindoh T, Chonan T, Sasaki H, Takishima T (1987). Effect of local vibration on ventilatory response to hypercapnia in normal subjects. *Bull. Eur. Physiopathol. Respir.*, <u>23</u>, 227-232.

Kryger M, Bode F, Antic R, Anthonisen N (1976). Diagnosis of obstruction of the upper and central airways. *Am. J. Med.*, <u>61</u>, 85-93.

Nishimaki C, Hida W, Miki H, Iwase N, Kikuchi Y, Inoue H, Takishima T (1988). Instability of extrathoracic airway during wakefulness affects sleep disordered breathing. *Am. Rev. Respir. Dis.*, <u>137</u>, A461.

Rajagopal KR, Abbrechet PH, Tellis CJ (1984). Control of breathing in obstructive sleep apnea. *Chest*, <u>85</u>, 174-180.

Takishima T, Sasaki T, Takahashi K, Sasaki H, Nakamura T (1972). Direct-writing recorder of the flow-volume curve and its clinical application. *Chest*, <u>61</u>, 262-266.

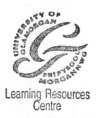

Learning Resources
Centre

Genioglossus and Inspiratory Pump Muscle Activity During Hypoxia, Hypercapnia and Sleep in Patients with Obstructive Sleep Apnea

S. Okabe, T. Chonan, W. Hida, M. Satoh,
O. Taguchi, Y. Kikuchi, H. Miki, N. Iwase
and T. Takishima

First Department of Internal Medicine, Tohoku
University School of Medicine, Sendai, Japan

ABSTRUCT

To examine the role of chemical drive in shaping the activity of the upper airway
and the inspiratory pump muscles during sleep in patients with obstructive sleep
apnea(OSA), we obtained electromyograms (EMG) of the genioglossus muscle (GG) and
inspiratory pump muscles (IPM) during hypoxia and hypercapnia in wakefulness and
non-REM sleep in six patients with OSA. Responses to hypoxia and to hypercapnia
were assessed by rebreathing in the supine position while awake. The sleep study
was conducted with the EMG electrodes placed in the same locations. The relationship between GG EMG and IPM EMG did not significantly differ between progressive hypoxia and hypercapnia during wakefulness. However GG EMG at a given level
of IPM EMG during apnea episodes was significantly greater than that obtained
during hypoxia and hypercapnia in wakefulness. This additional increase in GG
activity during apnea episodes may be due to mechanical drive induced by the
increase in intraluminal negative pressure of the upper airway.

KEYWORDS

Diaphragm; genioglossus muscle; hypercapnia; hypoxia; obstructive sleep apnea
syndrome; sleep.

INTRODUCTION

It has been suggested that in obstructive sleep apnea the inspiratory activity of
upper airway muscles diminishes at the onset of upper airway occlusion and passive collapse of the hypotonic pharynx occurs due to intraluminal negative pressure developed by the inspiratory pump muscles (Remmers et al., 1978). However,
it has been reported recently that inspiratory activity of the genioglossus
muscle occurs more frequently during sleep in patients with OSA than in control
subjects (Suratt et al., 1988) and that genioglossal EMG increases more than
diaphragmatic EMG during the latter half of the occulusive phase in patients with
OSA (Önal et al., 1982). The augmented upper airway muscle activity during OSA
has been explained by the compensatory mechanism to re-open the obstructed airway. However there is little information on the role of chemical drive in re-
cruiting upper airway muscles during the apneic phase in patients with OSA (Satoh
et al., 1989). In order to assess the possible role of chemical drive in modu-
lating upper airway and inspiratory pump muscle activity during obstructive

apnea, we measured the response of genioglossus (GG) and inspiratory pump muscle (IPM) activity during progressive hypoxia and hypercapnia in wakefullness, and during non-REM sleep in patients with OSA.

METHODS

The study was carried out in 6 male patients with OSA diagnosed by polysomnography. The average age of the group was 39.0+3.2 (mean+S.D.) and the average weight was 85.0+16.6kg. All were in a clinically stable condition and had no complications of lung disease or heart failure. The subjects apnea indices ranged between 38.9 and 86.0 episodes/hour. Responses to hypoxia at an end tidal PCO_2 of 45 torr and to hyperoxic hypercapnia were assessed by the rebreathing method while awake. The subject wore a noseclip and breathed through a mouthpiece connected to a rebreathing circuit in the supine position. End tidal PCO_2 and PO_2 were continuously monitored at the mouthpiece with a mass spectrometer (WSMR-1400, Westron) and arterial oxygen saturation was measured continuously with a pulse oximeter (Biox 3700, Ohmeda). In these hypoxic and hypercapnic tests, subjects rebreathed through a bag which contained a predetermined gas mixture: 25% O_2, 7% CO_2 in N_2 for the response to hypoxia and 7% CO_2 in O_2 for the response to hypercapnia. In the hypoxic test end-tidal PCO_2 was held constant (within 45+2 torr). GG EMG was measured with stainless steel wire electrodes inserted into the muscle percutaneously. IPM EMG was recorded with surface electrodes which were placed in the second intercostal space parasternally, or the seventh intercostal space at the mid-clavicular line. EMG signals were amplified, band-pass filtered, full-wave rectified and processed by "leaky" integrators. Peak integrated EMG activity was expressed as the percentage of the value at the lowest SaO_2 during the hypoxic test. The sleep study was performed in a quiet darkened room 1 or 2 hours after the last hypoxic or hypercapnic test with the EMG electrodes left in the same locations. The electroencephalogram and electrooculogram were recorded to determine sleep stages. Airflow at the nose and mouth was recorded with two thermistors. Thoraco-abdominal movement was measured with inductance plethysmographs which were placed at the level of mid-chest and umbilicus. Studies were performed in the supine position. Linear regression analysis was performed by the least squares method. All date are expressed as means+SD.

RESULTS AND DISCUSSION

Relationship between IPM and GG EMGs during progressive hypoxia and hypercapnia in wakefulness.

Both EMGs of IPM and GG showed phasic inspiratory activity in all patients examined and increased linearly with the decrease in arterial oxygen saturation (SaO_2) during progressive hypoxia and increase in end-tidal CO_2 fraction ($F_{ET}CO_2$) during progressive hypercapnia (Table 1). The response of EMG activity to hypoxia did not significantly differ between GG and IPM, nor did the response of EMG to hypercapnia differ significantly between GG and IPM. It has been reported that in normal volunteers the phasic inspiratory activity of the diaphragm and genioglossus muscles increases linearly with the decrease in SaO_2 during progressive hypoxia and with the increase in $F_{ET}CO_2$ during progressive hypercapnia (Onal et al., 1981). This is compatible with the data of the present study and suggests that during wakefulness the EMG response of GG and IPM to chemical stimuli is similar between normal subjects and patients with OSA.

The relationship between GG and IPM EMGs was compared between hypoxia and hypercapnia. The increase in GG EMG which accompanies a given increase in IPM EMG was 0.98+0.37 during hypoxia and 0.87+0.56 during hypercapnia and the two values were not significantly different. Bruce et al (1982) reported that the central chemoreceptor input preferentially increased phrenic nerve output, whereas peripheral

Table 1   Responses of IPM and GG EMGs to progressive hypoxia
(upper panel) and hypercapnia (lower panel)

		r	slope (units/%)
Hypoxia	IPM	0.85+0.13	-3.6+3.0
	GG	0.89+0.10	-3.9+1.7
Hypercapnia	IPM	0.94+0.02	36.1+15.3
	GG	0.80+0.13	29.3+12.1

chemoreceptor stimulation producred a greater increase in hypoglossal activity in anesthetized animals, but in awake animals genioglossal and diaphragmatic EMG responsed similarly during hypoxia and hypercapnia. Our data are compatible with the report on awake animals and suggest similar responsiveness of upper airway and chest wall inspiratory muscles to chemical stimuli.

Relationship between IPM and GG EMGs during sleep.

EMG activities during sleep were calculated from three consecutive pairs of apneic and postapneic ventilatory phases in each patient. In non-REM sleep both GG and IPM EMGs increased progressively during apneic episodes and the relationship between the two EMGs was linear (r = 0.78+0.05). The accentuation of GG activity which accompanied a given rise in IPM activity during non-REM sleep was 2.75+1.65 and significantly greater than that during hypoxia* and hypercapnia in wakefullness. GG activity at a given level of IPM EMG during apnea episodes was significantly greater than that obtained during awake hypoxic and hypercapnic tests. The additional increase in GG activity during apnea episodes may be due to mechanical drive induced by the increase in intraluminal negative pressure of the upper airway. Alternatively, it is also possible that IPM activity is inhibited at a given level of chemical stimulus through stimulation of the superior laryngeal nerve (Bellingham et al., 1989). The relative activation of genioglossus muscle against inspiratory pump muscles appears to be a non-chemical compensatory response to re-open the obstructed upper airway in patients with OSA.

REFERENCES

Bellingham, M.C., J. Lipski and M.D. Voss (1989). Synaptic inhibition of phrenic motoneurones evoked by stimulation of the superior laryngeal nerve. Brain Research, 486, 391-395.
Bruce, E.N., J. Mitra and N.S. Cherniack (1982). Central and peripheral chemoreceptor inputs to phrenic and hypoglossal motoneurons. J. Appl. Physiol., 53, 1504-1511.
Önal, E., M. Lopata and T. O'connor (1981). Diaphragmatic and genioglossal electromyogram responses to isocapnic hypoxia in humans. Am. Rev. Respir. Dis., 124, 215-217.
Önal, E., M. Lopata and T. O'connor (1982). Pathogenesis of apneas in hypersomnia-sleep apnea syndrome. Am. Rev. Respir. Dis., 125, 167-174.
Remmers, J.E., W.j. deGroot, E.K. Sauerland and A.M.Anch (1978). Pathogenesis of upper airway occulusion during sleep. J. Appl. Physiol., 44, 931-938.
Satoh, M., W. HIda, T. Chonan, H. Miki, N. Iwase, O. Taguchi, S. Okabe, Y. Kikuchi, H. Inoue and T. Takishima (1989). Role of hypoxic drive in the control of breathing during non-REM sleep in patients with obstructive sleep apnea. Am. Rev. Respir. Dis., 139, A81.
Suratt, P.M., R.F. Mctier and S.C. Wilhoit (1988). Upper airway muscle cativation is augmented in patients with obstructive sleep apnea compared with that in normal subjects. Am. Rev. Respir. Dis., 137, 889-894.

Section 3
RESPIRATORY MUSCLES
AND DYSPNEA

Involvement of Sensory and Motor Cortex in Human Respiratory Control

S.C. Gandevia

Department of Clinical Neurophysiology, Institute of
Neurological Sciences, The Prince Henry and Prince of
Wales Hospitals and School of Medicine, University of
New South Wales, Sydney, N.S.W. 2036, Australia

ABSTRACT

Based on electrophysiological studies in human subjects evidence is
presented to suggest that respiratory muscle afferents project to the
sensorimotor cortex, and that corticofugal projections can powerfully address
respiratory motoneurones via oligosynaptic pathways. These afferent and
efferent projections are similar to those documented for distal limb muscles.
Furthermore, these projections emphasize the likely importance of cortical
mechanisms in the control of human respiration.

KEYWORDS

Kinaesthesia; motor cortex; muscle spindle endings; respiratory muscles;
sensory cortex.

INTRODUCTION

The wide range of behavioural control of human respiration has long been
recognized. However, it has been difficult to describe the neural mechanisms
which permit this respiratory repertoire. This presentation provides a link
between some of the fundamental studies on rhythm generation posed early
in the Symposium and the behavioural and psychophysical studies reported
subsequently. One aim has been to determine whether basic neural
mechanisms available for control of human limb muscles are also available
for respiratory muscles. This has been approached in three ways. Firstly, do
muscle afferents innervating specialized receptors (muscle spindle endings
and Golgi tendon organs) project to the human cerebral cortex for both
respiratory and limb muscles? Secondly, is the human motor cortical output

capable of driving respiratory motoneurone pools in a relatively direct way? Finally, given that some sensory inputs involved in dyspnoea are unique (e.g. changes in blood gas tensions), are there other neural mechanisms involved in this sensation which do have a parallel with limb muscle kinaesthesia? Evidence is briefly reviewed below to indicate that all three questions can be answered in the affirmative.

Projections to the sensorimotor cortex by respiratory muscle afferents

Afferents from respiratory muscles have long been known to influence respiration although it is only recently than an interest in the projection of these afferents to the sensorimotor cortex has developed. Clearly, the electrophysiological demonstration of such a projection would be consistent with the postulated role for these afferents in kinaesthetic judgements about respiratory and truncal movements (e.g. Gandevia et al., 1981). Two approaches have been adopted to assess this possibility in human subjects. Davenport and colleagues (1986) examined averaged electroencephalographic changes following airway occlusion with a shutter. Complex cerebral evoked potentials were recorded following occlusion with a prominent positive wave at approximately 60 ms. If this were the first cortical activity produced by the complex afferent inputs associated with occlusion, its latency is relatively long, given that stimulation of mixed nerves at ankle level produces focal cerebral potentials at approximately 40 ms (e.g. Burke et al., 1981). We adopted an alternative strategy in which muscle afferents innervating one intercostal space were stimulated electrically with a near-nerve microelectrode in the mid-clavicular line (Gandevia and Macefield, 1989). The stimulus intensity was adjusted to produce a strong local contraction medial to the electrode with no cutaneous paraesthesiae. Although activating a limited number of respiratory muscle afferents such stimuli evoked cortical potentials averaged from scalp electrodes (Fig. 1). The amplitude of the response is similar to that for many other single limb muscles. The activity was maximal towards the midline, consistent with a projection to the medial region of the somatosensory "strip". The latency of the earliest detectable near-field activity was 20-25 ms, depending on the site and segmental level of intercostal nerve stimulation. One aspect of this cortical projection which may set it apart from that for limb muscles (see Gandevia and Burke, 1988; Macefield and Gandevia, 1989) is that its onset latency is relatively long, given the total conduction distance to the brain. This suggests that perhaps the *central* conduction time from respiratory (truncal) and even proximal upper limb muscles may be relatively longer than for distal muscles. These findings suggest that an oligosynaptic projection to the somatosensory cortex is present for respiratory as well as limb muscles. However, we do not yet know exactly which rapidly conducting muscle afferents contribute to the projection (i.e. muscle spindle or tendon organ afferents) or the sites and properties of the synaptic relays involved.

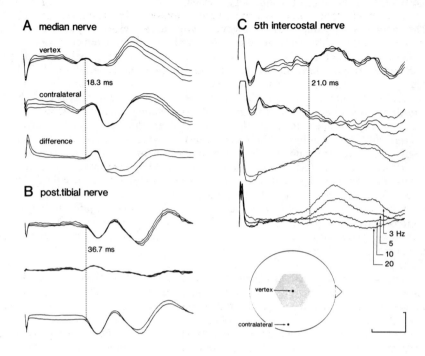

Fig. 1. Cerebral potentials evoked by transcutaneous stimulation of the median nerve at the wrist (A) and posterior tibial nerve at the ankle (B), and by intramuscular microstimulation of the fifth intercostal nerve (C). Negativity is shown upwards. Upper set of traces in each panel was recorded over the vertex and the second set over the 'hand area', contralateral to the side to which stimuli were delivered (see schematic diagram of head; the shaded area envelops usual recording montage). Reference electrode in contralateral earlobe. Each set has duplicate averages (n=512 in A and B, n=1024 in C) and the mean. Third set of duplicate traces represents near-field activity reconstructed from the difference potential between vertex and contralateral electrode sites. Onset of cortical potentials is defined from the difference potential and indicated by a vertical line. The initial cortical component of cerebral response to median stimulation is a focal negativity at the contralateral electrode (A); that to stimulation of posterior tibial nerve (B) and intercostal nerve (C) is a focal positivity and a negativity respectively, at the vertex. Lowest set of traces in C show the differential potentials as a function of stimulation frequency; the cortical potentials attenuate with increasing stimulus frequency. Amplitude calibration: 4 μV for A and B, 1 μV for C. Time calibration: 10 msec for A and C, 20 msec for B. (Reproduced with permission from Gandevia and Macefield, 1989).

Corticospinal actions on respiratory muscles

The nature of corticofugal pathways involved in respiratory motor control
has aroused less interest than those involved in limb movements (see Porter,
1985). The neurosurgical experience with motor cortical stimulation gave
little clue that it may markedly influence respiration (Penfield and Boldrey,
1937). The advent of non-invasive methods to activate the human
corticofugal output through the skull permitted a reinvestigation of this
question. Motor cortical stimulation using a single electrical stimulus with
the anode positioned towards the midline over the sensorimotor strip (i.e.
medial to the hand/arm representation) produces overt contraction of
respiratory and truncal muscles, especially when the muscles are already
contracting weakly (Gandevia and Rothwell, 1987; Gandevia and Plassman,
1989; Plassman and Gandevia, 1989). Such contractions occur following
single transcranial electrical stimuli although such stimuli can produce
multiple descending volleys through direct and transynaptic activation of
corticofugal cells (see Day *et al.*, 1987). These studies have revealed the
following properties for the corticofugal projection to human respiratory
muscles:

(i)   single cortical stimuli can produce a powerful drive to respiratory
muscles as judged by the duration and amplitude of the evoked muscle
action potentials and the size of the "pressure twitch";

(ii)   the latency of the cortically evoked EMG responses is relatively short,
with the central conduction time (from near the motor cortex to near the
motoneurone pool) being similar for respiratory and non-respiratory
muscles with motor pools at the same segmental level.

(iii)   the duration of the initial excitatory event within single abdominal
motoneurones (~1 ms) is the same as that for motoneurones of intrinsic hand
muscles (e.g. Day *et al.*, 1987).

(iv)   the cortical projection to respiratory muscles can still be demonstrated
during rebreathing when the chemical drive to breathe increases. The
overall projection may have similar potency during voluntary, rather than
chemically-driven respiration, at the same level of ventilation (Murphy et
al., 1990).

(v)   the one difference between the response to cortical stimulation for
limb and inspiratory muscles is that during breath-holding the amplitude of
cortically evoked responses declines progressively over 10-20 s for the
diaphragm whereas it remains constant for distal limb muscles (Gandevia *et
al.*, 1988).

Points (ii) and (iii) above form part of the argument that the human
corticospinal system may have evolved an oligosynaptic, possibly
monosynaptic, excitatory projection (Plassman and Gandevia, 1989). While
the techniques used for these studies are less direct than can be applied in

animal studies, they point to a need to reinvestigate this projection in sub-human primates. Indeed, Leyton and Sherrington (1917) in their detailed mapping of the motor cortex in the sub-human primates mention that stimulation at the appropriate locus produced contralateral chest or abdominal movements. Studies to date in the cat using electrophysiological and anatomical techniques have yielded no consensus about the role of corticospinal and corticoreticulospinal contributions to the "projection" (Lipski et al., 1986; Rickard-Bell et al., 1986; see also Planche, 1972; Aoki et al., this volume).

Further evidence for a powerful ability of volition to access respiratory motoneurones comes from the observation that the diaphragm can apparently be driven maximally during some voluntary respiratory tasks - such as a maximal inspiratory or maximal expulsive manoeuvre. This conclusion is based upon studies in which supramaximal phrenic nerve stimulation, interpolated during the attempted maximal effort fails to add to the voluntarily generated output from phrenic motoneurones (e.g. Bellemare and Bigland-Ritchie, 1984; Gandevia and McKenzie, 1985). While the studies in conscious human subjects using either transcranial cortical stimulation and phrenic nerve stimulation are limited in their capacity to prove the nature of the corticofugal connection with respiratory and truncal motoneurones, they emphasize the potency of the connection and its potential similarity with that to limb muscles.

Respiratory muscle kinaesthesia and dyspnoea

Many hypotheses have been put forward over the decades to isolate the mechanisms involved in the sensation of breathlessness or dyspnoea. Even if the definition of dyspnoea is restricted, for example, to a sensation of difficulty in breathing, then no *single* peripheral signal from the lung, chest wall or diaphragm will subserve it, nor will an isolated signal related to the central drive to breathe. Under specific circumstances it is probable that signals generated by intrapulmonary receptors (stimulated for example by histamine) and signals from peripheral and central chemoreceptors (for example in breath-holding) may contribute to respiratory sensations. Some mechanisms which have been established for respiratory muscle kinaesthesia include: (i) the likely contribution from respiratory muscle afferents to the detection of inspiratory loads (e.g. Gandevia et al., 1981) and (ii) the likely contribution from signals related to centrally-generated motor commands or effort (such as may occur during respiratory muscle weakness and changes in the relationship between muscle force and lung volume [e.g. Campbell et al., 1980]). While the latter mechanisms have clear parallels with kinaesthesia in limb muscles (for review see Gandevia, 1988), it is clear that other mechanisms may also be involved, either above or in combination with the above kinaesthetic mechanisms. For example, recent studies indicate that breathlessness may be increased when end-tidal CO_2 is elevated but other respiratory variables (including ventilation) are held constant (Adams et al., 1985; see also Banzett et al., 1989).

CONCLUSION

This presentation emphasizes neural mechanisms related to the "encephalization" of human respiration - in particular the powerful, oligosynaptic projections to and from the sensorimotor cortex involving respiratory and truncal muscles. Further studies may reveal the way in which these projections function during the variety of respiratory gymnastics performed in everyday activities.

ACKNOWLEDGEMENTS

Work in our laboratory is supported by the National Health and Medical Research Council and the Asthma Foundation of New South Wales. I am especially grateful to Drs. D.K. McKenzie and G. Macefield for their collaborations and comments on the manuscript.

REFERENCES

Adams, L., R. Lane, S.A. Shea, A. Cockcroft, and A. Guz (1985). Breathlessness during different forms of ventilatory stimulation: a study of mechanisms in normal subjects and respiratory patients. *Clin. Sci.*, 69, 663-672.

Banzett, R.B., R.W. Lansing, M.B. Reid, L. Adams, and R. Brown (1989). 'Air hunger' arising from increased PCO_2 in mechanically ventilated quadriplegics. *Respir. Physiol.*, 76, 53-68.

Bellemare, F. and B. Bigland-Ritchie (1984). Assessment of human diaphragm strength and activation using phrenic nerve stimulation. *Respir. Physiol.*, 58, 263-267.

Burke, D., N.F. Skuse and A..K. Lethlean (1981). Cutaneous and muscle afferent components of the cerebral potential evoked by electrical stimulation of human peripheral nerves. *Electroencephalogr. clin. Neurophysiol.*, 51, 579-588;

Campbell, E.J.M., S.C. Gandevia, K.J. Killian, C.K. Mahutte, and J.R.A. Rigg (1980). Changes in the perception of inspiratory resistive loads during partial curarization. *J. Physiol. (Lond.)*, 309, 93-100.

Davenport, P.W., W.A. Friedman, F.J. Thompson, and O. Franzen, (1986). Respiratory-related cortical potentials evoked by inspiratory occlusion in humans. *J. Appl. Physiol.*, 60, 1843-1848.

Day, B.L., J.C. Rothwell, P.D. Thompson, J.P.R. Dick and J.M.A. Cowan (1987). Motor cortex stimulation in intact man: II. Multiple descending volleys. *Brain*, 110, 1191-1209.

Gandevia, S.C. (1988). Neural mechanisms underlying the sensation of breathlessness: kinesthetic parallels between respiratory and limb muscles. *Aust. N.Z. J. Med.*, 18, 83-91.

Gandevia, S.C. and D. Burke (1988). Projection to the cerebral cortex from proximal and distal muscles in the human upper limb. *Brain*, 111, 389-403.

Gandevia, S.C., W.N. Gardner, B.L. Plassman and J.C. Rothwell (1988). Effects of motor cortical stimulation on human respiratory muscles during different tasks. *J. Physiol. (Lond.)*, 403, 77P.

Gandevia, S.C., K.J. Killian and E.J.M. Campbell (1981). The contribution of upper airway and inspiratory muscle mechanisms to the detection of pressure changes at the mouth in normal subjects. *Clin. Sci.*, 60, 513-518.

Gandevia, S.C. and G. Macefield (1989). Projection of low-threshold afferents from human intercostal muscles to the cerebral cortex. *Respir. Physiol.*, 77, 203-214.

Gandevia, S.C. and D.K. McKenzie (1985). Activation of the human diaphragm during maximal voluntary contractions. *J. Physiol. (Lond.)*, 367, 45-56.

Gandevia, S.C. and B.L. Plassman (1988). Responses in human intercostal and truncal muscles to motor cortical and spinal stimulation. *Respir. Physiol.*, 73, 325-338.

Gandevia, S.C. and J.C. Rothwell (1987). Activation of the human diaphragm from the motor cortex. *J. Physiol. (Lond.)*, 384, 109-118.

Leyton, A.S.F. and C.S. Sherrington (1917). Observations on the excitable cortex of the chimpanzee, orang-utan, and gorilla. *J. Exp. Physiol.*, 11, 135-222.

Lipski, J., A. Bektas and R. Porter (1986). Short latency inputs to phrenic motoneurones from the sensorimotor cortex in the cat. *Exp. Brain Res.*, 61, 280-290.

Murphy, K., A. Mier, L. Adams and A. Guz (1990). Putative cerebral cortical involvement in the ventilatory response to inhaled CO_2 in conscious man. *J. Physiol (Lond.)*, 420, 1-18.

Penfield, W. and E. Boldrey (1937). Somatic motor and sensory representation in the cerebral cortex of man as studied by electrical stimulation. *Brain*, 60, 389-443.

Planche, D. (1972). Effets de la stimulation du cortex cérébral sur l'activité du nerf phrénique. *Journal de physiologie*, 64, 31-56.

Plassman, B.L. and S.C. Gandevia (1989). Comparison of human motor cortical projections to abdominal muscles and intrinsic muscles of the hand. *Exp. Brain Res.*, 78, 301-308.

Porter, R. (1985). The corticomotoneuronal component of the pyramidal tract: corticomotoneuronal connections and functions in primates. *Brain Res.*, 10, 1-26.

Rickard-Bell, G.C., E.K. Bystrzycka and B.S. Nail (1986). Distribution of corticospinal motor fibres within the cervical spinal cord with special reference to the phrenic nucleus: a WGA-HRP anterograde transport study in the cat. *Brain Res.*, 379, 75-83.

Mechanoreceptors and Respiratory Sensation

Ikuo Homma, Arata Kanamaru and
Masato Sibuya

Department of Physiology, Showa University School of
Medicine, 1-5-8 Hatanodai, Shinagawa-ku, Tokyo 142,
Japan

ABSTRACT

Afferent activities from mechanoreceptors in the respiratory muscles are considered important in respiratory sensation. In this study, specific chest wall
vibration was applied to the upper inspiratory intercostal muscles and lower
expiratory intercostal muscles either in-phase with muscle contraction (upper
chest wall vibration during inspiration and lower during expiration), or out-of-
phase with contraction (upper during expiration and lower during inspiration).
In- and out-of-phase vibration induced cerebral evoked potentials. The source
generator producing these potentials was estimated by the dipole tracing method.
The source generator was located in the brainstem during in-phase vibration and
in the thalamus during out-of-phase vibration. During out-of-phase vibration,
subjects perceived the unpleasant sensation of dyspnea. These results suggest
that the generation of breathlessness may be strongly related to the thalamus.

KEYWORDS

In-phase vibration; out-of-phase vibration; breathlessness;
dipole-tracing method; brainstem; thalamus.

INTRODUCTION

The mechanism of respiratory sensation has been discussed for a long time.
Among various respiratory sensations, dyspnea has attracted the most attention,
as it is an important symptom in patients suffering from airway obstruction,
diffuse infiltrated lung, heart failure, pleural disorders and chest wall diseases. The sensation is a product of several steps including activation of
sensory receptors, transmission of the sensory activities to the central nervous
system, and activation of the higher center. Receptors that play a role in
respiratory sensation are mainly mechanoreceptors, which can be divided into two
groups according to their location. One group is located in the airway and the
afferent activities are transmitted to the brain via the vagal nerve. The other
group is located in the chest wall. The afferent activities from the chest wall
mechanoreceptors have been considered to be important for respiratory sensation
since the length-tension inappropriate theory was suggested to explain the generation of breathlessness (Campbell and Howell, 1963).

Vibration has been used to stimulate muscle mechanoreceptors. Many years ago it was reported that high frequency stretching of muscles stimulates receptors in the muscle spindle, especially muscle spindle primary endings (Granit and Henatch, 1956, Bianconi and Van Der Meulen, 1963). Sustained vibration applied to a human limb muscle induces a tonic contraction (Eklund and Hagbarth, 1966, Hagbarth and Eklund, 1966). This reflex is called tonic vibration reflex (TVR). Receptors operating in this reflex have been considered to be the muscle spindle primary endings.

The effect of vibration applied to the human chest wall was first reported by Gandevia and McCloskey (1976) using longitudinal sternal vibration. Homma et al. (1978) applied vibration more selectively either to the upper or the lower chest wall in man. In the thorax, only two regions have single-layered intercostal muscles. One region includes the second and third parasternal intercostal spaces where inspiratory muscle activities are recorded. The other region includes the seventh to tenth intercostal spaces at the anterior axillary line where expiratory activities are recorded (Taylor, 1960, Homma et al., 1978). Vibration, with frequency of 100 Hz and amplitude of about 1 mm, applied to the upper chest wall induces a sustained contraction in the underlying inspiratory intercostal muscles. Vibration applied to the lower chest wall induces a sustained contraction in the underlying expiratory intercostal muscles (Homma et al., 1978, Homma et al., 1981).

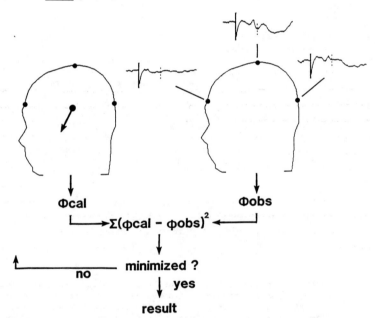

Fig. 1. The dipole tracing method.
Three recordings (right) showing stimulus-induced potentials at a specific latency were observed with electrodes placed in different areas of the scalp (defined as Φobs). A dipole current is assumed in the brain and the potential distribution yielded by the dipole on the scalp is calculated (defined as Φcal). The location of the dipole is shifted until the mean-squared deviation between Φobs and Φcal reach a minimum.

In-phase and Out-of-phase Vibration and Sensation

Short-span vibration was applied to the chest wall in phase with respiration. When vibration was applied to the upper chest wall during inspiration and to the lower chest wall during expiration, inspiratory and expiratory activities were augmented, respectively. Vibration applied to the upper chest wall during inspiration was called inspiratory in-phase vibration, and vibration applied to the lower chest wall during expiration was called expiratory in-phase vibration. Contrary to in-phase vibration, vibration applied to the upper chest wall during expiration and to the lower chest wall during inspiration was called out-of-phase vibration (Homma et al., 1978).

These phases in chest wall vibration yielded critical differences in the respiratory sensation they induced. During in-phase vibration, subjects perceived correctly that their respiratory movements increased in amplitude and the subjects did not perceive any unpleasant sensation. However, when vibration was applied out-of-phase with the contracting intercostal muscles, and thus the intercostal afferents were mismatched with the respiratory phase, the subjects experienced an unpleasant sensation of breathlessness (Homma et al., 1984).

A   **B**

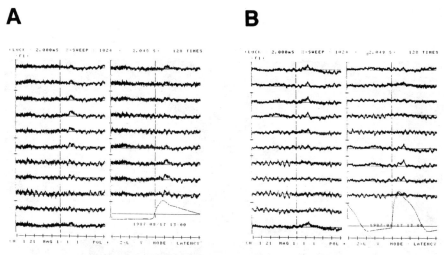

Fig. 2.   EEG waves recorded from 21 electrodes placed
          according to the 10-20 method were triggered at the
          onset of expiration and 128 potentials were
          averaged. In both A and B, the potentials in the
          left column were recorded from electrodes Fp1 and
          F3 to Oz and those in the right from Fp2 and F4 to
          Pz. Pz recording was replaced with the airflow
          recording; the upward deflection indicates expira-
          tion. Time marker at the bottom indicates 200
          msec/div. A: during in-phase vibration, B: during
          out-of-phase vibration.

Localization of the Source Generator in the Human Brain Associated with
Breathlessness

Recently Davenport et al. (1986) recorded respiratory related evoked potentials
elicited by airway occlusion from electrodes placed on the human scalp. And
even more recently, Gandevia and Macefield (1989) reported on cortical evoked
potentials elicited by electrical stimulation applied to human intercostal
nerves. These reports show that respiratory sensory information is transmitted
to the cortex. However, the relationship of sensory evoked potentials and subjective sensation, or the location of source generators has not been elucidated.

To estimate the location of the electric source generator in the human brain, a
dipole tracing method was developed (He et al., 1987, Homma et al., 1987). Fig.
1 shows the basic idea of the dipole tracing method. The potential distribution, measured from electrodes placed on the scalp, was defined as Φobs. A
dipole current was assumed in the brain, and a potential distribution that would
be seen on the scalp due to this dipole was calculated as Φcal. The location
of the dipole was shifted until the mean-squared deviation between the observed
and calculated potential distribution reached a minimum. The final dipole was
estimated to be the source generator of brain activity.

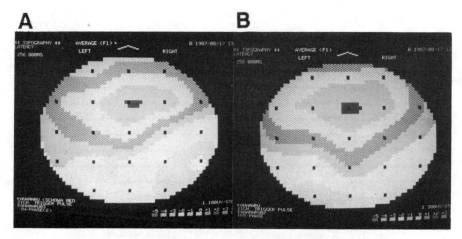

Fig. 3. Topography of the 21 potentials at 252 msec after
the onset of expiration observed during in-phase
vibration (A) and at 256 msec during out-of-phase
vibration (B). Dark spots in the center indicate
the highest voltage change.

Sixteen or twenty-one surface electrodes were placed on the scalp of the subjects according to the international 10-20 method for EEG. EEG wave, obtained
from each electrode, were triggered and averaged at the onset of expiration.
Triggering signals were obtained from a flowmeter attached to the mouthpiece and
128 wave potentials were averaged. In-phase or out-of-phase vibration was applied to the thorax while EEG potentials were recorded. Fig. 2A shows the averaged potentials of 128 breaths recorded from 21 electrodes during in-phase
vibration. A large positive potential can be seen 250 msec later than the trigger. Fig. 2B shows the averaged potential of 128 breaths during out-of-phase
vibration. A large positive wave can also be seen 250 msec after the trigger.
Topographies of the 21 potentials 256 msec after the onset of expiration showed
a large potential in almost the center of the cortex during both in- and out-of-
phase vibration (Fig. 3). These two topographies showed no differences. However, the location of source generator induced by in- and out-of-phase vibration
was different. The dipole of the wave obtained during in-phase vibration was
located deep in the brain. However, the dipole obtained during out-of-phase
vibration was located somewhat higher than the dipole induced by in-phase vibration. Fig. 4 shows the sagittal plane of an MRI image. The localization of the
source generators was superimposed on the MRI image. The source generator obtained during in-phase vibration corresponded to the brainstem and that obtained
during out-of-phase vibration corresponded to the thalamus.

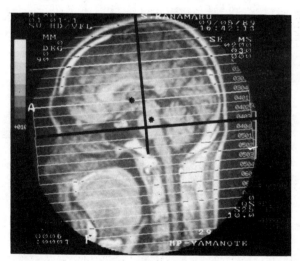

Fig. 4.   Calculated source generators superimposed on an MRI
          image. Two black dots indicate the location of the
          source generator obtained by the dipole tracing
          method. Lower: during in-phase vibration, upper:
          during out-of-phase vibration.

234   I. Homma et al.

In-phase and out-of-phase vibration induced different sensations. Illusive
sensation was induced and the subjects sensed breathlessness when muscle spindle
afferents from intercostal muscles were mismatched with the phase of contraction. The fact that the source generator was located in the thalamus during
out-of-phase vibration suggests that the generation of the unpleasant sensation,
breathlessness, may be strongly related to the thalamus as other genetic sensations have been shown to be.

          REFERENCES

Bianconi, R. and J. P. Van Der Meulen (1963). The response to vibration of the
    end organs of mammalian muscle spindles. J. Neurophysiol., 26, 177-190.
Campbell, E. J. M. and J. B. L. Howell (1963). The sensation of breathlessness.
    Brit. Med. Bull., 19, 36-40.
Davenport, P. W., W. A. Friedman, F. J. Thompson and O. Franzen (1986). Respi-
    ratory-related cortical potentials evoked by inspiratory occlusion in humans.
    J. Appl. Physiol., 60, 1843-1848.
Eklund, G. and K-E. Hagbarth (1966). Normal variability of tonic vibration re-
    flex in man. Exp. Neurol., 16, 80-92.
Gandevia, S. C. and D. I. McCloskey (1976). Changes in the pattern of breathing
    caused by chest vibration. Respir. Physiol., 26, 163-171.
Gandevia, S. C. and G. Macefield (1989), Projection of low threshold afferents
    from human intercostal muscles to the cerebral cortex. Respir. Physiol., 77,
    203-214.
Granit, R. and H. D. Henatch (1956). Gamma control of dynamic properties of
    muscle spindles. J. Neurophysiol., 19, 356-366.
Hagbarth, K-E. and G. Eklund (1966). Motor effects of vibratory muscle stimuli
    in man. In: Nobel Symposium I, Muscular Afferents and Motor Control. (R.
    Granit, ed.), Almqvist and Wiksell, Stockholm, pp. 177-186.
He, B., T. Musha, Y. Okamoto, S. Homma, Y. Nakajima and T. Sato (1987). Electirc
    dipole tracing in the brain by means of the boundary element method and its
    accuracy. IEEE Transactions on Biomedical Engineering, BME-34, 406-414.
Homma, I., G. Eklund, and K-E. Hagbarth (1978). Respiration in man affected by
    TVR contractions elicited in inspiratory and expiratory intercostal muscles.
    Respir. Physiol., 35, 335-348.
Homma, I., T. Nagai, T. Sakai, M. Ohashi, M. Beppu and K. Yonemoto (1981).
    Effect of chest wall vibration on ventilation in patients with spinal cord
    lesion. J. Appl. Physiol., 50 107-111.
Homma, I, T. Obata, M. Sibuya, and M. Uchida (1984). Gate mechanism in breath-
    lessness caused by chest wall vibration in humans. J. Appl. Physiol., 56, 8-
    11.
Homma, S., Y. Nakajima, T. Musha, Y. Okamoto and B. He (1987). Dipole-tracing
    method applied to human brain potentials. J. of Neurosci Methods. 21, 195-200.
Taylor, A. (1960). The contribution of the intercostal muscles to the effort of
    respiration in man. J. Physiol. , 151, 390-402.

Chest Wall Mechanisms in Respiratory Sensation

Murray D. Altose

Department of Medicine, Case Western Reserve
University, Cleveland, OH 44106, USA

ABSTRACT

The sensation of respiratory force corresponds in large part to
the sense of effort arising from corollary discharges of central
motor command signals. However, feedback from chest wall mechanoreceptors also plays a critical role in shaping respiratory
sensations. Chest wall vibration to activate muscle spindles
affects various sensations associated with breathing. Specific
cortical evoked potentials are associated with chest wall vibration suggesting that afferent impulses from chest wall muscle
receptors are transmitted to higher brain centers to directly
influence respiratory sensation. A role for chest wall receptors
in mediating certain respiratory sensations is also suggested by
the finding that when ventilation is voluntarily reduced below
spontaneously adopted levels, the intensity of dyspnea increases.
Limiting thoracic displacement or respiratory muscle force seems
to reduce some inhibitory feedback to either brain stem or cortical centers. Chest wall mechanoreceptor inputs and the resulting
sensation responses may be important in the behavioral control of
the level and pattern of breathing.

KEY WORDS

Respiratory sensation; dyspnea; chest wall vibration; respiratory
muscle mechanoreceptors; control of breathing.

INTRODUCTION

Breathing is controlled automatically by networks of neurons in
the brain stem that receive input from (a) chemoreceptors in the
blood and brain that are activated by changes in oxygen and
carbon dioxide tensions in the body from (b) mechanoreceptors in
the respiratory muscles, airways, lungs and chest wall that
monitor muscle tension, airflow, lung expansion and thoracic
excursions. Breathing is also under volitional control along
separate anatomical pathways from higher brain centers to spinal
motor neurons (Plum, 1970).

On a very short term basis, during vocalization or breathholding for example, behavioral systems can suppress and override the automatic control of breathing. There is also reason to believe that volitional or behavioral factors can also result in long term or persistent changes in the level and pattern of breathing (Sorli et al., 1978).

Purposeful volitional control of breathing requires that the higher brain is apprised of the state and condition of the respirtory muscles, the metabolic milieu and the mechanics of the ventilatory apparatus. With respect to breathing, however, little is known about sensory projections to the cerebral cortex. In recent years, psychophysical studies have established that sensory information from the respiratory system does reach cortical substrates for perception and volitional control of breathing.

                    PSYCHOPHYSICAL STUDIES

Studies of respiratory sensation have used techniques developed by psychophysicists to quantitate the sensory experience of various physical stimuli. In direct magnitude scaling, stimuli over a wide range of intensities are applied and the resulting subjective sensation responses can be expressed on a variety of different scales.

In rating scaling, the response is made by assigning a numerical value proportional to the magnitude of the sensation. If one stimulus is perceived to be twice a intense as another, it is assigned twice the numerical value. Alternatively, in cross modality matching, the sensation response is expressed by adjusting some other signal such as the force on a dynamometer in response to changes in the perceived intensity of the test stimulus. Visual analog scaling is another form of cross modality matching where line length serves as a the response continuum.

Ratio scaling has shown that the respiratory sensations of force and displacement are similar to other sensory modalities in that a constant percentage change in stimulus magnitude produces a constant percentage change in sensation level. There is a power function relationship between stimulus magnitude (S) and sensation response (R) according to the psychophysical power law:

$$R = K S^n$$

where K is a constant and n is the exponent describing the rate of growth of sensation as the stimulus increases (Stevens, 1957).

Scaling studies have been performed that involve the magnitude estimation of a wide range of easily discernible external elastic and resistive ventilatory loads. When breathing against ventilatory loads of increasing magnitude, there is a progressive increase in sensation intensity and the relationship between load magnitude and the resulting sensation follows the psychophysical power law (Altose and Cherniack, 1981). The intensity of the sensation during loaded breathing, however, is not strictly a function of the added elastance or resistance. It appears that load sensation is preferentially based on the level and duration

of the forces generated by the respiratory muscles during loaded breathing (Killian et al., 1982).
Force sensation can be mediated by feedback of afferent signals from muscle receptors or by corollary discharges of central nervous system motor command signals. Afferent signals of muscle tension and motor command signals can be separately and independently quantitated in the assessment of both limb and respiratory muscle force (McCloskey et al., 1974). Normally, there is a close relationship between the level of motor command to muscle and the resulting muscle tension and both signals seem to contribute to kinesthetic sensibility (McCloskey, 1978).

Studies of the perception of inspired volume also suggest that sensory information from the respiratory muscles is of primary importance in the subjective assessment of thoracic displacement (Wolkove et al., 1981). The perceived magnitude of a change in tidal volume is greater during ventilatory loading and less during artificial passive ventilation as compared to normal active breathing (DiMarco et al., 1982).

The ability to quantitate the magnitude of an added ventilatory loads is critically dependent on the integrity of the central nervous system processing of separate signals of respiratory force and displacement. Both in healthy elderly subjects and in patients with chronic obstructive lung disease, the exponents for the magnitude scaling of ventilatory loads are reduced, but the separate sensations of respiratory force during inspiratory efforts against a closed airway and of inspired volume during free breathing from functional residual capacity remain unaffected (Tack et al., 1982, Gottfried et al., 1985).

EFFECTS OF CHEST WALL VIBRATIONS

It has long been considered that feedback of afferent signals from mechanoreceptors in the respiratory muscles is important in respiratory sensation. The length-tension hypothesis of Campbell and Howell (1963) first suggested a primary role of muscle spindles in mediating the sensation of dyspnea. More recently, Homma et al. (1984) have shown that vibration of the upper rib cage during inspiration and of the lower thorax during expiration, to activate muscle spindles, results in illusions of chest expansion and deflation, respectively. Conversely, out-of-phase vibration of the upper chest during exhalation or of the lower thorax during inspiration produces an uncomfortable sensation of dyspnea. Homma et al. (1988) went on to demonstrate evoked potentials in the brain following muscle spindle stimulation by chest wall vibration.

RESPIRATORY RELATED CORTICAL EVOKED RESPONSES

The recording of evoked potentials over the brain has been used to characterize the pathways between sensory end organs in the ventilatory apparatus and the somatosensory cortex. Davenport et al. (1986) have demonstrated measurable evoked potentials over the scalp of awake humans following brief early and mid-inspiratory airway occlusions. Scalp potentials following airway occlusion include a positive peak at about 60 msec, a negative peak at about 110 msec and second positive peak at about 180 msec. They are thought to result from the initial activation of inspiratory muscle afferents. However, the latency of the initial cerebral peak is longer than that elicited by electrical stimulation of peripheral nerve fibers (Yamada et al., 1985). This appears to be explained by different methods of stimulation. Airway occlusion involves the application of a load opposing the contraction of the respiratory muscles. The reference point is the departure of mouth pressure from control levels but this may not precisely correspond to the actual activation of inspiratory muscle mechanoreceptors with high thresholds.

The respiratory related evoked potentials elicited by airway occlusion can be recorded over both cerebral hemispheres (Revelette and Davenport, 1990), suggesting bilateral projections of respiratory related sensory information to the somatosensory cortex. The observation that the peak amplitude of the evoked response following airway occlusion is greater over the left cerebral hemisphere than the right points to a specialization of the left somatosensory cortex in the perception of increases in inspiratory impedance.

A recent report by Gandevia and Macefield (1989) also provides clear evidence for a direct projection to the human cerebral cortex of low-threshold muscle afferents from the parasternal and lateral intercostal muscles.

EFFECTS OF VOLITIONAL CHANGES IN VENTILATION

A role for chest wall receptors in mediating the sensation of dyspnea is further suggested by the findings that the intensity of dyspnea increases, at a given chemical drive, when ventilation is voluntarily constrained below the spontaneously adopted breathing level. In the study of Chonan et al. (1987) normal subjects rated their sensation of dyspnea as PCO_2 increased during free breathing and during rebreathing while ventilation was voluntarily maintained at a constant baseline level. The effects on dyspnea of voluntary reduction in the level of ventilation at a constant PCO_2 were also evaluated. At a given PCO_2, constraining ventilation resulted in an increase in dyspnea and the accentuation in the intensity of dyspnea correlated closely with the degree to which tidal volume was reduced.

Either muscle spindles or tendon organs may be responsible for the increase in dyspnea when ventilation is constrained. Tendon organs are force receptors, and with increases in muscle tension, their firing rate increases. When tidal volume is constrained, inspiratory muscle force is reduced resulting in less central respiratory inhibition by tendon organ afferents. With a consequent increase in central respiratory motor command, the sense of effort and the sensation of dyspnea would increase. Alternatively, changes in the firing rate of muscle spindles produced by constraining tidal volume could mediate the sensation of dyspnea through a direct action on higher brain centers. The importance of chest wall receptors in mediating dyspnea when ventilation is constrained is further supported by our recent finding that vibration of the chest wall to stimulate respiratory mechanoreceptors substantially reduced the severity of dyspnea that re-

sults when ventilation is reduced below spontaneously adopted
levels (Altose et al., 1989).

BEHAVIORAL CONTROL OF BREATHING

Behavioral influences transmitted through neural pathways involving somatomotor and limbic forebrain structures are important in
the control of volitional respiratory acts including verbal
communication and emotional expression. Behavioral factors
shaped by the sensations associated with the act of breathing may
also be involved in adjusting the level and pattern of breathing
particularly in patients with lung disease. For example, dyspnea
may produce habitual or learned changes in ventilatory pattern
that serve to minimize the intensity of the sense of effort or
discomfort. This is in keeping with a model of respiratory
regulation, proposed by Poon (1989) that the control of breathing
patterns is determined by a balance between prevailing chemical
drive and a propensity of the controller to reduce respiratory
effort.

Recent studies by Chonan et al. (1990) have shown that a constant level of chemical drive, the sensation of difficulty in
breathing intensifies when ventilation is either voluntarily
raised or lowered from the spontaneously adopted level even when
PCO_2 and PO_2 remains unchanged. Similarly at a constant level of
minute ventilation respiratory sensations grow when the breathing
frequency is either voluntarily increased or decreased from the
spontaneously adopted level. This is consistent with the possibility that the level and pattern of breathing are regulated at
least in part, to minimize the sensations of respiratory effort
and discomfort.

There is reason to believe that the extent of behavioral adjustments in breathing pattern depends on the perceptual sensitivity
of respiratory sensation. In a group of normal subjects, Katz-
Salamon et al. (1989) determined the perceptual responses to
changes in inspired volume and also measured the ventilatory
responses to breathing through dead space of 1100 ml. and against
an elastic load of 20 cmH_2O. There was a significant negative
correlation between the exponents for the magnitude scaling of
inspired volume and the changes in tidal volume from resting
ventilation to that during dead space breathing against the
elastic load. Subjects with the highest exponents demonstrated
the smallest changes in tidal volume

Similar findings were reported by Oliven et al. (1985) in a group
of patients with moderately severe chronic obstructive lung
disease. They demonstrated that those patients with the highest
exponents for the magnitude scaling of respiratory force had the
greatest reductions in tidal volume during external ventilatory
loading and following methacholine induced bronchoconstriction.
These findings suggest that enhance perceptual sensitivity and a
high level of sensation lead to a decrease in respiratory neuromotor output so as to diminish the sense of discomfort and minimize breathlessness.

REFERENCES

Altose, M.D., and N.S. Cherniack (1981). Respiratory sensation
and respiratory muscle activity. Adv. Physiol. Sci., 10, 111-
119.
Altose, M.D., I,. Syed, and L. Shoos (1989). Effects of chest
wall vibration on the intensity of dyspnea during constrained
breathing. Proc. Int. Union Physiol. Sci. 17, 288.
Campbell, E.J.M., and J.B.L. Howell (1963). The sensation of
breathlessness. Br. Med. Bull., 19, 36-40.
Chonan, T., M.B. Mullholland, N.S. Cherniack, and M.D. Altose
(1987). Effects of voluntary constraining of thoracic displace
ment during hypercapnia. J. Appl. Physiol., 63, 1822-1828.
Chonan, T., M.B. Mulholland, M.D. Altose, and N.S. Cherniack
(1990). Effects of changes in level and pattern of breathing on
the sensation of dyspnea. J. Appl. Physiol. In Press.
Davenport P.W., W.A. Freedman, F. J. Thompson, and O. Franzen
(1986). Respiratory-related cortical potentials evoked by
inspiratory occlusion in humans. J. Appl. Physiol., 60, 1843-
1848.
DiMarco, A.F., D.A. Wolfson, S.B. Gottfried, and M.D. Altose
(1982). Sensation of inspired volume in normal subjects and
quadriplegic patients. J. Appl. Physiol, 53, 1481-1486.
Gandevia, S.C., and G. Macefield (1989). Projection of low
threshold afferents from human intercostal muscles to the cere
bral cortex. Respir. Physiol, 77, 203-214.
Gottfried, S.B., S. Redline, and M.D. Altose (1985). Respiratory
sensation in chronic obstructive pulmonary disease. Am. Rev.
Respir. Dis., 132, 954-959.
Homma, I., A. Kanamaru, and M. Sibuya (1988). Proprioceptive
chest wall afferents and the effects on respiratory sensation.
In:Respiratory Psychophysiology. (C.von Euler and M. Katz-
Salamon, ed). pp. 161-166. Stockton Press, New York.
Homma, I. T. Obata, M. Sibuya and M. Uchida (1984). Gate mecha
nism in breathlessness caused by chest wall vibration in humans.
J. Appl. Physiol., 56, 8-11.
Katz-Salamon, M., I. Syed, L. Shoos, and M.D. Altose (1989).
Respiratory response to elastic loading during dead space
breathing. Proc. Int. Union Physiol. Sci., 17, 175.
Killian, K.J., D.D. Bucens, and E.J.M. Campbell (1982). Effects
of breathing patterns on the perceived magnitude of added loads
to breathing. J. Appl. Physiol., 52,578-584.
McCloskey, D.I. (1978). Kinesthetic sensibility. Physio. Rev.,
58,763-820.
McCloskey, D.I., P. Ebeling, and G. M. Goodwin (1974). Estima-
tion of weights and tensions and apparent involvement of a
"sense of effort". Exp. Neurol., 42, 220-232.
Oliven, A., S.G. Kelsen, E.C. Deal, and N.S. Cherniack (1985).
Respiratory pressure sensation: Relationship to changes in
breathing pattern in patients with chronic obstructive lung
disease. Am. Rev. Respir. Dis., 132, 1214-1218.
Plum, F. (1974). Cerebral control of breathing. In:Ventilatory
and Phonatory Control Systems, (J. Wyke, ed.), pp. 208-217.
Oxford University Press, London.
Poon, C.S. (1989). Effects of inspiratory resistive load on
respiratory control in hypercapnia and exercise. J. Appl.
Physiol., 66, 2391-2399.
Revelette, W.R., and P.W. Davenport (1990). Effects of timing of
inspiratory occlusion on cerebral evoked potentials in humans.
J. Appl. Physiol., 68, 282-288.

Sorli, J., A. Grassino, G. Lorance, and J. Milic-Emili (1978).
Control of breathing in patients with chronic obstructive lung
disease. Clin. Sci. Mol. Med., 54, 294-304.
Stevens, S.S. (1975). On the psychophysical law. Psychol. Rev.,
64, 153-181.
Tack, M., M.D. Altose, and N.S. Cherniack (1982). Effect of
aging on the perception of resistive ventilatory loads. Am.
Rev. Respir. Dis., 126, 463-467.
Wolkove, N., and M.D. Altose, S.G. Kelsen, P.G. Kondapalli and
N.S. Cherniack (1981). Perception of changes in breathing in
normal human subjects. J. Appl. Physiol.,50, 78-83.
Yamada, T., M. Machida, and J. Tippin (1985). Somatosensory
evoked potentials. In:Evoked Potential Testing: Clinical
Applications. (J.H. Owen and H. Davis, ed.). pp. 109-158.
Grune and Straton, New York.

Dyspnea Sensation During Dead Space Breathing

Y. Kikuchi, H. Miki, O. Taguchi,
C. Shindoh, W. Hida, T. Chonan, M. Satoh,
S. Okabe and T. Takishima

First Department of Internal Medicine, Tohoku
University School of Medicine, Sendai 980, Japan

ABSTRACT

We examined the relationship between dyspnea sensation and several ventilatory
parameters including oxygen consumption of the respiratory muscle (V_{O_2}resp) in
normal subjects during incremental dead space loading induced hyperventilation
with and without inspiratory resistive load until the task was no longer
tolerated. In both the control and resistive loaded study, V_{O_2}resp increased
with an increase in minute ventilation (MV). Although both V_{O_2}resp and the
sensation of dyspnea at the same level of MV increased with an increase in
resistance, the relationship between V_{O_2}resp, occlusion pressure ($P_{0.15}$) and the
sensation of dyspnea did not differ among control, 10, and 20 $cmH_2O/l/sec$
resistive loaded breathing. To further examine these relationships, we also
measured the effect of a 1 liter-decrease in end-expiratory lung volume during
both dead space and 20 $cmH_2O/l/sec$ inspiratory resistive loaded breathing. We
found that endurance time was increased 2-4 times and V_{O_2}resp at the same level
of ventilation was decreased. Dyspnea sensation was correlated with MV, and
this relationship did not change with a lowered FRC. Dyspnea sensation was also
correlated with V_{O_2}resp but, in contrast, the relationship did change as FRC was
lowered. These results show that the ventilatory command signal is closely
related to the dyspnea sensation and that, although V_{O_2}resp is also related to
the sensation at the same lung volume, it does not uniquely determine the
sensation if lung volume changes. We also found that the quality of the
sensation changed relatively quickly at some point during dead space loaded
breathing. This change was usually followed by a rapid increase in frequency
and a decrease in tidal volume. The subjects felt insufficient inflation
compared to their efforts but this was not due to respiratory muscle fatigue nor
hypercapnia.

KEYWORDS

Loaded breathing; resistance; oxygen consumption of the respiratory muscle; lung
volume; breathing pattern; behavioral control of breathing.

INTRODUCTION

Dyspnea, or breathlessness, is an important cause of suffering and disability in

patients with chronic obstructive pulmonary disease and pulmonary fibrosis.
Dyspnea is a complex sensation and almost surely represents several different
types of sensation. Although the mechanisms leading to dyspnea are far from
clear, Harrison (Harrison, 1950) proposed some 40 years ago the interesting
concept that the sensation of dyspnea arises in the respiratory muscles and can
be likened to the pain of intermittent claudication or angina pectoris. After
him, Levinson and Cherniack (Levinson and Cherniack, 1968) showed that, in
patients with severe chronic obstructive pulmonary disease, the oxygen cost of
breathing is exceedingly high and that, during exercise the additional
consumption of oxygen by the respiratory muscles required to produce an increase
in ventilation may be the rate limiting step in exercise. However, whether the
oxygen consumption of the respiratory muscles is related to the sensation of
dyspnea has not yet been determined.

In the present study, we first examined the relationship between oxygen
consumption of the respiratory muscles and the sensation of dyspnea during dead
space and inspiratory resistive loaded breathing. Second, we examined the
question of the effect of end expiratory lung volume on the relation of dyspnea
to ventilatory parameters. Finally, we examined whether the quality of the
sensation changed during graded increased ventilation.

METHODS

Figure. 1 shows a block diagram of the experimental set-up. The apparatus
consists of three parts; one is a flow measuring system with pressure and gas
sampling parts, the second is an expandable dead space, and the third is a
spirometer. In the flow measuring system, inspiratory and expiratory lines were
separated by a Hans-Rudolph valve. An electrically controlled solenoid valve
was connected to the inspiratory side of the line to obtain occlusion pressure
($P_{0.15}$). Expired volume was obtained from integration of mouth flow. Mouth
pressure was measured with a Validyne differential pressure transducer (MP-45)
and expired CO_2 fraction ($F_{ET}CO_2$) was measured with a mass-spectrometer. The
expandable dead space consisted of a long piece of corrugated plastic tubing
functioning as a bellows. The volume of the dead space was gradually increased
by an electrical motor at a constant speed of 100 ml/min with an inspiratory
resistive load, or 200 ml/min without resistance. Dead space volume was changed
from 1 liter to 3 liter at these two rates. Oxygen consumption of the
respiratory muscles was measured with the spirometer attached to the distal end
of the dead space. The dead space and the spirometer were initially filled with
pure oxygen. Expired CO_2 was absorbed by soda lime in the spirometer circuit.
The slope of the spirometer volume at end-expiration is a measure of overall
$\dot{V}_{O_2}$. Changes in that slope reflect increases in $\dot{V}_{O_2}$ of the respiratory muscles.
Lung volume changes were measured with abdominal and rib cage Respitrace belts
and monitored on a storage oscilloscope. The sensation of dyspnea was measured
on a visual analog scale (VAS) which was displayed on the storage oscilloscope.
The two ends of the scales were labeled "none at all" and "most intense
imaginable" and were numbered from 0 to 100.

Five well trained normal subjects were studied. The subject sat on a chair with
the respitrace belts. After quiet breathing, dead space and inspiratory
resistance were added and the volume of the dead space was gradually increased
at a constant speed, until the task was no longer tolerable. We found that
usually ventilation increased sufficiently with increasing dead space volume so
that end-tidal CO_2 did not increase very much. However, to exclude possible CO_2
effects, if the subject's end-tidal CO_2 rose to 7 %, he was asked to voluntarily
increase his ventilation gradually. During these measurements, the subject was
asked to maintain FRC at the control level by watching the oscilloscope. In the
first series of experiments, three measurements were made; one was with no added
resistance, the others were with inspiratory resistances of 10 and 20

Experimental Block Diagram

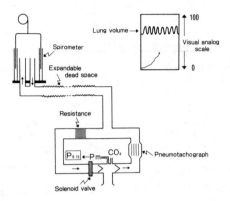

Fig. 1. Experimental block diagram.

$cmH_2O/l/sec$. In the second series of experiments, we examined the effects of a decrease in lung volume on the relation between oxygen consumption of the respiratory muscles and the sensation of dyspnea. For this purpose the subjects were asked to perform the expanding dead space rebreathing maneuver with the high inspiratory resistive load, but this time at an end expiratory volume one liter below control FRC. During these measurements we also examined changes in the quality of the sensation.

RESULTS

Dyspnea Sensation and the Respiratory Muscle Oxygen Consumption

Respiratory muscle oxygen consumption increased with an increase in minute ventilation during dead space rebreathing, with and without an inspiratory resistive load. The magnitude of increased oxygen consumption increases with the magnitude of the resistance at the same level of ventilation. However, there was no significant differences between the three values of peak oxygen consumption obtained when the subjects felt the maximal sensation of dyspnea during control or with either of the resistive inspiratory loads.

This sensation of dyspnea increased almost linearly with an increase in minute ventilation. However, the mean value of VAS was significantly increased with an increase in resistance at the same level of ventilation. On the other hand, although the sensation increased with an increase in $P_{0.15}$, the relationship between the sensation and $P_{0.15}$ did not differ among the magnitudes of resistance used. The sensation of dyspnea increased with an increase in oxygen consumption during dead space rebreathing. Table 1 shows the mean values of overall oxygen consumption at the same level of VAS in five subjects with and without an inspiratory resistance. $\dot{V}_{O2}$ did not differ among the magnitudes of resistances at the same level of VAS.

Table 1. Mean values (+SE) of the overall oxygen consumption
during FRC breathing with and without resistance at
several VAS levels.

VAS	$\dot{V}_{O2}$ (ml/min)		
	Control	R=10	R=20
30	227.6+6.2	202.8+16.3	224.4+20.6
50	277.0+19.1	279.6+24.3	274.0+32.3
70	324.8+26.1	346.2+35.3	322.8+40.5
90	385.2+36.6	403.2+49.9	395.8+50.2

Values are mean+SE (N=5). VAS, visual analog scale score.

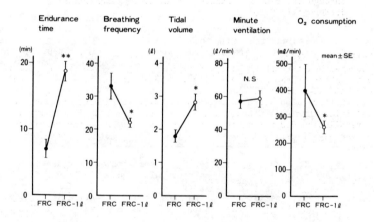

Fig. 2. Effects of the lung volume during dead space and
inspiratory resistance on the endurance time,
breathing frequency, tidal volume, minute
ventilation and oxygen consumption at the end of
the task. Values are mean+SE of five subjects.
* p<0.05, ** p<0.01, NS= not significant.

Effects of Decreased FRC on $\dot{V}_{O2}$ and Dyspnea.

Figure 2 shows the endurance time, breathing frequency, tidal volume, minute

Table 2. Comparison of the increases in respiratory muscle
oxygen consumption during resistive loaded
breathing between FRC and FRC-1 liter.

Ventilation	Respiratory Muscle $\dot{V}_{O2}$ (ml/min)	
	at FRC	at FRC-1 liter
60 % MV	47.6±17.5	30.8±12.8*
80 % MV	99.6±26.3	53.0±15.8*
100 % MV	197.0±41.4	81.0±16.9*

Values are mean±SE (N=5). The increased oxygen consumption
of the respiratory muscle was obtained as the difference
from the initial value of FRC breathing through the heavy
inspiratory resistance (R=20). MV (minute ventilation) was
expressed as the percent values of the minute ventilation
when the subject felt the maximal sensation at FRC breathing
through the same resistance. * indicates significantly
different ($p<0.05$).

ventilation, and oxygen consumption changes at the end of the task when the
subjects breathed through the inspiratory resistance (R=20) with end expiratory
volume at FRC or at FRC minus one liter. The endurance time was markedly
increased at FRC-1 liter by about 2 times, compared to that at FRC. The
breathing pattern also differed between the two. Breathing frequency was lower
at FRC-1 liter than at FRC and tidal volume was higher at FRC-1 liter. However,
minute ventilation did not differ. Oxygen consumption of the respiratory
muscles was significantly lower at FRC-1 liter breathing, compared to FRC
breathing.

Table 2 shows the mean values of the increased oxygen consumption of the
respiratory muscles at the same levels of minute ventilation. The oxygen
consumption of the respiratory muscles was obtained as the difference from the
initial value of FRC breathing. This result shows that, at FRC-1 liter
breathing, the oxygen consumption of the respiratory muscles was markedly
decreased compared to that at FRC breathing.

Although the dyspnea sensation also increased with an increase in the
respiratory muscle oxygen consumption at FRC-1 liter breathing through the high
inspiratory resistance, the relationship of the sensation to oxygen consumption
of the respiratory muscles was significantly different from FRC breathing.
However, the relationship of dyspnea to minute ventilation was not strongly
influenced by changes in end expiratory volume.

Changes in the Quality of the Sensation

When the subject increased ventilation toward his maximal level during dead

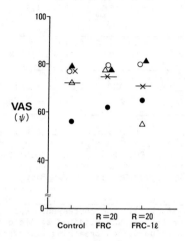

Fig. 3.   The values on the dyspnea index scale at which the
          subjects felt that the quality of their sensation
          changed. Each symbol corresponds to one subject.

space breathing with and without inspiratory loads, the quality of the sensation
changed relatively quickly at some point. The quality of the sensation usually
changed at relatively similar dyspnea index values in the individual. Figure 3
shows the values on the dyspnea index scale at which subjects felt that the
quality of their sensation changed. These dyspnea index scores at the
transition seemed to be characteristic of the individual, and independent of the
magnitude of the resistance and lung volume. The change in the quality was
usually felt around the peak tidal volume in the same series and followed by a
rapid increase in frequency and a decrease in tidal volume. This point was
reached at a wide variety of end inspiratory lung volumes. Also, hypercapnia
was not associated with this phenomenon. Peak inspiratory mouth pressure did
not decrease beyond the transitional point.

DISCUSSION

In the first experiment, we found that, during gradually increasing dead space
and resistive loaded breathing, there was a unique relationship among the
sensation of dyspnea, the oxygen consumption of the respiratory muscle, and
occlusion pressure. This relation was not affected by inspiratory resistive
loading from 0 to 20 $cmH_2O/l/sec$, when FRC was maintained. Because occlusion
pressure is usually thought of as an index of the motor command signal from the
respiratory center, this finding can be interpreted as meaning that, even when
breathing with an inspiratory resistance, the sensation of dyspnea is tightly
coupled with the motor command signal. This is similar to results previously
reported work by Killian et al. (Killian et al., 1984) and supports the current
concept of the mechanisms contributing to dyspnea. Moreover, this result also
implies that the sensation of dyspnea is tightly coupled with the respiratory

muscle oxygen consumption, at least in these experimental conditions.

In the second experiment, we found that, when the subjects breathed with gradually increasing dead space and resistance 20 at FRC-1 liter, endurance time increased and the oxygen consumption of the respiratory muscles at a given ventilation decreased compared to values obtained while breathing at FRC. The oxygen consumption of the respiratory muscles was not uniquely related to the sensation, when lung volume changed. These results suggest that, although the oxygen consumption was correlated to the sensation of dyspnea at FRC breathing, it may be not a primary determinant of the sensation of dyspnea. If it is assumed that oxygen consumption of the respiratory muscles reflects motor command signals, these results suggest that other factors in addition to motor command signals also contribute to dyspnea.

We found the quality of the sensation changed relatively quickly at some point during incremental dead space loaded breathing. The dyspnea index values were relatively similar, and independent of the magnitude of the resistance and lung volume. Most subjects complained of insufficient inflation compared to their expectation at any given effort. Because end inspiratory lung volumes were widely different at these transitional points between control and states with resistances, limiting mechanical factors of the lung or chest wall do not contribute to this observation. Also, because peak inspiratory mouth pressure did not decrease even after these points and $F_{ET}CO_2$ did not increase (less than 7%), this phenomenon was not due to respiratory muscle fatigue nor hypercapnia. Although the precise mechanisms were not clarified, the finding that the frequency of breathing rapidly increased and tidal volume decreased after the quality changed, suggests that changes in the sensation of dyspnea are associated with behavioral changes in the pattern of breathing.

In conclusion, among the many possible contributors to dyspnea, our results at FRC breathing seem to be consistent with the notion that motor command signals are a primary determinant of the sensation of dyspnea. However, in extending these experiments to lower lung volumes, the dyspnea sensation versus oxygen consumption relationship changed. To the extent that oxygen consumption of the respiratory muscles reflects motor command signals, other factors in addition to motor command signals also contribute to dyspnea. Our data from the qualitative studies confirm the description of dyspnea as a complex of sensations, rather than a single phenomenon, and suggest that different mechanisms, including behavioral modifications of the pattern of breathing, may be involved at different levels of perceived discomfort.

REFERENCES

Harrison, T. E. (1950) Principles of Internal Medicine (T. E. Harrison, Ed.). Philadelphia, Blakiston, pp. 111-119.
Killian, K. J., S. C. Gandevia, E. Summers, and E. J. M. Campbell (1984). Effect of increased lung volume on perception of breathlessness, effort, and tension. J. Appl. Physiol., 57: 686-691.
Levinson, H. and R. M. Cherniack (1968). Ventilatory cost of exercise in chronic obstructive pulmonary disease. J. Appl. Physiol., 25: 21-27.

Effect of Expiratory Muscle Fatigue on Sense of Effort During Expiratory Loading

S. Suzuki, J. Suzuki, T. Ishii and T. Okubo

The First Department of Internal Medicine, Yokohama
City University School of Medicine, Yokohama 232,
Japan

ABSTRACT

We have examined whether fatigue of the expiratory muscle, i.e., the abdominal
muscle, may account for changes in the sense of effort during expiratory
threshold loading in normal subjects. The respiratory effort sensation was
scored using a modified Borg scale, and expiratory muscle fatigue was assessed
from changes in the maximum static expiratory pressure (PEmax) and from changes
in both the centroid frequency (fc) and high- to low-frequency power ratio (H/L
ratio) of the abdominal muscle electromyogram (EMG). Expiratory threshold
loading (mouth pressure, 60% of PEmax at FRC and duty cycle = 0.5) was continued until exhaustion or for 30 min, and was repeated 15 min after the end of
the first expiratory loading. The endurance time of the second loading was
shorter than that of the first loading. PEmax before the second run was lower
than in the control. The maximum static mouth pressure during expiratory
loading (PEmaxload) decreased initially and remained to be decreased. The
decrease in PEmaxload during the second run was greater than that during the
first. Both fc and the H/L ratio decreased initially and then remained constant. The Borg score rose with time and the second run showed a greater
increase in the Borg score than the first. At the early stage of loading, a
given increase in Borg score was associated with a decrease in the H/L ratio,
but further increase in Borg score was not accompanied by a further decrease in
the H/L ratio toward the end of loading. There was no appreciable difference
in the relation between Borg score and H/L ratio between the first and second
runs. The relation between Borg score and PEmaxload also showed a similar
change. We conclude that an increase in respiratory effort sensation during
expiratory loading is merely associated with expiratory muscle fatigue, and
that the latter is not a unique cause of the former.

KEYWORDS

Expiratory muscle; muscle fatigue; respiratory sensation; threshold load; Borg
scale.

INTRODUCTION

Weakness of the respiratory muscle, increased ventilation, and increased impedance of the total respiratory system are the most common circumstances under

which dyspnea occurs. The sensory mechanism in the limb skeletal muscle is thought to involve conscious awareness of the outgoing motor command (McCloskey et al., 1974). In the respiratory system, an increase in motor output can be expected whenever the peripheral muscle is weakened or fatigued. However, the relationship between sensation of dyspnea and the presence of inspiratory muscle fatigue is controversial. Gandevia et al. (1981) found a progressive increase in the sense of effort during continuous maximal inspiration. During non-fatiguing contractions of the respiratory muscle, the sense of effort is reported to be heightened when either the magnitude or duration of inspiratory pressure increases (Altose et al., 1982; Killian et al., 1982). Supinski et al. (1987) found that the sense of effort during loaded breathing increased progressively as fatigue of the inspiratory muscle produced by threshold loading became progressively severe. However, the intensity of the sense of effort varied as a function of the pattern of pressure development. Bradley et al. (1986) showed that the severity of inspiratory effort sensation during resistive loading is independent of the development of diaphragmatic fatigue, but is directly related to inspiratory intrathoracic pressure.

On the other hand, in chronic obstructive pulmonary disease (COPD), work of breathing is increased on expiration, as well as on inspiration (McIlory and Christie, 1954). Expiratory muscle fatigue develops in COPD, although the magnitude of the fatigue is lower than that of the inspiratory muscle (Rochester et al., 1979). In our previous study of expiratory muscle fatigue, we found that expiratory resistive loading induces expiratory fatigue. Therefore, we hypothesized that the sense of effort during expiratory loading may be related to muscle fatigue.

To examine this hypothesis, two successive trials of expiratory threshold loaded breathing were performed with a 15-min interval allowed for recovery. The second run was done to evaluate the effect of the expiratory muscle fatigue. At each run, expiratory muscle fatigue and respiratory sensation were examined with time. Thus, we analyzed the relationship between expiratory muscle fatigue and the sense of effort during expiratory threshold loaded breathing.

METHODS

Seven healthy male subjects were studied. All were non-smokers with normal spirometry, and were prohibited from taking coffee or other beverages containing caffeine. Informed consent was obtained from all participants. During loaded breathing, airflow was measured using a Fleisch pneumotachograph and a differential pressure transducer (Validyne MP-45, CA), and tidal volume was obtained by integration of the airflow signal. Mouth pressure was monitored with a differential pressure transducer (Validyne MP-45 250 mmHg) connected to the tap of the mouthpiece. The end-tidal carbon dioxide concentration was monitored by a mass spectrometer (WSMR-1400, Westron Co., Chiba, Japan).

The respiratory muscle power was evaluated in terms of maximum static mouth pressure, which was obtained by maximally expiring against the closed valve. The maximum expiratory pressure (PEmax) was measured at total lung capacity (TLC) and functional residual capacity (FRC). The maximum respiratory pressure measurements were repeated until reproducible control measurement values were obtained. To evaluate respiratory fatigue, the pressure measurements were done at 5, 10 and 15 min following the end of threshold loading. During the loading, we measured the maximum static expiratory pressure (PEmaxload) every 1 min at end-expiratory volume and evaluated it by comparison with the control value measured at about 1 liter above FRC, since in a preliminary study, the increase in FRC during loading was estimated to be about 1 liter.

The electromyogram (EMG) activity of the abdominal muscle was recorded from

surface electrodes placed between the anterior iliac crest and the umbilicus.
EMG signals were measured through a preamplifier (Model 1253A, San-ei, Tokyo)
and band-pass filtered (FV-664, NF Electronic Instruments). The EMG signal was
analyzed by Fast Fourier Transform (FFT). The centroid frequency (fc) and
high- to low- frequency power ratio (H/L ratio) of the EMG were obtained according to Sellick et al. (1985). Both fc and the H/L ratio were expressed a
percentage of the average value for the first 5 breaths. Time course of fc and
the H/L ratio was obtained every one minute during loading.

To evaluate respiratory sensation, a category scale, a 10-point modified Borg
scale, was used (Borg, 1982; Jones et al., 1985). The subject was asked to
indicate, by pointing, the position on the scale that represented magnitude of
the respiratory effort required at the time of the estimate. Sensory estimates
were made after the first 30 s of each run to serve as the control value, and
then every 1 min until the subject was no longer able to reproduce the target
mouth pressure.

We modified the coil spring of the Threshold valve (Threshold Inspiratory
Muscle Trainer, Healthscan Products Inc., USA). The threshold load device was
connected to the expiratory port of a two-way valve, through which the subject
breathed air by supporting the cheeks with both hands while wearing a noseclip.
The magnitude of threshold was set at 60% of control PEmax at FRC by adjusting
the length of the coil spring. The breathing cycle was 15 breaths/min and the
duty cycle was 0.5.

Protocol

After the control measurement of PEmax, expiratory threshold loaded breathing
was started. The subject was asked to continue for 30 min or until exhaustion.
Visual feedback of the mouth pressure signal displayed on the oscilloscope was
used to constrain the breathing frequency to 15 breaths/min and expiratory
duration to 2.0 s. After a 15-min recovery from the first run, PEmax was
measured, and then the second run, using the same expiratory threshold load,
was started in the same way as for the first run. During the loaded breathing,
PEmaxload, Borg score, EMG and end-tidal CO_2 concentration were assessed every
1 min.

All signals were recorded on electromagnetic data tape (XR-510, Teac, Tokyo)
and on an eight-channel strip-chart recorder (Rectigraph 8K, San-ei NEC). All
data were expressed as mean±SE. Statistical analysis was done using two-way
analysis of variance (ANOVA) for comparison of the two curves, and t-test for 2
values.

RESULTS

The Borg score increased progressively with time and a great variety was observed in the time course of the score among the subjects. In the second run,
all subjects had a higher Borg score than in the first run (p<0.05)(Fig. 1).
In both the first and second runs, two subjects were able to complete the full
30-min expiratory threshold loading. The endurance time of the other 4 subjects who were not able to complete the loading was shorter in the second run
than in the first run (1st and 2nd run, 12.0±3.3 and 8.5±3.5 min, respectively).

The centroid frequency of the first run decreased by 8.2±1.1% immediately after
the start of loading (P<0.01) and remained decreased (Table 1). The second run
also showed a similar decrease. The H/L ratio showed a change similar to that
of the centroid frequency and the decrease immediately after the start of
loading was 25.2±5.2% (p<0.01).

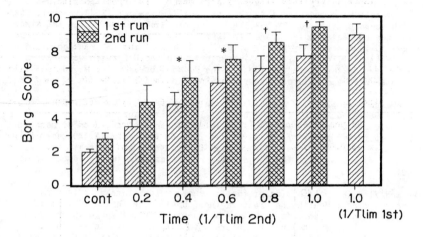

Fig. 1. Borg score for the 1st and 2nd runs. Note that the
score for the 2nd run is higher than that for the 1st.
*p<0.05, †p<0.01; comparison between 1st and 2nd runs.

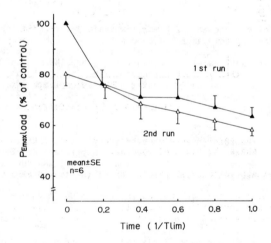

Fig. 2. PEmaxload during loading. PEmaxload values are
expressed as percentages of the PEmax at 1 liter
above FRC. The 1st curve is significantly different
from the 2nd (p<0.01, ANOVA).

The PEmaxload during loaded breathing decreased progressively with time (Fig.
2). At the end of loading the decrease was $63.2 \pm 3.4\%$ (P<0.05). In the second
run, the decrease in PEmaxload during loading was greater than that in the
first run (P<0.01 by ANOVA).

The control PEmax before loading was 171 ± 21 cmH_2O at TLC and 133 ± 11 cmH_2O at
FRC, and was thus within our normal limits. At 15 min after the end of the

TABLE 1. Centroid frequency (fc) and H/L ratio of abdominal EMG.

		control	Time (1/Tlim)				
			0.2	0.4	0.6	0.8	1.0
fc	1st run	100	$91.8 \pm 1.1^{\dagger}$	$90.2 \pm 1.9^{\dagger}$	$91.5 \pm 2.2^{\dagger}$	$91.3 \pm 1.0^{\dagger}$	$91.9 \pm 2.8*$
	2nd run	95.4 ± 1.7	91.0 ± 2.1	$90.6 \pm 1.9*$	$90.5 \pm 1.9*$	$90.3 \pm 1.6*$	$89.2 \pm 2.4*$
H/L	1st run	100	$74.8 \pm 5.2^{\dagger}$	$69.3 \pm 9.2^{\dagger}$	69.0 ± 6.7	$66.7 \pm 7.5^{\dagger}$	$68.7 \pm 15.2^{\dagger}$
	2nd run	81.2 ± 6.4	$67.7 \pm 8.1*$	$66.2 \pm 7.6*$	65.5 ± 9.7	63.3 ± 10.4	$59.3 \pm 9.8*$

Values are means$\pm$SE of percentages of the control at the 1st run.
Time is expressed as a ratio to endurance time (Tlim) of each run.
*$p < 0.05$, † $p < 0.01$ compared with the control of each run.

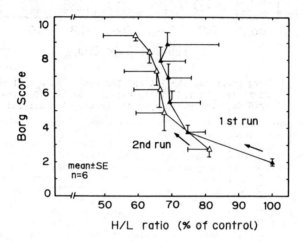

Fig. 3. The relationship of Borg score to H/L ratio. Arrow
shows the start of loading.

first run, PEmax decreased by 10% at TLC ($p < 0.02$) and 13% at FRC ($p < 0.01$).

In the first run, the end-tidal CO_2 concentration was observed to rise by 1-2%
in the last few minutes in 4 of 6 subjects. In the second run, a further one
subject showed a rise in CO_2 concentration, in addition to the above 4 subjects.

Figure 3 shows the relationship between the Borg score and the H/L ratio. At
the initial stage of the first run, a given increase in Borg score was associated with a large decrease in the H/L ratio, although after the mid-stage of
loading the Borg score increased further while there was only a small decrease
in the H/L ratio. The curve of the second run showed almost the same trace as
that for the first, although the second curve was shifted slightly upward, i.e.
toward a higher Borg score, and to the left. Furthermore, the Borg score
versus the PEmaxload curve showed a similar relationship to that of the Borg
score versus H/L ratio.

DISCUSSION

In the present study, we demonstrated that respiratory sensation during expiratory threshold loading increased progressively with time. The changes observed in expiratory muscle power and EMG during loading suggested that expiratory muscle fatigue might occur. In the second run, before which muscle fatigue already existed, the magnitude of the increase in Borg score was consistently greater than that in the first. Therefore, expiratory muscle fatigue may play a substantial role in the respiratory sensation during expiratory threshold loading. However, at the latter stage of loading, a further increase in the intensity of the respiratory sensation was not associated with an increase in expiratory muscle fatigue in terms of respiratory pressure and the EMG. It is thus possible that expiratory muscle fatigue may not always be responsible for the development of increased respiratory sensation during expiratory threshold loading.

In inspiratory muscle fatigue (Bradley et al., 1986), the Borg score is reported to be closely related to intrathoracic pressure, but not to fatigue of the diaphragm. In the present study, the expiratory pressure measured at the mouth was kept constant at 60% of each individual's PEmax (threshold) throughout the loading. Therefore, mouth pressure, i.e. intrathoracic pressure, does not seem to influence the sense of effort during expiratory threshold loading. Furthermore, in the study of Bradley et al. (1986), the duration of loading was only 10 breaths, which corresponded almost to the first one minute of our study. In the first 1-5 min of our study, changes in the H/L ratio and fc were progressive and the Borg score increased sharply. Therefore, it is not possible to compare the present data with theirs.

We evaluated expiratory muscle fatigue on the basis of maximum static expiratory muscle pressure during loading (PEmaxload) and after the end of the loading (PEmax), and from power spectral analysis of the EMG. During loading, both PEmaxload and EMG analysis showed development of expiratory muscle fatigue. Early in the loading, muscle fatigue, shown by a decrease in PEmaxload, appeared, but in the latter stage, any further decrease in PEmaxload was small. On the other hand, a maximum sustained contraction of skeletal muscle produces a progressive decrease in the output of force (Bigland-Ritchie et al., 1978). Further, Gandevia et al. (1981) showed that maximum inspiratory pressure during sustained maximal inspiration decreased in the latter stage of contraction. However, the duration of muscle contraction in the latter studies was less than 60 s, and thus markedly different from that in the present study. Further, time course of PEmaxload in the present study was different from that in the above studies. Meanwhile, EMG measured on the skin between the anterior iliac crest and the umbilicus may come from the rectus abdominis muscle. The fact that there were no further decreases in expiratory pressure and EMG parameters may mean that abdominal muscles other than the rectus abdominis muscle might contribute much more to maintaining a high abdominal pressure, resulting in no further decrease of PEmaxload.

The Borg score rose progressively to a maximum with time, and expiratory muscle fatigue was increased as shown by changes in PEmaxload and EMG. This suggests that a given relationship might exist between expiratory muscle fatigue and sense of effort during expiratory threshold loading. However, the relationship between Borg score and the H/L ratio or PEmaxload was not linear. In the initial stage of loading, Borg score increased linearly with a decrease in the H/L ratio or PEmaxload, but in the latter stage it increased further without any substantial change in the latter parameters. This suggests that factors other than expiratory muscle fatigue might contribute to the development of a heightened sense of effort. On the other hand, end-tidal CO_2 concentration was observed to increase in the last few minutes in 4 of 6 subjects. Subjects either able or unable to complete the 30-min loading showed a rise of CO_2 concentration. In the second run, all subjects except for one who completed the loading showed a rise of CO_2 concentration during the latter stage of loading. It is possible that in the latter stage, the rise of CO_2 concentration might increase the sense of effort to some extent, the rise in CO_2 perhaps being produced in turn by a decrease in ventilation due to muscle fatigue. In the latter stage, expiratory muscle fatigue might advance further, although neither EMG nor PEmaxload indicated further muscle fatigue.

In the second run, the Borg score started from a value equal to or slightly higher than that in the first run and was significantly higher throughout the loading that in the first run. Although the decreased PEmaxload in the first run recovered to some extent before the start of the second run, the expiratory muscle power (PEmax) showed a substantial decrease. During the second run PEmaxload decreased to a greater extent than during the first run. This suggests that fatigue of the expiratory muscle may have been more severe in the second run than in the first. Thus, it is possible that greater respiratory muscle fatigue produces a more increase in the sense of effort. Furthermore, the curve of Borg score vs. H/L ratio or PEmaxload for the first run showed almost the same trace as that in the second run, although the second run shifted it slightly upward and to the left. The increase in muscle fatigue like that seen in the second run may be responsible for the enhanced respiratory sensation.

REFERENCES

Altose, M.D., A.F. Dimarco, S.B. Gottfried, and K.P. Strohl (1982). The sensation of respiratory muscle force. Am. Rev. Respir. Dis. 126, 807-811.
Bigland-Ritchie, B., D.A. Jones, G.P. Hosking, and R.H.T. Edwards (1978). Central and peripheral fatigue in sustained maximum voluntary contractions of human quadriceps muscle. Clin. Sci. Mol. Med. 54, 609-614.
Borg, G.A.V. (1982). Psychophysical bases of perceived exertion. Med. Sci. Sports Exercise 14, 377-381.
Bradley, T.D., D.A. Chartrand, J.W. Fitting, K.J. Killian, and A. Grassino (1986). The relation of inspiratory effort sensation to fatiguing patterns of the diaphragm. Am. Rev. Respir. Dis. 134, 1119-1124.
Gandevia, S.C., Killian, and E.J.M. Campbell (1981). The effect of respiratory muscle fatigue on respiratory sensations. Clinical Science 60, 463-466.
Jones, G.L., K.J. Killian, E. Summers, and N.L. Jones (1985). Inspiratory muscle force and endurance in maximum resistive loading. J. Appl. Physiol. 58, 1608-1615.
Killian, K.J., D.D. Bucens, and E.J.M. Campbell (1982). Effect of breathing patterns on the perceived magnitude of added loads to breathing. J. Appl. Physiol. 52, 578-584.
Macklem, P. T (1988). Respiratory sensation and pattern of respiratory muscle activation during diaphragm fatigue. J. Appl. Physiol. 65, 2182-2189.
McCloskey, D.I., P. Ebeling, and G.M. Goodwin (1974). Estimation of weight and tensions and apparent involvement of a "Sense of Effort". Exper. Neurol. 42, 220-232.
McIlory, M.B., and R.V. Christie. The work of breathing in emphysema (1954). Clin. Sci. 13, 147-154.
Rochester, D.F., N.M. Braun, and N.S. Arora (1979). Respiratory muscle strength in chronic obstructive pulmonary disease. Am. Rev. Respir. Dis. 119(2), 151-154.
Sellick G.C., A. Mazar, and M.J. Belman (1985). Changes in diaphragmatic EMG spectra during hyperpneic loads. Respir. Physiol. 61, 137-152.
Supinski, G.S., S.J. Clary, H. Bark, and S.G. Kelsen (1987). Effect of inspiratory muscle fatigue on perception of effort during loaded breathing. J. Appl. Physiol. 62, 300-307.

Chest Wall Distortion and Dyspnea

K. Yoshino and K. Konno

The First Department of Internal Medicine, Tokyo
Women's Medical College, 8-1, Kawada-cho,
Shinjuku-ku, Tokyo 162, Japan

ABSTRACT

The chest wall is composed of three main parts: the diaphragm, the
rib cage, and the abdomen. During quiet breathing, the rib cage
and addomen can move independently with a single degree of freedom
in a normal subject (Konno and Mead, 1967). In other words, any
part within either the rib cage or abdomen can move in the same
direction and no distortion of the chest wall will be observed.

Out-of-phase motion of various parts of the chest wall can be seen
in hemiplegic patients, in neonates during REM sleep, and in
patients with emphysema (Campbell, 1969). Inward motion of the
abdomen during the inspiratory phase occurs in severe respiratory
failure (Ashutosh et. al., 1975; Sharp et. al., 1977) and
respiratory muscle fatigue (Roussos and Macklem, 1976) can be seen
even during quiet breathing. Most of the patients with such out-
of-phase motion of the chest wall will complain of dyspnea. Based
on these clinical observations, our study investigated the
relationship between chest wall distortion and dyspnea.

SUBJECTS AND METHODS

The subjects were three males. Chest wall distortion was produced
by the new breathing maneuver which is transdiaphragmatic pressure
(Pdi) zero breathing.

During this maneuver, the subject tries to maintain a tidal volume
similar to that during quiet breathing while keeping Pdi as near as
possible to zero until it is impossible to continue further. The
experimental design is shown in Fig. 1.

The changes in Pdi were monitored on an oscilloscope, so that the
subject could watch the Pdi tracing during the experimental period.
Pleural pressure, flow, and tidal volume were recorded. In
addition, the electrical activity of the sternomastoid (Est),
parasternal intercostal muscles (Eic), diaphragm (Edi) and
abdominal muscles (Eab) was recorded. Chest wall configuration was
evaluated using a magnetometer. Dyspnea was graded according to
the Borg score (Borg, 1982) and the experiment was carried out in

the standing position.

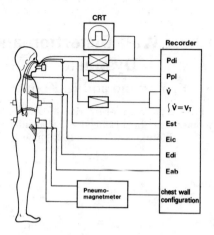

Fig. 1. Diaphragm to measure during Pdi=0
         breathing maneuver. Pdi: transdia-
         phragmatic pressure; Ppl: pleural
         pressure; V: flow; V : tidal volume;
                             T
         Est, Eic, Edi and Eab: electrical
         activity of sternocleidomastoid, para-
         sternal intercostal muscle, diaphragm
         and abdomen, respectively.

The physiological characteristics of Pdi=0 breathing were as
follows: 1) Only the inspiratory accessory muscles were utilized;
2) Pleural pressure was the only driving pressure producing
ventilation; and 3) It was possible to produce paradoxical motion
of the rib cage and abdomen.

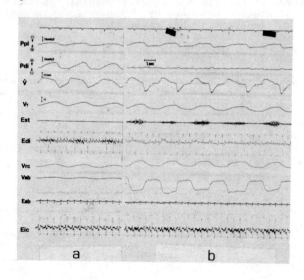

Fig. 2.   Changes in the measured parameters
during quiet breathing (a) and Pdi=0
breathing (b). Vrc and Vab: volume of
rib cage and abdomen calibrated by
isovolume maneuver.

Figure 2 shows an example of Pdi=0 breathing. Although the tidal
volume was maintained at the same level as during quiet breathing,
neither Pdi nor any diaphragmatic electrical activity was observed.
Marked paradoxical motion of the rib cage and abdomen was noted,
and also an increase in parasternal intercostal muscle and
sternomastoid activity was shown. Figure 3 shows the changes of
chest wall configuration displayed in a Konno-Mead diagram (Konno
and Mead, 1967) during quiet breathing and Pdi=0 breathing.

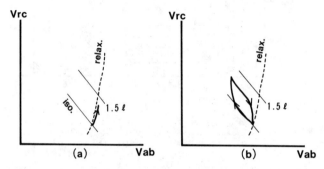

Fig. 3.   Chest wall configuration on the Konno-
Mead diagram during quiet breathing (a)
and Pdi=0 breathing (b). relax: relaxation line; iso: isovolume line.

Marked paradoxical motion of the rib cage and abdomen during Pdi=0
breathing can be observed. Changes of chest wall configuration
were evaluated not only by the anteroposterior (a-p) motion of the
rib cage and abdomen but also by the lateral motion of the rib
cage, as shown in Fig. 4.

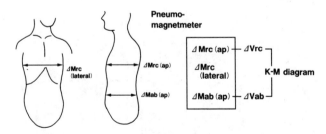

Fig. 4.   Diagram to measure the chest wall con-
figuration.ΔMrc(ap) and Δ Mab(ap):
change of anteroposterior motion of rib
cage and abdomen; Δ Mrc(lateral): change
of lateral motion of rib cage; Vrc and
Vab: volume of rib cage and abdomen calibrated by isovolume maneuver.

RESULTS

The relationship between the changes in a-p motion of the rib cage and the Borg score is shown in Fig. 5.

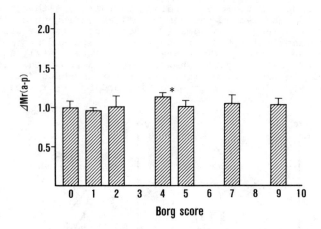

Fig. 5. Relationship between the change in
         anteroposterior (a-p) motion of rib
         cage and Borg score. A-p motion is
         expressed relative to initial in Borg
         score 0. *: p<0.01.

The a-p motion of the rib cage is standardized by the same tidal volume and is expressed by the change in a-p motion of the rib cage (Δ Mrc(ap)). As shown in Fig. 5, no change in a-p motion was observed even at higher Borg scores. The relationship between the changes in lateral motion of the rib cage and the Borg score is shown in Fig. 6.

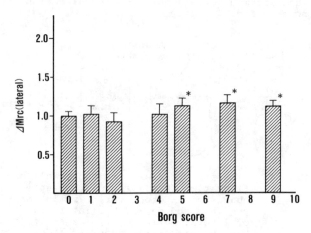

Fig. 6. Relationship between the change in
         lateral motion of rib cage and Borg

score. Lateral motion is expressed
relative to the initial value in Borg
score 0. *: p<0.01.

Lateral motion is also standardized the same tidal volume and is
expressed by the change in lateral motion of rib cage (Δ
Mrc(lateral)). As Borg score increased, a parallel increase in
lateral motion of the rib cage was observed. The relationship
between the changes in the integrated electrical activity of the
parasternal and intercostal muscles and the Borg score is shown in
Fig. 7.

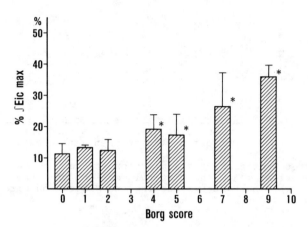

Fig. 7. Relationship between the change in
         integrated electrical activity of
         parasternal intercostal muscle.
         *: p<0.01.

The integrated IMG was normalized by its value during maximal
inspiratory effort at FRC. A marked increase in electrical
activity was observed as the Borg score increased.

Thus, our findings can be summarized as follows: 1) During Pdi=0
breathing, there was marked distortion within the rib cage, i.e.,
no change in a-p motion but a relative increase in lateral motion
as the Borg score increased; and 2) There was inappropriate a-p
motion of the rib cage for a given electrical activity of the
parasternal intercostal muscles.

Two clinical cases are presented below:

Case 1: The patient was a 71-year-old male with emphysema and
abdominal laxity produced by previous surgery. Lung function tests
showed the following: %VC - 73%; %FEV$_1$ - 31%; %TLC - 128%; Cst(1) -
0, 39L/cmH$_2$O; and %DL$_{CO}$ - 62%. He complained of dyspnea even when
performing ordinary daily activities.

The left panel of Fig. 8 shows the changes in gastric pressure
(Pga), Pdi, flow, tidal volume and chest wall configuration of this
patient during quiet breathing. The right panel shows the changes
in the measured parameters after the abdomen was restricted with an
elastic bandage.

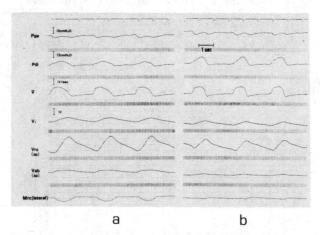

a   b

Fig. 8. The change in the measured parameters
         during quiet breathing (a) and after
         compressing the abdomen with elastic band.

During quiet breathing, the a-p motion of the rib cage (Vrc(ap))
was   paradoxical   to   the   lateral   motion   of   the   rib   cage
(Mrc(lateral)), but after bandaging, no distortion within the rib
cage was observed.

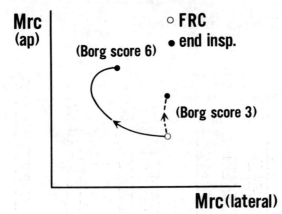

Fig. 9. Change of the regional motion of the
         rib cage. Solid line: with elastic band;
         dotted line: without elastic band.

Figure 9 is a diagram showing rib cage distortion in relation to
the Borg score. The a-p motion of the rib cage is expressed on the
ordinate and the lateral motion on the abscissa.   The   solid   line
indicates no abdominal bandaging and the broken line indicates
abdominal bandaging.   As shown in Fig. 9, the marked   distortion
within the rib cage was greatly reduced after bandaging and at the
same time the Borg score was reduced from 6 to 3.

Case 2: The patient was a 47-year-old male with COPD. In this patient, an increase in the Borg score was produced by step-wise increases in inspiratory resistance loading. After a particular load had been applied, the subject rested for long enough to avoid any effect of inspiratory muscle fatigue on the following loading test.

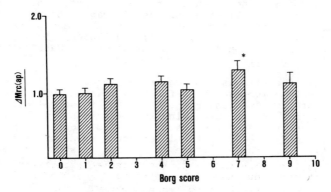

Fig. 10. Relationship between the change in a-p
motion of rib cage and Borg score.
A-p motion is expressed relative to the
initial value in Borg score 0.
*: p<0.01.

Figure 10 shows the relationship between changes in the a-p motion of the rib cage and the Borg scores. No change in a-p motion was observed even at higher Borg scores.

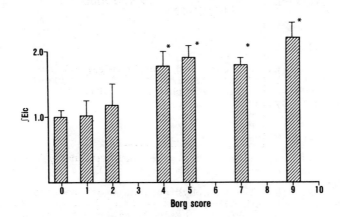

Fig. 11. Relationship between the change in
integrated electrical activity of
parasternal intercostal muscle. Integrated electrical activity is expressed
relative to the initial value in Borg
score 0. *: p<0.01.

Figure 11 shows the relationship between changes in the electrical

activity of the parasternal intercostal muscles and the Borg score.
A parallel increase in EMG was seen with higher Borg scores.

DISCUSSION

The intercostal muscles are known to be rich in spindles (Derenne
et. al., 1978) and these can be involved in reflex arcs mediating
functions like stabilization of the rib cage (Duron, 1973; von
Euler, 1974; Shannon and Zechman, 1972), the perception of
respiratory movement (Duron, 1973; von Euler, 1974), and the
control of postural and antigravitational tone (Massion et. al.,
1960; Meulders et al.).

We found that out-of-phase motion of the rib cage, i.e., a-p motion
versus lateral motion, was significantly related to a sensation of
shortness of breath during Pdi=0 breathing in normal subjects, as
well as during quiet breathing in a patient with emphysema,
abdominal laxity and one case of COPD during incremental
inspiratory loading. Since the intercostal spindles participate in
stabilization of the rib cage, rib cage distortion apparently
stimulates the spindles, and their increased discharge produces the
sensation of dyspnea.

In 1963, Campbell and Howell proposed the new concept that the
sensation of dyspnea was related to an inappropriateness of the
volume achieved for a given tension developed by the muscles.

Our study showed that there was an inappropriate a-p motion of the
rib cage for the extent of the electrical activity of the
parasternal intercostal muscle during Pdi=0 breathing in normal
subjects and in a patient with COPD when incremental inspiratory
loading was applied. Thus, this inappropriate electrical activity
may stimulate the intercostal spindles, and result in a sensation
of dyspnea.

CONCLUSION

Distortion of the rib cage and inappropriate a-p motion for the
extent of the electrical activity of the parasternal intercostal
muscles both seem to stimulate the intercostal spindles and produce
a sensation of dyspnea.

REFERENCES

Ashutosh, K., R. Gilbert, J.H. Auchincloss and D. Peppi (1975).
    Asynchronous breathing movements in patients with obstructive
    pulmonary disease. Chest, 67, 553.
Borg, G.A.V. (1982). Psychophysical basis of perceived exertion.
    Med. Sci. Sports Exercise, 14, 377-381.
Campbell, E.J.M. (1969). Physical signs of diffuse airways
    obstruction and lung distension. Thorax, 24, 1.
Campbell, E.J.M. and J.B.L. Howell (1963). The sensation of
    breathlessness. Br. Med. Bull., 19, 36.
Derenne, J-Ph., P.T. Macklem and Ch. Roussos (1978). The
    respiratory muscles: mechanics, control, and pathophysiology,
    Part 1-3. Am. Rev. Respir. Dis., 118, 119-601.
Duron, B. (1973). Postural and ventilatory functions of intercostal
    muscles. Acta Neurobiol. Exp., 33, 355.

Konno,   K. and J. Mead (1967). Measurement of the   separate   volume
changes   of   rib   cage and abdomen   during   breathing.   J.   Appl.
Physiol., 22, 407.
Massion, J., M. Meulders and J. Colle (1960). Fonction   posturale
des muscles respiratoires. Arch. Int. Physiol., 68, 314.
Meulders,   M., J. Massion and J. Colle (1960). Influence du   lobe
anterieur   du cervelet sur l'activite tonique   et   respiratoire
des muscles intercostaux. Arch. Ital. Biol., 98, 430.
Roussos, C.S. and P.T. Macklem (1976). Response of the   respiratory
muscles to fatiguing loads. Am. Rev. Respir. Dis., 113, 200.
Shannon,   R.   and F.W. Zechman (1972). The   reflex   and   mechanical
response   of   the   inspiratory muscles to an   increased   airflow
resistance. Respir. Physiol.,, 16,   51.
Sharp,   J.T., N.B. Goldberg, W.S. Druz, H.C. Fishman and   J.   Danon
(1977).   Thoracoabdominal   motion   in   chronic   obstructive   lung
disease. Am. Rev. Respir.   Dis., 115, 47.
von   Euler, C. (1974). On the role of proprioceptors in   perception
and execution of motor acts with special reference to   breathing.
In: Loaded   Breathing   (L.D. Pengelly, A.S.   Rebuck   and   E.J.M.
Campbell, ed.), p. 139,   Ontario, Longman Canada, Ltd.

Phrenic Nerve Stimulation in Myasthenia Gravis

A. Mier

Department of Medicine, Charing Cross Hospital,
Fulham Palace Road, London W6 8RF, UK

ABSTRACT

Repetitive supramaximal stimulation at frequencies of 3 to 5 Hz is commonly performed to detect abnormal neuromuscular transmission of an affected peripheral nerve in patients with suspected myasthenia gravis (Ozedmir and Young, 1976). Such patients often complain of dyspnea, but little is known about phrenic nerve function in this condition. Since the diaphragm is the main muscle of inspiration and may be affected in myasthenia gravis, the present studies were performed to determine whether abnormalities of neuromuscular transmission could be detected during phrenic nerve stimulation.

KEYWORDS

Dyspn ea; diaphragm

Thirteen patients with myasthenia gravis and exertional dyspnea were studied. Investigations were also performed on 15 controls - 10 normal subjects and 5 patients with diaphragm weakness not due to myasthenia gravis. The phrenic nerves were stimulated supramaximally in the supraclavicular region with surface electrodes first at 1 Hz and then at 3 Hz. The amplitude of diaphragm muscle action potentials was recorded with surface electrodes in the 7th or 8th inter-costal space, during stimulation in the supine posture at resting end expiration.

Diaphragm muscle action potentials varied between 0.8 and 1.4 mV during stimulation at 1 Hz. No decrement was seen in diaphragm muscle action potentials in any of the control subjects when stimulation frequency was increased to 3 Hz. By contrast, 5 patients with myasthenia gravis showed a consistent characteristic decrement in diaphragm muscle action potentials at 3 Hz; this was demonstrated on both sides in 3 patients and on one side in two. Recovery occurred within 3 seconds when stimulation frequency returned to 1 Hz. No decrement was seen during stimulation of either nerve in the other 8 patients with myasthenia gravis.

Therefore abnormalities of neuromuscular transmission were detected during repetitive phrenic nerve stimulation at 1 to 3 Hz in a proportion of patients with myasthenia gravis who complained of dyspnea. This appears to be a useful and simple test for assessing diaphragmatic involvement in such patients with

A. Mier

myasthenia gravis.

REFERENCES

Ozedmir, C. and Young, R. (1976). The results to be expected from electrical testing in the diagnosis of myasthenia gravis. Am. N.Y. Acad. Sci., 174, 203-22.

Concurrent Depression of Respiratory and Antigravity Muscle Activities by Stimulation of the Pontine Dorsal Tegmentum in Decerebrate Cats

K. Kawahara, Y. Nakazono, Y. Yamauchi
and Y. Miyamoto

Department of Information Engineering, Yamagata
University, Yonezawa 992, Japan

ABSTRACT

The tonic electrical stimulation of the midpontine dorsal tegmentum in decerebrate
cats resulted in the concurrent suppression of the tonic discharges of bilateral
hindlimb extensor muscles and the rhythmic discharges of diaphragmatic activity.
This short report reviews the detailed properties of such stimulus effects on
postural tone and respiration.

KEYWORDS

Postural tone; respiration; midpontine tegmentum; decerebrate cat.

INTRODUCTION

In the acute precollicular-postmammillary decerebrate cats, stimulation of the dorsal
part of the caudal tegmental field (DTF) in the pons along the midline results in
long-lasting suppression of extensor muscle tone (Mori et al., 1982). During the
course of our investigation on locomotor-respiratory coupling during locomotion in
the mesencephalic cats, we have found that DTF stimulation used for reducing the
decerebrate rigidity not only elicits long-lasting suppression of postural tone but
also suppresses the diaphragmatic activity (Kawahara et al., 1988a). In this report,
we have analyzed the DTF-elicited suppressive effects on postural tone and
respiration, and presumed the possible neural mechanisms responsible for such
characteristic suppressive effects.

METHODS

Cats of either sex were surgically decerebrated at the precollicular-postmammillary
level under halothane anesthesia. Electromyograms (EMG) were recorded by
implanting bipolar electrodes made of thin copper wires into the bilateral soleus
muscles and the diaphragm. Bipolar recording of the external intercostal and the
hypoglossal nerve activities were also performed by implanting thin copper wires.
End-tidal Pco_2 was monitored with an infrared gas analyzer and recorded. DTF
stimulation consisted of a rectangular pulse of 0.2 ms duration at 50 pulses/s
with an intensity of 50 – 70 µA. At the end of each experiment, the amimals were
deeply anesthetized (pentobarbital sodium, i.v.) and sacrificed.

K. Kawahara *et al.*

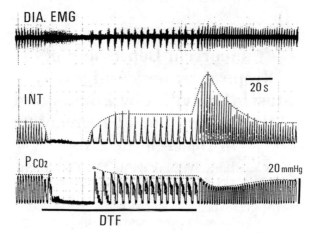

Fig. 1.   Recovery of respiratory movements during stimulation.
DIA EMG, diaphragmatic EMG; INT, integrated DIA EMG;
Pco_2, CO_2 tension of expired air.   (Modified From
Kawahara et al., 1988a)

POSTURAL AND RESPIRATORY SUPPRESSION

The midline DTF stimulation suppressed the extensor muscle tone as well as the
diaphragmatic activity (Kawahara et al.,1988a; 1988b).   The reduced or abolished
tonic discharges of the bilateral soleus muscles did not recover to the prestimulus
level even after stimulation ended.   In contrast, the rhythmic discharges of the
diaphragm, once strongly suppressed by DTF stimulation, gradually recovered in spite
of the continuation of the stimulation.   DTF stimulation also suppressed the tonic
and rhythmic discharges of the external intercostal muscle activity (Kawahara et
al., 1989b).   In addition to the above two kinds of respiratory muscle activities,
DTF stimulation suppressed the activity of the hypoglossal nerve innervating the
genioglossus nuscle (Kawahara et al.,1989a).   The tonic discharges of the hypoglossal nerve was depressed by DTF stimulation and the decreased nerve activity
persisted after stimulation ended.

RECOVERY OF RESPIRATION DURING STIMULATION

The respiratory movements resumed in spite of the continuation of DTF stimulation
(Fig. 1).   In this animal, DTF stimulation resulted in apnea for more than 30 s.
After that, the respiratory movements gradually resumed and became stable at the
later part of DTF stimulation. The characteristic features of such stable respiration are summarized as follows: (1) The respiratory frequency was smaller than
the prestimulus frequency.   (2) The peak amplitude of the integrated diaphragmatic
EMG was greater than that before stimulation.   (3) The end-tidal Pco_2 was kept at
almost the same level as before stimulation.

MECHANISMS RESPONSIBLE FOR RECOVERY OF RESPIRATION

Figure 2 shows a schematic model to explain the recovery process of respiratory
movements during DTF stimulation.   The existence of the rebound augmentation of
respiratory movements at the end of DTF stimulation (Fig.1) suggested that DTF-
elicited suppressive effects on respiration was not abolished but continued to
operate during the entire period of stimulation (top trace in Fig. 2). If this is

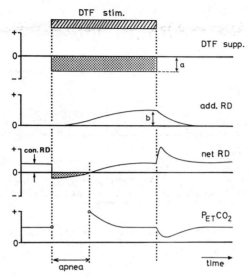

Fig. 2. Schematic model for recovering process of respiration.
add. RD, additional respiratory drive; net RD, sum-
mation of respiratory drives; con. RD, control RD.

the case, the strong respiratory drive to overcome the exerted inhibition must be
brought about during stimulation. This respiratory drive is termed here as the
additional respiratory drive (add.RD). When the respiratory depression induced
by DTF stimulation is just compensated with the additional RD, the minute
ventilation may be kept at almost the same value as before stimulation, and consequently the end-tidal Pco_2 was kept at the same level as before stimulation. we
hypothesize that DTF-elicited inhibition of respiration immediately returns to a
zero level, but the additional RD does not. This difference in the decay time
course may produce the rebound augmentation of respiratory movements.

This work was supported by a grant from the Ministry of Education and Culture of
Japan (01570055).

REFERENCES

Kawahara, K., Y. Nakazono, S. Kumagai, Y. Yamauchi and Y. Miyamoto (1988a).
  Parallel suppression of extensor muscle tone and respiration by stimulation of
  pontine dorsal tegmentum in decerebrate cat. Brain Res., 473, 81-90.
Kawahara, K., Y. Nakazono, S. Kumagai, Y. Yamauchi and Y. Miyamoto (1988b).
  Neuronal origin of parallel suppression of postural tone and respiration elicited by stimulation of midpontine dorsal tegmentum in decerebrate cat. Brain Res.,
  474, 403-406.
Kawahara, K., Y. Nakazono, S. kumagai, Y. Yamauchi and Y. Miyamoto (1989a).
  Inhibitory influences on hypoglossal neural activity by stimulation of midpontine
  dorsal tegmentum in decerebrate cat. Brain Res., 479, 185-189.
Kawahara, K., Y. Nakazono and Y. Miyamoto (1989b). Depression of diaphragmatic
  and external intercostal muscle activities elicited by stimulation of midpontine
  dorsal tegmentum in decerebrate cats. Brain Res., 491, 180-184.
Mori, S., K. Kawahara, T. Sakamoto, M. Aoki and T. Tomiyama (1982). Setting and
  resetting of level of postural muscle tone in decerebrate cat by stimulation of
  brain stem. J. Neurophysiol., 48, 737-748.

Nasal Receptors Responding to Temperature and Pressure Changes in the Nose

H. Tsubone

Department of Animal Environmental Physiology,
Faculty of Agriculture, The University of Tokyo,
Bunkyo-ku, Tokyo 113, Japan

ABSTRACT

This study demonstrated that the ethmoidal branch of the trigeminal nerve contains fibers connected to nasal 'cold' and 'pressure' receptors. Nasal 'cold' receptors were stimulated by inhalation of cold air and inhibited with warm air passing through the nose. Nasal 'pressure' receptors were activated by nasal occlusion performed at end-expiration when the nose was subjected to negative pressure.

KEYWORDS

Trigeminal nerve; nose; nasal receptors; temperature; pressure; upper airway

MATERIALS AND METHODS

Single unit, as well as whole nerve, afferent activity was recorded from the ethmoidal nerve, in a total of 45 anesthetized rats breathing through the nose or a tracheostomy.

Nasal 'Cold' Receptors

In 14 rats breathing through the nose, cold($0{\sim}15°C$), room($22{\sim}26\ °C$) and warm air($30{\sim}45\ °C$), and in some rats nasal occlusion were applied into the nose through a facemask(volume=2ml).
In 11 rats breathing through a tracheostomy, a constant airflow($100{\sim}300$ ml/min) with cold, room and warm air mentioned above were passed through the nose with an inspiratory direction.

Nasal 'Pressure' Receptors

In 15 rats breathing through the nose, nasal occlusion was performed at end-expiration and/or end-inspiration by closing the facemask. In other 5 rats breathing through a tracheostomy, maintained negative($-0.1{\sim}-3.7$ kPa) and positive($0.8{\sim}3.0$ kPa) pressures were applied to the isolated upper airway. In these rats, tracheal occlusion was also applied at end-expiration.

RESULTS

Forty endings were identified as 'cold' receptors which were stimulated by cooling and inhibited by warming to the nose during nasal breathing. Nineteen of the 40 'cold' receptors discharged spontaneously with 1-8 spikes in each respiratory cycle during nasal breathing of room air while others were silent until the rat was exposed to cold air. Such effect of temperature on the ethmoidal afferent was also seen in its whole nerve activity as shown in Fig. 1. Fifty-five of 85 'cold' receptors tested were activated by constant airflow with room and cold air but inhibited with warm air which were applied to the isolated upper airway.

Twenty-two endings were identified as 'pressure' receptors which were activated by nasal occlusion when the upper airway was subjected to negative pressure(mean peak pressure, -0.1~-3.7 kPa). During three consecutive nasal occlusions, mean pressure threshold to stimulate these receptors was -0.73, -0.87 and -0.96 kPa(n=22) at the 1st, 2nd and 3rd inspiratory effort, respectively. All the 12 fibers tested for maintained pressures were clearly stimulated by negative pressure(Fig. 2). Only three of them were also stimulated by positive pressure. All of the 'pressure' receptors were not stimulated by tracheal occlusion which induced an augmentation of activity in alae nasi as well as other upper airway muscles.

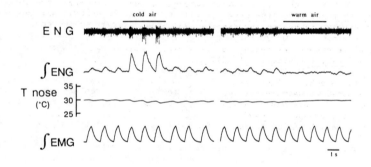

Fig. 1. Nasal 'cold' receptors stimulated by cold air(left panel) but not by warm air(right panel).

DISCUSSION

Pressure, flow(or temperature) and drive(or respiratory muscle activity) have been thought as major elements to stimulate sensory endings in respiratory mucosa and/or submucosa in the upper airway. In fact, some nervous receptors concerned with these sensory stimuli have been recorded in the dog larynx: 'pressure', 'cold' and 'drive' receptors(Sant'Ambrogio, et al., 1983). The present study evidenced that the nose has also 'cold' and 'pressure' receptors. The nasal 'cold' receptors might be contribute to some respiratory reflexes such as inhibitory effects of breathing including a prolongation of T_E, increase of nasal flow resistance and bronchoconstriction or bronchodilation(Widdicombe, 1988; Mathew and Sant'Ambrogio, 1988), and the nasal 'pressure' receptors might be involved in maintaining upper airway patency when the nose is occlusive(van Lunteren, et al., 1984, Mathew, 1984).

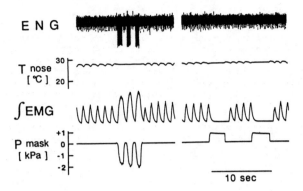

Fig. 2. Nasal 'pressure' receptor responded to negative
pressure(left panel) but not to positive
pressure(right panel).

REFERENCES

Mathew, O. P.(1984). Upper airway negative-pressure effects on respiratory
activity of upper airway muscles. J. Appl. Physiol., 56, 500-505.
Mathew, O. P. and F. B. Sant'Ambrogio(1988). Laryngeal reflexes. In:
Respiratory function of the upper airway(O. P. Mathew and G. Sant'Ambrogio eds.
), Lung biology in health and disease, 35, pp.259-302.
Sant'Ambrogio, G., O. P. Mathew, J. T. Fisher and F. B. Sant'Ambrogio(1983).
Laryngeal receptors responding to transmural pressure, airflow and local muscle
activity. Respir. Physiol., 54, 317-330.
van Lunteren, E., W. B. Van de Graaff, D. M. Parker, J. Mitra, M. A. Haxhiu, K.
P. Strohl and N. S. Cherniack(1984). Nasal and laryngeal reflex responses to
negative upper airway pressure. J. Appl. Physiol., 56, 746-752.
Widdicombe, J. G.(1988). Nasal and pharyngeal reflexes. In: Respiratory
function of the upper airway(O. P. Mathew and G. Sant'Ambrogio eds.), Lung
biology in health and disease, 35, pp.233-258.

Reflex Activities of Upper Airway Muscles During Nasal Occlusion in Anaesthetized Dogs

O. Kaminuma and H. Tsubone

Department of Animal Environmental Physiology,
Faculty of Agriculture, The University of Tokyo,
Bunkyo-ku, Tokyo, 113, Japan

ABSTRACT

The present study confirms the considerable augmentation in the activity of upper airway dilating muscles, alae nasi(AN) and posterior cricoarytenoid muscles(PCA), during nasal occlusion. It was also elucidated that during such reflexes the contribution of superior laryngeal nerve is greater in PCA than in AN in the activation of these muscles. In the latter muscle(AN), the lack of volume feedback in lung might be a major factor to stimulate it during nasal occlusion.

KEYWORDS

Nasal occlusion; tracheal occlusion; diaphragm; alae nasi; posterior cricoarytenoid muscle; superior laryngeal nerve; electromyogram; airway receptors.

MATERIALS and METHODS

In order to apply the nasal and tracheal occlusions a small mask was constructed around the nose and a cannula with two side arms was placed in the trachea below the larynx in nine anaesthetized and spontaneously breathing dogs. Nasal and tracheal occlusions were performed at end-expiration for three consecutive breathings by inflating balloons which were placed in the nose-mask and tracheal cannula. These occlusions were repeated three times or more before and after the both sides of the superior laryngeal nerves(SLNs) were sectioned. In all experiments, electromyograms(EMGs) from diaphragm(DIA), alae nasi(AN) and posterior cricoarytenoid muscle(PCA), esophageal(Peso) and intratracheal(Ptr) pressure were recorded(Fig. 1).

RESULTS and DISCUSSION

During nasal occlusion, the extrathoracic airway(Ptr) was subjected to negative pressure, i.e., -2.46, -2.83, and -3.15 kPa(n=30) at the 1st, 2nd and 3rd inspiratory effort, respectively. Peak DIA activity increased 28.3, 48.5 and 68.3% from the control before occlusion, respectively.
During nasal occlusion Peak AN and PCA activities increased 295, 718, 1260% and

175, 251, 330% from the control before nasal occlusions, respectively. Such result indicate that the increase of EMG activity was much larger in Peak AN than that in Peak PCA. Peak PCA activity was significantly larger in nasal occlusion than tracheal occlusion(P<0.05), though Peak AN activity also tended to be greater in nasal occlusion than tracheal occlusion. These results indicate that a marked enhancement of upper airway dilating muscle activities is induced by nasal occlusion. These reflexes have been considered to contribute in maintaining upper airway patency(van Lunteren et al. , 1984, Sant'Ambrogio, et al. , 1985).

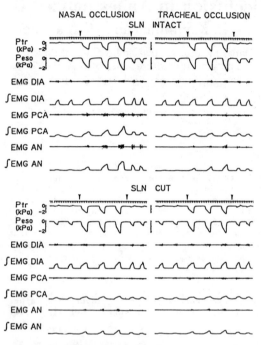

Fig. 1. Reflex responses of upper airway dilating muscles and diaphragm during nasal and tracheal occlusions before and after the section of SLNs.

Furthermore, it was elucidated that the effect of enhancement of AN activity was considerable even if the occluded airway did not include the larynx and nose.
The augmented activity in PCA during nasal occlusion was largely diminished by sectioning both the SLNs, while the augmented AN activity was less diminished by such elimination of laryngeal afferents(Fig. 2). Therefore, laryngeal component is considerably important in activation of PCA, while it is not necessarily a predominant factor on AN. In the latter muscle, the lack of volume feedback in lung might be a major factor to stimulate it.
Inspiratory time(T_I) was markedly prolonged and mean inspiratory slope(Peak DIA/T_I) decreased in nasal occlusion, whereas these changes were maximum in the first inspiratory effort. These respiratory effects attributable to negative pressure in the upper airway would protect the airway from its abrupt collapse(Mathew, 1984).
It has been known that some mechanoreceptors sensitive to pressure changes are present in the upper airway, larynx(Sant'Ambrogio, et al., 1983; Tsubone et al. 1987), pharynx(Hwang, et al., 1984) and nose(Tsubone, 1989). Although these

receptors have been divided into two groups, either 'negative' or 'positive' pressure receptor, a great number of receptors were identified as 'negative' pressures in the dog and cat larynx and also in the rat nose. These receptors activated by negative pressure have been considered to play an important role on the airway protective reflexes during upper airway occlusion(Mathew and Sant'Ambrogio, 1988).

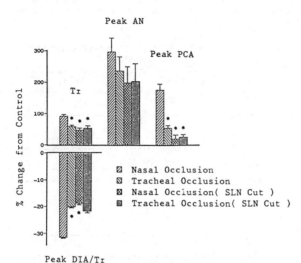

Fig. 2. Changes in inspiratory time(T_I), Peak AN and PCA activities and mean inspiratory slope(Peak DIA/T_I, by nasal and tracheal occlusions before and after the section of SLNs.
* ; Differences are significant(P<0.05 ; Student's t-test, comparison with nasal occlusion before SLNs cut).

REFERENCES

Hwang,J-C., W.M.St.John and D.Bartlett,Jr.(1984). Receptors responding to changes in upper airway pressure. Respir. Physiol., 55, 355-366.
Mathew,O.P. (1984). Upper airway negative-pressure effects on respiratory activity of upper airway muscles. J. Appl. Physiol.: Respirat. Environ. Exercise Physiol., 56(2), 500-505.
Mathew,O.P. and F.B.Sant'Ambrogio (1988). Laryngeal reflexes. In: Respiratory function of the upper airway(O.P.Mathew and G.Sant'Ambrogio, Eds.), pp.259-302.
Sant'Ambrogio,F.B., O.P.Mathew, W.D.Clark and G.Sant'Ambrogio (1985). Laryngeal influences on breathing pattern and posterior cricoarytenoid muscle activity. J. Appl. Physiol., 58(4), 1298-1304.
Sant'Ambrogio,G., O.P.Mathew, J.T.Fisher and F.B.Sant'Ambrogio (1983). Laryngeal receptors responding to transmural pressure, airflow and local muscle activity. Respir. Physiol., 54, 317-330.
Tsubone,H., O.P.Mathew and G.Sant'Ambrogio (1987). Respiratory activity in the superior laryngeal nerve of the rabbit. Respir. Physiol., 69, 195-207.
Tsubone,H. (1989). Nasal 'pressure' receptors. Proceedings of XXXI I.U.P.S. Congress, Helsinki, Finland, 9-14, July.
van Lunteren,E., W.B.van DE Graaff, D.M.Parker, J.Mitra, M.A.Haxhiu, K.P.Strohl and N.S.Cherniak (1984). Nasal and laryngeal reflex responses to negative upper airway pressure. J. Appl. Physiol., 56(3), 746-752.

Dilator Nares Activity in Relation to Obstructive Sleep Apnea

K. Asakura, Y. Nakano, T. Shintani and
A. Kataura

Department of Otolaryngology, Sapporo Medical
College, Sapporo, Japan

ABSTRACT

We evaluated the activities of dilator nares EMG,and also submental EMG during
sleep in three patients with obstructive sleep apnea syndrome. Both EMG
activities showed periodic changes which proved to be correlated with each
other(r=0.85). Apnea and hypopnea episodes always occurred at the nadir of
these periodic changes. The activities of dilator nares EMG, as well as
submental EMG, at the nadir of these periodic changes were significantly lower
during REM(Rapid Eye Movement) sleep than non-REM sleep and also significantly
lower during obstructive apnea than hypopnea. These EMG activities were also
revealed to be correlated positively with the decrease in SaO2 level, and
negatively with the duration time of obstructive apnea.

KEYWORDS

Obstructive sleep apnea syndrome, Dilator nares EMG, Submental EMG, Sleep stage,
SaO2

INTRODUCTION

Several studies have demonstrated the respiration related contraction of the
nasal mucosa, and also the respiration related activity of dilator nares(
Asakura et al., 1986, 1987; Strohl et al.,1980), which cause an increase in
size of the nasal cavities and then decrease in the nasal airway resistance
during early inspiration(Strohl et al., 1982). An increase in nasal airway
resistance causes the pharyngeal pressure to decrease during inspiration,
thereby increasing the tendency for this airway to collapse. Both structual
changes of the nasal cavity, such as septal deviation, and neuromuscular changes
which cause nasal obstruction may play an important role in pathogenesis of
obstructive sleep apnea syndrome . In this study, we evaluated the activity of
dilator nares EMG(Electromyography), as well as submental EMG, during sleep in
patients with this syndrome .

MATERIALS and METHODS

Three adult patients with obstructive sleep apnea syndrome were included in this study. The activity of dilator nares EMG and submental EMG were examined simultaneously during sleep study. Each EMG activity was integrated and was expressed as the percent ratio to the maximum activity recorded during sleep. The comparison of EMG activity during apnea-hypopnea was made by using the EMG activity at the nadir of each periodic change. A continuous recording of SaO_2 was made using a percutaneous oximeter(Biox3700,Ohmeda) and the changes of the tidal volumes were also recorded using a computerized system of respiratory inductive plethysmograph(Respigraph, Nimus).

RESULTS

Dilator narcs EMG activity, as well as submental EMG activity, involved periodic changes during sleep in all patients. The activity of dilator nares EMG proved to be correlated with those of submental EMG activity (r=0.85). Hypopnea-apnea episodes always occurred at the nadir of each periodic change of respiratory activity. When the relationship with a sleep stage was examined, the EMG activity of both submental and dilator nares revealed to be significantly weaker during the REM sleep stage than the non-REM(table 1). The occurrence of obstructive sleep apnea was also more frequent during REM sleep.

Table1. Relationship of EMG activity and sleeping stage.

	Dilator nares EMG(%)	Submental EMG(%)	Apnea occurence
non-REM sleep	25.3+17.9*	17.3+ 7.9	18/36(50%)**
REM sleep	3.6+ 3.8	6.1+ 7.4	10/11(91%)

*Each EMG value represented percent ratio to the Maximum activity.
**Prevalence of apnea at the nadir of periodic respiration.

Table 2. Relationships between severity of airway
obstruction and EMG activities.

	Dilator n. EMG (%)	submental EMG (%)	SaO_2 (%)	Apnea duration (sec)
Hypopnea	15.1+ 7.9	53.0+17.7	80.8+ 9.2	–
Apnea-Hypopnea	5.7+ 6.3	38.6+24.0	70.6+15.6	26.6+17.0
AH-2	7.0+ 6.9	50.0+20.7	78.0+ 8.6	18.5+ 7.6
AH-1	3.0+ 3.7	15.1+ 7.8	55.5+16.1	43.2+19.0

Using a computerized Respigraph system , any decrease of tidal volume less than 25 % of control respiration for more than 12 seconds was prescribed as apnea-hypopnea(AH). As shown in table 2, the dilator nares EMG activity, as well as submental EMG activity at the nadir of periodic respiration, was significantly lower during AH hypopnea periods than hypopnea periods. Among the AH episodes, those with paradoxical respiratory movements of thorax and abdomen were denoted AH-1 and distinguished from other AH episodes(AH-2). AH-1 was thought to be accompanied by more complete obstruction of the upper respiratory tract than AH-2 which included central type apnea. As indicated in table 2, the activities of dilator nares EMG and submental EMG were significantly lower during AH-1 than AH-2. SaO_2 level was significantly lower and apnea duration was significantly longer in APNEA 1 than APNEA 2. The coefficiency value between dilator nares EMG vs SaO2, dilator nares EMG vs apnea duration, submental EMG vs SaO2, and submentalEMG vs apnea dutration were 0.40, -0.41, 0.66 and -0.63, respectively.

DISCUSSION

EMG activities of digastrics and genioglossus were reported to be different during REM and non-REM sleep and closely related to the occurence of occulsive sleep apnea (Remmers et al. 1978; Onal et al., 1982a, 1982b).
In this study, we also noted that the dilator nares EMG activity was closely related to the sleeping stage and occurence of upper airway obstruction in the patients with obstructive sleep apnea syndrome. It was reported that the frequency of apneic episodes in patients with pollinosis increased significantly during their affected season(McNicholas et al., 1982). Dayal(1985) reported that surgical correction of anterior sited septal deviation reduced the severity of obstructive sleep apnea. So, any decrease in activity of the dilator nares during sleep might facilitate the obstructive sleep apnea syndrome, especially in the patients with organic nasal obstruction.

REFERENCE

Asakura K., K. Hoki, A. Kataura, T. Kasaba and M. Aoki (1986).   Respiration-related movements of the nose in dogs.
    Acta Otolaryngol.(Stockh)   , 101, 122-128.
Asakura K, K. Hoki, A. Kataura, T. Kasaba and M.Aoki (1987).   Spontaneous nasal oscillations in dog - a mucosal expression of   the respiration-related activities of cervical sympathetic nerve.
    Acta Otolaryngol.(Stockh), 104, 533-538.
Dayal V.S. and E.A. Phillipson (1985). Nasal surgery in the   management of sleep apnea. Ann. Otol. Rhinol. Laryngol., 94, 550- 554.
McNicholas W.T., S. Tarlo, P. Cole, N. Zamel, R. Rutherford, D.   Griffin and E.A. Phillipson(1982). Obstructive apnea during sleep   in patients with seasonal allergic rhinitis. Am. Rev. Resp.   Dis., 126, 625-628.
Onal E., M. Lopata and T. O'connor(1982a). Pathogenesis of apnea in hypersomnia-sleep apnea symdrome. Am. Rev. Respir. Dis., 125,   167-174.
Onal E., and M. Lopata(1982b). Periodic breathing and the   pathogenesis of occulusive sleep apneas. Am. Rev. Respir. Dis., 126,   676-680.
Remmers J.E., W.T. DeGroot, E.K. Sauerland and A.M. Anch(1978).   Pathogenesis of upper airway occlusion during sleep. J. Appl.   Physiol., 44, 931-938.
Strohl K.P., M.J. Hensley, M. Hallett, N.A. Saunders and R.H.   Ingram Jr(1980). Activation of upper airway muscles before onset   of inspiration in normal humans. J. Appl. Physiol., 49, 638-642.
Strohl K.P., C.F. O'cain and A.S. Slutsky(1982). Ala nasi   activation and nasal   resistance in healthy subjects. J. Appl.   Physiol., 52, 1432-1437.

Different Course in the Phase-related Fluctuation of the High-frequency Oscillation in the Phrenic and Cranial Nerve Activities in Rabbits

F. Kato, K. Takano, Y. Tsukamoto,
N. Kimura and T. Hukuhara, Jr.

Department of Pharmacology II, Jikei University School
of Medicine, Minato-ku, Tokyo 105, Japan

ABSTRACT

Phase-related fluctuation of the high-frequency oscillation (HFO) in the efferent discharges of the phrenic and vagus nerves was quantitatively analyzed in rabbits. The consistency of the fluctuation in the frequency of the HFO components in these nerve activities within inspiratory phase supports the view that the HFO is originated in a common network whose activity is deeply modulated by the respiratory rhythm. In contrast, the time course of the mean square values for the amplitude of HFO components differed prominently between the phrenic HFO and cranial HFO. It is suggested that the frequency and strength of the inspiratory motoneuronal synchronization are separately determined.

KEYWORDS

Phrenic nerve; vagus nerve; high-frequency oscillation; time series analysis; Fourier analysis; respiratory center; respiratory muscles; neural network

INTRODUCTION

Synchronized inspiratory (I) discharges of the motor nerve fibers of the phrenic nerve at about 70-130 Hz (Cohen, 1973) also appear with considerably high coherence in the inspiratory motor activities of the cranial nerves involved in the phasic control of the upper airway resistance (Kato et al., 1987). The functional significance of the HFO, therefore, is supposed to lie in the efficient maintenance of respiratory movements through the central coordination of the musculature contraction (Kato et al., 1987; Webber, 1989). To elucidate the neural process underlying the formation of HFOs in the phrenic and vagus nerve activities, the fluctuation patterns of these HFOs within respiratory cycles were quantitatively compared.

METHODS

Experiments were performed on ten vagotomized rabbits anesthetized with ether and paralyzed with gallamine and maintained by artificial ventilation. Concentration of the CO_2 in the expired gas and the arterial blood pressure were monitored continuously to check that the animal was normoventilated. The efferent discharges of the bilateral phrenic and vagus nerves were simultaneously recorded on a magnetic tapes. Afterwards, the nerve activities were reproduced and converted to a digital signal for consecutive 30 respiratory cycles. After detection of onset of the I phase for each neural breath, power spectral densities for the nerve activities from 0 to 200 Hz were estimated from the 160-ms data windows which were taken every 50 ms step from I onset of respective cycle and ensemble-averaged for 30 cycles.

By means of nonlinear least-squares method developed by the authors (Kato et al., 1987), the following parameters representing the oscillating state of the HFO were quantitatively estimated: 1) mean square value, an estimate for the total amount of the HFO component within the data window, 2) peak-frequency, an estimate for the modal and mean oscillating frequency of the HFO, and 3) half-value width, an estimate for spatiotemporal variation of the oscillating frequency of the HFO.

RESULTS

Figure 1 shows a typical result illustrating changes in the three parameters for the HFOs in the bilateral phrenic and vagus nerve discharges within I phase. The peak-frequencies for the HFOs in these four nerve activities fluctuated consistently with each other in the course of the I phase: a slight drop in the first about 1/4 portion of the I phase to the lowest and a elevation towards the highest at the terminal of the I phase (Fig. 1, top).

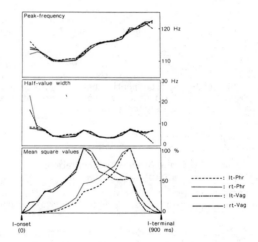

Fig. 1. Variations in the course of the respiratory cycle in the peak-frequency, the half-value width and the mean square values. Abscissa, time from the onset of I phase (ms). It-Phr, rt-Phr, It-Vag and rt-Vag represents changes in the HFOs in the left phrenic, right phrenic, left vagus and right vagus nerve activities, respectively. Total respiratory cycle duration was 1.84 ±0.04 s (mean±S.D.) and the end-tidal concentration of CO_2 was 3.5% for this animal.

In contrast, the changes in the mean square values of the phrenic and vagus HFOs in the course of the I phase differed from each other depending on the kind of the nerve: the mean square value for the vagus HFO rose more rapidly than the phrenic HFO at the I onset and peaked at the middle of the I phase, whereas that for the phrenic HFO peaked at about 2/3 of the mean I time from the I onset (Fig. 1, bottom). Differences between the activities derived from the right and left nerve trunks were not recognized. Mean square values of the HFO components in these nerve activities were consistently estimated to be zero for the data windows within expiratory phases. Similar and consistent results were observed in other nine rabbits, though the range of the fluctuation of the peak-frequency within the I phase differed slightly among each rabbit.

DISCUSSION

The phase-related fluctuations in the peak-frequency and the mean square values for the HFO in the phrenic nerve activity are in accordance with our earlier studies using similar analytical techniques (Kato et al., 1986), which clearly showed that the oscillating state of the HFO-generating network is profoundly modified by res-piratory-modulated inputs. The present study succeeded in quantitative description of the changes in the HFOs in the simultaneously recorded phrenic and vagus nerve activities in the course of the I phase. The consistency in the fluctuation of the peak-frequency and the half-value width for the phrenic and vagus HFO within I phase provides a strong support to the hypothesis proposed by Wyss (1955) that the HFOs in these nerve activities are originated in a common neural mechanism in the brain stem which might be designated as "the common HFO-generator".

In contrast to the frequency, fluctuations within phase in the amount of the HFO output represented by the mean square values differed prominently between the phrenic and the vagus nerve activity. This dissimilarity is not contradictory to the previous observations by Cohen (1975) where the integrated I bursts in the phrenic and recurrent laryngeal nerves were compared in spontaneously breathing cats. As HFOs might be inherently involved in and mainly contribute to the central control of respiratory movements, this regional heterogeneity might be related to the dif-ference in the functional role of the HFOs in these motor nerve activities in the coordinated respiratory behaviors.

Though the neuronal mechanism for the generation and formation of HFO is still unclear, it is reasonable to imagine that the activity of the "common HFO-gene-rator", whose oscillating state is phasically modified by the respiratory-rhythmic in-puts, would define the phase and frequency of the HFO-locked firing of the neurons in the premotor and/or motor pool organizations separately from the neuronal mechanisms determining the amplitude of the final motor outflow of the respective nerve conveyed to respiratory-related musculature.

Supported partly by the Ministry of Education, Science and Culture, Japan, Grant-in-Aid for Developmental Scientific Research, No. 01870012 and by the Science Re-search Promotion Fund of Japan Private School Promotion Foundation (1988).

REFERENCES

Cohen, M.I. (1973). Synchronization of discharge, spontaneous and evoked, between inspiratory neurons. Acta Neurobiol. Exp., 33, 189-218.
Cohen, M.I. (1975). Phrenic and recurrent laryngeal discharge patterns and the Hering-Breuer reflex. Amer. J. Physiol., 228, 1489-1496.
Kato, F., Y. Fujisaki, N, Kimura, K. Takano and T. Hukuhara, Jr. (1986). Variation of high frequency oscillations in the phrenic nerve activity in the course of one respiratory cycle. J. Physiol. Soc. Jpn, 48, 381.
Kato, F., N. Kimura, K. Takano and T. Hukuhara, Jr. (1987). Quantitative spectral analysis of high frequency oscillation in efferent nerve activities with respiratory rhythm. In: Respiratory Muscles and Their Neuromotor Control (G. C. Sieck, S.C. Gandevia and W.E. Cameron, eds), pp. 263-267, Alan R. Liss, New York.
Webber, C.L., Jr. (1989). High-Frequency oscillations within early and late phases of the phrenic neurogram. J. Appl. Physiol., 66, 886-893.
Wyss, O.A.M. (1955). Synchronization of inspiratory motor activity as compared be-tween phrenic and vagus nerves. Yale J. Biol. Med., 28, 471-480.

Different Effects of Halothane and Enflurane on Diaphragmatic Contractility *in vivo*

Tetsuo Kochi, Toru Ide, Shiro Isono,
Tadanobu Mizuguchi and
Takashi Nishino

Department of Anesthesiology, Chiba University School
of Medicine and the Department of Anesthesiology,
National Cancer Center Hospital, 1-8-1, Inohana,
Chiba, 280, Japan

ABSTRACT

To examine the effects of volatile anesthetics on the contractile performance of diaphragm, we determined the force-frequency relations of canine diaphragm in vivo under halothane (n=6) or enflurane (n=6). Force-frequency relationship was obtained by applying various frequencies of electric stimulation to bilateral phrenic nerves and measuring the transdiaphragmatic pressure (Pdi) developed at functional residual capacity against an occluded airway. In animals anesthetized with enflurane Pdi significantly decreased with 50 and 100 Hz stimulation in the presence of increasing MAC value. By contrast, with halothane there was no difference of Pdi at any stimulation frequencies during any of the three levels of anesthesia. On the other hand, there was no statistical difference between Pdi-frequency relationships during 1 MAC of halothane and enflurane in 8 animals. From these results, we conclude that halothane does not impair diaphragmatic contractility any more than enflurane does, and enflurane decreases force generation of the diaphragm at high stimulation frequencies in dose related fashion.

KEYWORDS

Contractility; Diaphragm; Force-frequency relationship; Transdiaphragmatic pressure; Anesthetics; Halothane; Enflurane

INTRODUCTION

Recently Aubier et al. (1981a, b, 1984, 1986) have developed a method to assess the contractility of diaphragm in vivo and have examined the effects of various pharmacological agents on the fatigued diaphragm. In this connection, little information is available so far regarding the effects of various anesthetics on the contractility of the diaphragm in vivo. Accordingly, we examined the effects of halothane and enflurane on diaphragmatic function in mechanically ventilated dogs.

MATERIALS AND METHODS

Twelve mongrel dogs were anesthetized in the supine position with thiopental 15 mg/kg intravenously, with anesthesia being maintained with either halothane (n=6) or enflurane (n=6). The animals were tracheotomized and mechanically ventilated throughout the experiments. Transdiaphragmatic pressure (Pdi) was determined as the difference between esophageal and abdominal pressures recorded by the two balloon-catheter systems. During a given study period, Pdi (cmH_2O) was recorded during electrical stimulation of the phrenic nerve at different frequencies (10, 20, 50, and 100 Hz) while the airway was occluded at end-expiratory lung volume.

Diaphragmatic contractility was assessed during three levels of anesthesia in each animal, namely 1, 1.5, and 2MAC of either halothane or enflurane, each after 1 hour of steady state conditions. The sequence of changing anesthetic level was randomized between animals. In addition, in 8 of 12 dogs, the relationship between Pdi and frequency of stimulation was also assessed during 1 MAC of halothane and enflurane at the end of the first protocol. This was done by changing anesthetic either from halothane to enflurane (n=4) or from enflurane to halothane (n=4). Statistical analysis was performed using two way analysis of variance and the Tukey's test.

RESULTS

Table 1 demonstrates the values of Pdi at stimulation frequencies of 10, 20, 50, and 100 Hz under three levels of anesthesia in both groups.

Table 1. Values of Pdi at various stimulation frequencies of phrenic nerve at three levels of halothane and enflurane anesthesia.

	$Pdi\ (cmH_2O)$			
	10 Hz	20 Hz	50 Hz	100 Hz
Halothane group				
1 MAC	18.8±5.2	35.9±5.8	44.8±6.1	45.4±6.1
1.5 MAC	18.8±4.5	37.5±4.6	44.3±5.0	44.4±5.1
2 MAC	18.4±4.2	37.0±5.2	44.9±6.7	44.9±6.8
Enflurane group				
1 MAC	12.5±2.5	27.3±3.0	37.4±4.7	34.0±4.4
1.5 MAC	12.7±2.5	28.6±3.0	32.7±3.3	21.0±5.0**
2 MAC	11.0±2.1	22.8±3.3[+]	25.3±4.1[**,+]	14.1±3.8[**,+]

(** $p<0.01$ vs 1 MAC, + $p<0.05$ vs 1.5 MAC)

Halothane

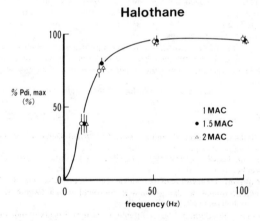

Fig. 1. Force-frequency response curves of the diaphragm at three levels of halothane anesthesia. o, •, and △ denote the values at 1, 1.5, and 2 MAC. Each point represents average data (± SEM).

Enflurane

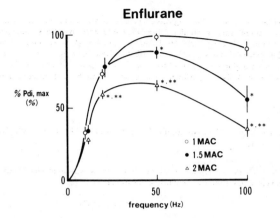

Fig. 2. Force-frequency response curves of the diaphragm at three levels of enflurane anesthesia. * and ** represent statistical difference (* p < 0.01 vs 1 MAC, ** p < 0.01 vs 1.5 MAC). For definitions see Fig. 1 legends.

Figures 1 and 2 depict the force-frequency relationships in the halothane (Fig. 1) and enflurane (Fig. 2) groups. Values of Pdi were expressed in % of maximum Pdi obtained in each animal. It is apparent from Fig. 2 that enflurane exerts a dose dependent decrease of diaphragmatic force generation at higher stimulation frequencies of 50 and 100 Hz. Enflurane at 2 MAC also decreased tension development at 20 Hz stimulation more than it did at 1 and 1.5 MAC. By contrast, halothane did not affect force generating properties at any stimulation frequencies. Although Pdi of enflurane tended to be less than that of halothane at 1 MAC at the range of frequencies between 20 and 100 Hz, the Pdi-stimulation frequency relations obtained in 8 animals at 1 MAC of halothane and enflurane were essentially identical and the difference was not statistically significant.

CONCLUSION

We conclude that increasing enflurane concentrations produce a progressive decreases in force generation of canine diaphragm in response to higher frequencies of stimulation. By contrast, increasing halothane concentrations do not affect diaphragmatic contractile properties, at least in the range of MAC maltiples used in the present experiments.

REFERENCES

Aubier, M., Farkas, G., De Troyer, A., Mozes, R. and Roussos, C. (1981a). Detection of diaphragmatic fatigue in man by phrenic stimulation. J. Appl. Physiol., 50, 538-544.
Aubier, M., Trippenbach, T. and Roussos, C. (1981b). Respiratory muscle fatigue during cardiogenic shock. J. Appl. Physiol., 52, 499-508.
Aubier, M., Viires, N., Murciano, D., Medrano, G., Lecocguic, Y. and Pariente, R. (1984). Effects and mechanism of action of terbutaline on diaphragmatic contractility and fatigue. J. Appl. Physiol. 56, 922-929.
Aubier, M., Viires, N., Murciano, D., Seta, J.P. and Pariente, R. (1986). Effects of digoxin on diaphragmatic strength generation. J. Appl. Physiol. 61, 1767-1774.

Diaphragmatic Shortening During Vomiting

T. Abe, S. Hua, H. Sato, N. Kusuhara,
M. Tanaka and T. Tomita

Department of Medicine, School of Medicine, Kitasato
University, 1-15-1, Kitasato, Sagamihara, Kanagawa 228,
Japan

ABSTRACT

In lightly anesthetized and spontaneously breathing dogs, we investigated the diaphragm shortening during vomiting. Results: 1) illustrate that segmental shortening is a function of both segmental electrical activity and surrounding pressures; and 2) suggest that crural function may not be homogeneous for both medial and lateral portions.

KEYWORDS

Diaphragm; Vomiting; Electromyogram; Costal; Crural.

INTRODUCTION

It has been reported that there is no electrical activity in the medial part of the crural segment of the canine diaphragm during vomiting (Monges et al. 1978). The focus of our study was how the diaphragm works during vomiting.

METHODS

We studied 8 mongrel dogs (ranging in weight from 12.5 to 29.0 kg). Anesthesia was induced with an intravenous injection of thiopental sodium and small additional doses were given to maintain a constant, light level of anesthesia. The animals breathed spontaneously during the measurements. The diaphragm length was measured during room air breathing, occluded breathing, progressive hypercapnea, and vomiting. Electromyographic (EMG) activity of the diaphragm and abdominal pressure were also measured. Diaphragmatic shortening was measured by piezoelectric transducers (Newman et al. 1985) fixed onto the left costal, the medial, and the lateral parts of the left crural segments. Vomiting was induced with intravenous injection of apomorphine.

RESULTS

During progressive hypercapnia, diaphragmatic shortening and EMG activity increased in all parts of the diaphragm (Fig. 1, Fig. 2). During vomiting: 1)

abdominal pressure increased dramatically (Fig. 3); 2) in the costal segment, EMG
activity and shortening increased; 3) in the medial part of the crural segment,
EMG activity decreased or disappeared and the crural segment lengthened; 4) in
the lateral part of the crural segment, EMG activity increased, however crural
segmental length was variable.

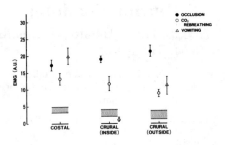

Fig. 1.   EMG activity of the diaphragm (Edi). During
occluded breathing and CO_2 rebreathing, peak
diaphragmatic Edi increased significantly ($P<0.01$)
in all three parts of the diaphragm compared to
room air breathing. During vomiting, Edi
increased significantly in costal segment ($P<0.01$)
and lateral part of crural segment ($P<0.05$),
however, Edi did not increase in medial part of
crural segment. Bars; SE. Dotted area; mean$\pm$SE
during room air breathing.

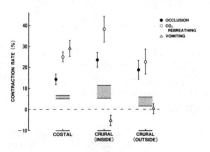

Fig. 2.   Diaphragmatic shortening. During occluded
breathing and CO_2 rebreathing, diaphragmatic
shortening increased significantly ($P<0.01$) in all
three parts of the diaphragm compared to
room air breathing. During vomiting, shortening
increased significantly ($P<0.01$) in costal
segment; in medial part of crural segment, the
diaphragm significantly ($P<0.05$) lengthened; and
in lateral part of crural segment, shortening did
not change significantly. Bars; SE. Dotted area;
mean$\pm$SE. Negative value for contraction means
lengthening.

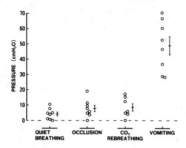

Fig. 3. Abdominal pressure change. During vomiting, abdominal pressure increased dramatically. Bars; mean+SE.

DISCUSSION

These results suggest that during vomiting: a) contraction of the costal diaphragm contributes to an increase in abdominal pressure; b) lengthening of the medial part of the crural diaphragm allows relaxation of lower portion of the esophagus; and c) coordination of costal and crural segments facilitates regurgitation of gastric contents. These results: 1) illustrate that segmental shortening is a function of both segmental electrical activity and surrounding pressures; and 2) suggest that crural function may not be homogeneous for both medial and lateral portions.

REFERENCES

Monges, H., J. Salducci and B. Naudy (1978). Dissociation between the electrical activity of the diaphragmatic dome and crura muscular fibers during esophageal distension, vomiting and eructation. An electromyographic study in the dog. J. Physiol., Paris, 74, 541-554.

Newman, S., J. Road, F. Bellemare, J. P. Clozel, C. M. Lavigne, and A. Grassino (1984). Respiratory muscle length measured by sonomicrometry. J. Appl. Physiol.: Respirat. Environ. Exercise Physiol. 56: 753-764.

Activity of the Respiratory Muscles During Cough

I. Kobayashi, T. Kondo, H. Suzuki, Y. Ohta and H. Yamabayashi

Department of Medicine, School of Medicine, Tokai
University, Isehara, Kanagawa, 259-11, Japan

ABSTRACT

We studied the electrical activity of the respiratory muscles during cough on
anesthetized and tracheostomized 12 dogs.

Expiratory activities were observed in the inspiratory muscles during cough.
The costal part of the diaphragm (N=7) and the external intercostal (EIC)
muscles (N=3) were observed. Expiratory activity developed approximately 50
msec after the termination of the preceding inspiratory activities. In
contrast, expiratory muscles, i.e., internal intercostal (IIC) muscle and
transversus abdominis (TA) muscle, were active only during expiratory phase of
cough. These activities developed approximately 30 msec after the termination
of the diaphragmatic inspiratory activity. Expiratory activities of
inspiratory muscles developed significantly later than that of expiratory
muscles (P<0.01).

KEYWORDS

Cough; diaphragm; expiratory activity; medullary inspiratory neuron; PIIA

METHOD

The experiments were carried out on 12 mongrel dogs weighing 10-14 kg. The
animals were anesthetized with pentobarbital sodium. Light anesthesia was
maintained with intraperitoneal dial-urethan. Each animal was tracheostomized
and placed in the supine position. Respiratory flow, pleural pressure (Ppl),
gastric pressure (Pg) and the electrical activity of the intercostal muscles,
diaphragm and abdominal muscles were measured. Electrodes for diaphragmatic
measurements were inserted in the costal part of the diaphragm by laparoscope
to avoid injury to the abdominal wall (Kondo et al., 1988).

The electrical activity of respiratory muscles was studied under following
conditions: (1) quiet breathing, (2) cough during quiet breathing,(3)
hypercapnia induced by breathing with CO_2-mixed air (end-tidal CO_2
concentration of 7%). Cough was provoked by gentle mechanical stimulation of
the tracheal mucosa with a fine polyethylene catheter.

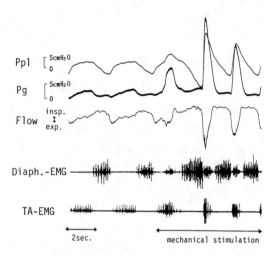

Fig. 1. Activity of the respiratory muscles during quiet breathing
and cough. Ppl: pleural pressure, Pg: gastric pressure,
Diaph.: diaphragm TA: transversus abdominis.
Cough is characterized by abrupt increase in Ppl and Pg.
The diaphragm is active during expiratory phase of cough
(7/12 dogs). There is a short silent interval between the
inspiratory and expiratory diaphragmatic activities.

RESULT

Fig. 1 shows a recording during quiet breathing and cough. During quiet
breathing, the diaphragm is active only during inspiration. On the other hand,
expiratory muscles (TA) are active only during expiration. When the trachea
was stimulated mechanically, cough is characterized by abrupt increase in Ppl
and Pg. There is no preparatory inspiration in the first cough. In the second
and third cough there is a preparatory inspiration. In these responses, the
diaphragm is active during inspiratory and early-expiratory phases. There is a
short silent interval between the inspiratory and expiratory activities in
the diaphragm.   The first cough lacks preparatory inspiration, but the
diaphragm is active during the expiratory phase in both. In contrast, all
the expiratory muscles are active only during expiratory phase of cough. We
observed this type of expiratory activity in diaphragm in 7 of 12 dogs.
When the respiratory center is stimulated by hypercapnia, no expiratory
activity develops in the diaphragm.
We also analyzed the response of another inspiratory muscle, the external
intercostal (EIC) muscle during cough. EIC is also active during the
expiratory phase as well as during inspiratory phase of cough. We observed
the expiratory activity of EIC in 3 of 6 dogs.   Expiratory activity of EIC
does not develop during hypercapnia.

We defined the short silent intervals as the time from the termination of
diaphragmatic inspiratory activity to the onset of expiratory activity of
individual respiratory muscles.   The silent interval for diaphragm is
52.9±24.6 msec (S.D.) and that for EIC is 51.1±20.5 msec. Thus the expiratory
activity of both inspiratory muscles developed synchronously. The silent
interval for IIC is 34.3±13.0 msec and that for TA is 27.8±15.2 msec.

These intervals of diaphragm and EIC are not statistically significant. In contrast, the onset of expiratory activity in inspiratory muscles are significantly later than that of expiratory muscles ($P < 0.01$ by paired t-test).

DISCUSSION

The phrenic activity during expiratory phase of cough has been observed in the crural part of the diaphragm in human subjects (Agostoni et al., 1960) and in the costal part of the diaphragm in experimental animals (Tomori and Widdicombe, 1969). We observed the expiratory activity of costal part of the diaphragm in 7 of 12 dogs. These results are comparable to those reported by Tomori and Widdicombe. They found that this expiratory activity was derived from activity of spinal motoneurons. However in our present investigation, the expiratory activities of inspiratory muscles during cough were not necessarily preceded by inspiratory activity. Furthermore, the expiratory activity of the inspiratory muscles developed significantly later than that of the expiratory muscles. This finding suggests that the commands driving these inspiratory activities are different from those for expiratory muscles.

Jakus et al.(1985) reported that the firing frequency of the inspiratory neurons in the medulla was increased during inspiratory phase of cough; however in their report, medullary inspiratory activity remained at the early-expiratory phase of cough. This suggests that the medullary inspiratory neurons are to some extent responsible for this expiratory activity. The physiological role of the phrenic expiratory activity during cough is yet unclear. There are short silent intervals between inspiratory and expiratory phrenic activities. This may indicate that the expiratory activity during cough is different from the post-inspiratory inspiratory activity (PIIA).

REFERENCES

Kondo, T., Suzuki, H., Ohta, Y., Yamabayashi, H.(1988). An EMG analysis on regulation of the diaphragm and abdominal muscles. Tohoku J. Exp. Med., 156, Suppl., 43–55

Agostoni, E., Sant'Ambrogio, G., Del Portillo Carrasco, H. (1960). Electromyography of the diaphragm in man and transdiaphragmatic pressure. J. Appl. Physiol., 15, 1093–1097

Tomori, Z., Widdicombe J.G. (1969).Muscular, bronchomotor and cardiovascular reflexes elicited by mechanicalstimulation of the respiratory tract. J. Physiol., 200, 25–49

Jakus, J., Tomori, Z., Stransky, A. (1985).Activity of bulbar respiratory neurones during cough and other respiratory tract reflexes in cats. Physiol. Bohemosolov., 34, 127–136

A Case of Neuroleptics-induced Respiratory Dyskinesia

K. Honda, M. Yaginuma, R. Horikoshi,
Y. Kaneko, M. Kaneko and H. Kumashiru

Department of Neuropsychiatry, Fukushima Medical
College, Hikarigaoka 1, Fukushima-shi 960, Japan

ABSTRACT

It is known that respiratory disturbances derived from extrapyramidal reactions can often occur with long -term use of neuroleptics. This is one of the symptoms of tardive dyskinesia, and since it causes involuntary movement of the respiratory muscles, it is called respiratory dyskinesia(RD). In this study, we report a patient with continued episodes of dyspnea after long-term use of neuroleptics who was admitted repeatedly to the ICU with dyspnea.

KEYWORD

Respiratory dyskinesia, tardive dyskinesia, neuroleptics, respiratory acidosis, Meige's syndrome

RESPIRATORY DYSKINESIA

Tardive dyskinesia is a syndrome of various involuntary movements after prolonged neuroleptic treatment or withdrawal. In this syndrome, BLM(bucco-lingo-masticatory)dyskinesia or trunkal dyskinesia is commonly seen, on the other hand, neuroleptics-induced RD has been very rarely reffered. Our case showed that RD produced life-threatening ventiratory disturbances with respiratory acidosis and this state required intensive respiratory control in ICU. RD has almost improved with palliative neuroleptic treatment, but Meige's syndrome (Blepharospasm-Oromandibular dystonia)has been lasting. It was concluded that RD with respiratory acidosis may become very severe and may be transformed into other types of neuroleptics associated tardive syndrome.

CASE REPORT (Fig. 1)

Mr.T ; 69year-old-man, print engineer. Diagnosis; manic depressive psychosis. Present history; Subsequent to the death of his mother, the patient initially entered a depressive state and then changed to a manic state, and was admitted. In 1973, the patient was admitted again for manic state and after that he had been treated as an outpatient with neuroleptics including haloperidol. From approximately 1985 to 1986 the patient developed frequent blephalospasm and extention of the tongue, and eventually mild dyspnea appeared.In April 1987, administration of the drugs (14.5mg of haloperidol and 0.5mg of triazoram at the time) was discontinued. From June 1987, dyspnea and chest discomfort began to occur before sleep and the patient was admitted to the ICU of this hospital on June 26 for acute respiratory failure. The patient has respiratory acidosis at the time of admission, but with administration of O_2 and artificial respiration the symptoms improved. Any remarkable abnormalities were not found in the ECG, chest Xp, brain CT, and the Swan-Ganz catheter test during the period of admittance. After discharge in July 1986, the same kind of respiratory distress and dyspnea reoccurred and emergency admittance was needed 6 days later. During the previous period of admittance, involuntary movements of the. mouth, tongue and eyelids continued even after relief of the dyspnea and tests taken during admittance to the ICU indicated the unlikeliness of cardiopulmonary causes,and therefore the patient was referred to the psychiatric department. Since the neurological signs of oral, buccal, mandibular, laryngeal, and RD were noted, he was given continuous administration of 150mg of sulpiride and 5mg of diazepam. Improvement was seen to a certain degree, but the various dyskinesias, the irregular breathing pattern, and the frequent -shallow ventilation persisted. In April 1988, mild manic state occurred and the patient was admitted to our ward. While fully realizing the risk of aggravated respiratory disturbance, a small dosage of neuroleptics was administered. Treatment with 3mg of timiperone, 120mg of tioridazine, 30mg of levomepromazine before sleep, and 3mg of trihexyphenidyl improved the BLM dyskinesia, RD, and blepharospasm, but the bilateral ptosis which was noted from the time of admittance, continued.Respiration after discharge has been within normal limits.

Fig. 1.   Clinical Course of This Case

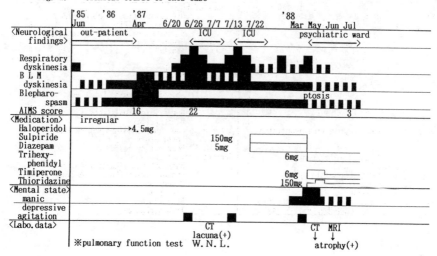

DISCUSSION

Diagnosis

Weiner and Casey et al have reported on the existence of RD. The reasons for equating our case of respirator disturbance with that state is; ①Discontinuance of long-term neuroleptics therapy brought on respiratory disturbance that became milder with careful re-administration of neuroleptics and the course of symptoms wer generally parallel to that of other dyskinesias. ② There were no signs of cardiopulmonary injury or a gross organic brain lesion. However, with CT and MRI, the possibility of dyskinesia being caused by brain atrophy or central nervous degeneration due to aging cannot be excluded. ③The respiratory disturbance occured durir resting periods and was not pronounced during sleep or conversation. It worsened during times of psychological tension.

Clinical feature----comparison of this case with reported cases   (Table. 1)

Including this case, since Weiner, 12 cases of neuroleptics-induced RD have been reported. The ages were 30 to 70 with an average age of 55.7±12.4 years. There were 6 males and 6 females, showing no sex difference. Concerning the psychiatric diseases for which neuroleptics were prescribed, there were 5 cases of schizophrenia, 4 cases of affective disorder, and 3 cases of neurosis as there was no specificity of the diseases. All patients had a history of long-term neuroleptics therapy and haloperidol was the most common p -RD drug in 6 cases, chlorpromazine being next. There was a high incidence of BLM, trunk and limb dyskinesia as neuroleptic associated tardive syndrome(Jeste, 1986), and the inicial symptom was RD in 3 of the 12 cases The interval from iniciation of drug therapy to the occurrence of RD was from 1 to 24 years and the average was 10.3±9.1 years. Concerning the activating cause of the RD, there were 6 cases of discontinuance or decrease in dosage of neuroleptics and 6 cases of continued drug administration. There was RD other than tardive dyskinesia in all cases and the symptoms were generally consistent with RD but as in this cases, other types of dyskinesia occurred (Meige's syndrome). The examination of blood gas analysis at the time of RD revealed 4 cases of respiratory alkalosis, and 3 cases of respiratory acidosis as the latter was the mos severe. In our case, during the period of exacerbated RD, there was respiratory acidosis and marked dyspnea as there was a near respiratory failure state and as a result treatment in the ICU was necessary. As treatment for the RD, butyrophenone neuroleptics were used in 4 cases, phenothiazine neuroleptics in 4 cases reserpine in 4 cases, etc, and good results have been obtained.

Prognosis

Casey et al and Goswami et al have reported patients with respiratory acidosis and life-threatening respiratory dyskinesia. Our case is almost similar and although the general condition of the patient is bein maintained with the re-administration of neuroleptics, there is a possibility that the effect of re-administration is only temporary. There is a possibility that there will be worsened dyskinesia, parkinsonism or other dyskinesias including Meige's syndrome and there remains the problem of possible psychiatric symptoms, extrapyramidal side effects and threat to life from those problems.

Table 1. Summary of Case Reports of Neuroleptics Induced Respiratory Dyskinesia (N=12)

Age	Mean 55.7 ± 12.4y (30 ~ 70y)		Causes of RD		
Sex	Female 6 , Male 6		Discontinuation or decreasing		
Diagnosis	Schizophrenia	5	of neuroleptics		6
	MDI	4	Taking neuroleptics continuously		6
	Neurosis	3	Dyskinesia symptoms except RD		
Previous medication			Mouth		9
	Neuroleptics(unknown)	1	Limb		9
	Haloperidol	6	Trunk		8
	Phenothiazines		Tongue		7
	Chlorpromazine	4	Face		7
	Thioridazine	2	Abdominal muscle, Chest wall		5
	Trifluoperazine	2	Laryx		3
	Trihexyphenidyl	2	Upper intestinal tract		1
	Li, l-dopa	1	Blepharospasm		3
Firstly appeared neuroleptics associated			Arterial blood gases findings before therapy		
tardive syndrome			Respiratory alkalosis		4
	BLM	4	Respiratory acidosis		3
	Respiratory system	3	Current medication		
	Trunk, Limb	4	Butyrophenones(haloperidol etc)		4
	Abdominal muscle	1	Phenothiazines(Chlorpromazine etc)		4
	Blepharospasm	1	Reserpine		2
	Unknown	1	Diazepam		2
Dration from medication till RD appearance			Benztropine		2
	Mean 10.3 ±9.1y (1 ~ 24y)		Trihexyphenidyl		1

CONCLUSION

① We have reported a case of severe respiratory dyskinesia occuring after the discontinuance and decrease in dosage of long-term neuroleptics administration.
② In this instance the respiratory dyskinesia included respiratory acidosis which required treatment in the ICU. In order to relieve the problem, neuroleptics were used and good results in respiratory control were obtained.
③ During the course, the respiratory dyskinesia and other tardive dyskinesias were generally similar but after relief of the RD, neuroleptics induced Meige's syndrome remained.
④ This study indicated the necessity of administering drugs with full knowledge of psychiatric symptoms and the various types of neuroleptic associated tardive syndromes that cause respiratory dyskinesia and sometimes have a life-threatening prognosis.

REFERENCES

Casey, D.E. , P. Rabins (1978). Tardive dyskinesia as a life-threatening illness Am J Psychiatry 135:4, 486-488
Chiang, E.C. , W.M. Pitts and M.R.Garcia (1985). Respiratory dyskinesia: Review and case reports. J CLIN PSYCHIATRY 46:6, 232-234
Faheem, A.D. , D.R. Brightwell , G.C.Burton and A. Struss (1982). Respiratory dyskinesia from prolonged neuroleptic use: Tardive dyskinesia? Am J Psychiatry 139:4, 517-518
Goswami, U. and S.M. Channabasavanna (1985). On the lethality of acute respiratory component of tardive dyskinesia. Clin Neurol Neurosurg. Vol.87-2, 99-102
Jeste, D.V. (1989). Pathophysiology and management of tardive dyskinesia. Jpn. J. Psychopharmacol. 9: 12
Kaneko, Y. and H. Kumashiro (1986). Levodopa-induced respiratory disturbance --Its pathophysiology--. Medicine and Biology. 113(1): 55-58
Kaneko, Y. and H. Kumashiro (1987). Levodopa and respiratory abnormality with reference to dyskinesia. Medicine and Biology. 114(2): 117-120
Steen, S.N. (1976). The effects of psychotropic drugs on respiration. Pharmac. Ther. B, Vol. 2, 717-741
Weiner, W.J. , G.G. Christopher and H.L. Klawans (1978). Respiratory dyskinesias: extrapyramidal dysfunction and dyspnea. Annals of Internal Medicine. 88: 327-331

Breath-holding Sensation — Respiratory Muscle Activity and Breathlessness Sensation

K. Fujieda, S. Okubo, H. Morinari and M. Harasawa

Department of Respiratory Diseases, Tokyo Teishin Hospital, 2-14-23, Fujimi, Chiyoda-ku, Tokyo 102, Japan

ABSTRACT

We examined the relationship between breathlessness sensation and electromyogram(EMG) activity of respiratory muscle during voluntary breath holding. Six normal male subjects were studied. Sensation of breathlessness was assessed by modified Borg scale. Relationship between EMG activity and breathlessness sensation was compared among three different conditions of breath holding. Continuous increase of EMGic and EMGsm during breath holding up to the breaking point was observed. This was assosiatd with the outward displasement of rib cage. Activity of EMGic and EMGsm rather than EMGdi was closely related with breathlessness sensation. We conclude that breath-holding sensation is more directly related to rib cage muscle activity rather than diaphragmatic activity.

KEYWORDS

Breath holding; breathlessness; respiratory muscle activity; diaphragm; rib cage muscle; electromyogram.

INTRODUCTION

It has been suggested that distress sensation during breath holding mainly arises from diaphragmatic contraction (Eisel,1968; Noble,1971). However, there is some evidence that respiratory effort sensation is related to rib cage muscle activity during loaded breathing (Bradlay, 1986; Ward,1988). These reports suggest that different respiratory muscles induce different sensation during breath holding and resistive loaded breathing. However, breath holding is considered to be extremely loaded breath with infinite resistance. In this study we examined EMG activity of respiratory muscles and sensory score of breathlessness during

breath holding in normal man to assess the contribution of
respiratory muscles activity to distress sensation during breath
holding. We also examined the effect of chest wall geometry and
lung volume on the sensation.

METHOD

Each subject hold their breath under three different conditions;
(1) at FRC without rib cage restriction, (2) with restriction
of rib cage and (3) without retriction of rib cage at about the
same lung volume as (2). Sensation of breathlessness was assessed
by modified Borg scale (scale 0 to 10). Integrated EMG of
diaphragm (EMGdi), parasternal intercostal muscle (EMGic) and
sternocleidomastoid muscle (EMGsm) were evaluated. Chest wall
geometry was measured by Konno-Mead diagram using magnetometer.

RESULTS

During breath holding at FRC,
muscle activity appeared after
some silent period and became
greater up to breaking point.
There was continuously
increasing activity of EMGic and
EMGsm which was accompanied by
increase of A-P diameter of rib
cage. These activities
correlated well with sensory
score. However, it was not the
case with EMGdi. Under the
condition of restriction of rib
cage EMGic and EMGsm activiies
were as same as at FRC. Fig.1
shows comparison of EMG activity
between two of the three
different conditions at the same
sensation. In EMGic, activity
was almost constant and the
points were located near the
identical line. EMGsm also
distributed near the line. This
indicates that the consistancy
of relation between EMG activity
of rib cage muscles and breath-
holding sensation was not
affected by the change of
geometry of chest wall and lung
volume. However, in case of
EMGdi, distribution of points
deviated markedly from the line
as shown in the bottom panel
of Fig.1.

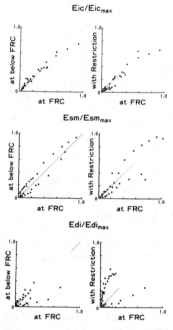

Fig.1.
Comparison of EMG activity be-
ween the two different conditions at the same sensation.
Solid diagonal line at 45° represents line of identity.

DISCUSSION

The results of our study suggest that parasternal intercostal and sternocleidomastoid muscle activity are more directly related to breath-holding sensation than that of diaphragm. During breath holding, diaphragm and accessory muscles were activated by different manner. In rib cage muscles, two types of activity were observed. One is continuous or tonic activity which is accompanied with gradual expansion of rib cage. Another is periodic and phasic activity which synchronizes with intermittent activity of EMGdi. Periodic isovolume displacement of rib cage and abdomen might be due to these phasic activity. Furthermore, in spite of activation of rib cage muscles, rib cage moved inward when EMGdi was active. It is well accepted that rib cage muscles have non-ventilatory function; stabilization of the chest wall. Continuous and increasing activity of EMGic and EMGsm may be one of the reflections of this function. Thus, rib cage muscles possibly act both as non-ventilatory and ventilatory muscle during breath holding. In contrast, diaphragm contracts only for inspiratory action. Non-ventilatory function of rib cage muscles during breath holding seems to increase the length of diaphragm which would be very favorable for diaphragm to contract effectively just after the breaking point.

REFERENCES

Bradley,T.D., D.A.Chartrand, J.W.Fitting, K.J.Killian and A.Grassino (1986). The relation of inspirartory effort sensation to fatiguing patterns of the diaphragm. Am. Rev. Respir. Dis.,134, 1119-1124.
Eisele,J., D.Trenchard, N.Burki and A.Guz (1968). The effect of chest wall block on respiratory sensation and control in man. Clin. Sci., 35, 23-33.
Noble,M.I.M., J.H.Eisele, H.L.Frankel, Wendy Else and A.Guz (1971). The role ofthe diaphragm in the sensation of holding the breath. Clin. Sci., 41, 275-283.
Ward,M.E., D.Eidelman, D.G.Stubbing, F.Bellmare and P.T.Macklem (1988). Respiratory sensation and pattern of respiratory muscle activation during diaphragm fatigue. J.Appl.Physiol., 65 (5), 2181-2189.

Dyspnea and Inspiratory Muscle Fatigue During Exercise in Patients with Chronic Obstructive Pulmonary Disease

H. Matsushita, S. Fujimoto, N. Kurihara
and T. Takeda

The First Department of Internal Medicine, Osaka City
University Medical School, 1-5-7 Asahimachi,
Abeno-ku, Osaka 545, Japan

ABSTRACT

Role of inspiratory muscle fatigue in the genesis of dyspnea in the patients with
chronic obstructive pulmonary disease(COPD) has yet to be fully studied. The purpose of the present study is to investigate possible relationship between respiratory muscle fatigue and sensation of dyspnea during exercise in eight COPD patients.
Six of them showed diaphragmatic fatigue during exercise. With diaphragmatic fatigue, these patients were extremely dyspneic. Five of the six with diaphragmatic
fatigue showed sternomastoid muscle fatigue, which preceded diaphragmatic fatigue.

KEYWORDS

Respiratory muscles; dyspnea.

INTRODUCTION

For patients with chronic obstructive pulmonary disease, the chief problem in their
daily life is exertional dyspnea. Recently the possibility has been raised sensory
information from the inspiratory accessory and rib cage muscle may be important
sources. But the role of inspiratory muscle fatigue in the genesis of dyspnea in
COPD patients has yet to be fully studied. The purpose of the present study is to
investigate possible relationship between respiratory muscle fatigue during exercise
and sensation of dyspnea in patients with severe COPD.

Table 1. Pulmonary Function and Blood Gas levels in 8 Patients
with Chronic Obstructive Pulmonary Disease

	$FEV_{1.0}$ liters	$FEV_{1.0}/FVC$ %	RV liters	RV/TLC %	%D_{LCO} %	Pdi_{max} cmH_2O	$Paco_2$ torr	Pao_2 torr
Mean	0.62	40.2	3.31	62.3	48.8	43.3	45.4	74.8
S.D.	0.15	8.2	0.89	9.5	19.1	19.8	10.7	9.3

$FEV_{1.0}$,forced expired volume in 1 s; $FEV_{1.0}/FVC$,ratio of $FEV_{1.0}$ to forced vital
capacity; RV,residual volume; RV/TLC,ratio of RV to total lung capacity;
%D_{LCO},carbon monoxide diffusing capacity in percentage of predicted normal;
$Paco_2$,arterial CO_2 pressure; Pao_2,arterial O_2 pressure.

METHODS

Subjects. Eight males with severe COPD, whose mean age($\pm$S.D.) was 64$\pm$7 years, were studied. Mean values for pulmonary-function indexes and blood gases are listed in Table 1.

Protocol of exercise test. Our protocol was started with a 3-min rest, which was followed by graded stage treadmill exercise. Each stage of exercise lasted for 3 min. During stage 1, the treadmill was kept horizontal and its speed was set at 0.75 mile/h. Subsequently the treadmill speed was increased by 0.25 mile/h and its elevation by 4% at each time of stage advance. A 10-point modified Borg scale for the intensity of breathlessness was displayed in front of the patients during exercise, and they were allowed to stop exercise at a maximum breathlessness.

Measurements. Transdiaphragmatic pressure(Pdi) was measured using double balloon catheters, which were placed in the esophagus and stomach and connected to differential pressure transducers. Pdi was obtained as a quotient of electrical subtraction: gastric pressure minus esophageal pressure(Pes). Maximal Pdi(Pdi$_{max}$) and maximal Pes (Pes$_{max}$) were measured during a maximal inspiratory effort from FRC against an occlusion.

The diaphragmatic EMG(EMGdi) was recorded via a silver wire esophageal electrodes located between the two balloons. The sternomastoid muscle EMG(EMGsm) was recorded from the surface electrodes. These electrodes were connected to EMG amplifier assemblies. The output of the EMG amplifier assembly was passed through a 20-500 Hz bandpass filter, then it was transmitted to the analog-to-digital converter. All signals were sampled at a rate of 1024Hz and subsequently processed on a microcomputer for power spectral density analysis. Electrocardiographic signal was removed by a cross-correlation technique reported by Levine. The H/L ratio is the ratio of power in the frequency band of 150-350 Hz to that in the frequency band of 20-47 Hz. The H/L ratio at the first 10 seconds of the stage 1 exercise was assigned a value of 100% and used as a control value, and a 20% fall of H/L ratio was construed as meaning inspiratory muscle fatigue. Integrated EMG activity was mean activity of rectified EMG signal during inspiration. Control value of integrated EMG activity was the largest signal recorded during Pdi$_{max}$ maneuvers. Minute ventilation(VE), oxygen uptake, carbon dioxide production and respiratory rate were measured by use of a respiromonitor(MINATO RM300). Tension-Time index was the result of multiplying mean Pdi/Pdimax by Ti/Ttot. Work rate of the diaphragm(Wdi) was calculated from integration of the result of multiplying Pdi by respiratory flow rate.

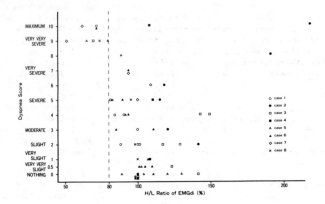

Fig. 1.   Relationship between Respiratory Effort Sensation
and H/L Ratio of EMGdi during Exercise

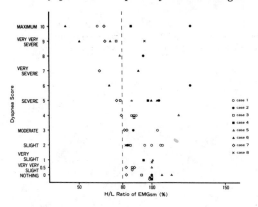

Fig. 2. Relationship between Respiratory Effort Sensation
and H/L Ratio of EMGsm during Exercise

RESULTS

Fig. 1 shows relationship between respiratory effort sensation and H/L ratio of diaphragmatic EMG during treadmill exercise. Six of eight COPD patients showed diaphragmatic fatigue, but the other two patients showed no sign of diaphragmatic fatigue. In the patients who showed diaphragmatic fatigue, they were extremely dyspneic(Borg score 9 or 10) at diaphragmatic fatigue. Fig. 2 illustrates relationship between respiratory effort sensation and H/L ratio of sternomastoid muscle EMG during exercise. In five out of six patients with diaphragmatic fatigue, sternomastoid muscle fatigue was encountered prior to diaphragmatic fatigue. Table 2 is the summary of relationship between the Borg scale and measurements of respiratory muscle function. There were high correlations between the Borg scale and VE/maximal voluntary ventilation(MVV), Pes/Pes$_{max}$ and integrated EMGsm activity.

Table 2. Correlation between the Borg Scale and Measurements
of Respiratory Muscle Function

	rs	p value
Integrated EMGdi activity	0.43	0.0006
H/L ratio of EMGdi	-0.40	0.0017
Integrated EMGsm activity	0.58	<0.0001
H/L ratio of EMGsm	-0.45	0.0004
Pes/Pes$_{max}$	0.57	<0.0001
Pdi/Pdi$_{max}$	0.38	0.0039
TTdi	0.37	0.0035
Wdi	0.33	0.0101
VE/MVV	0.67	<0.0001

rs, rank-difference coefficient of correlation of Spearman.

CONCLUSIONS

We have found that during treadmill exercise in COPD patients the activity of sternomastoid muscle is correlated with intensity of dyspnea. But they had very strong respiratory sensation once diaphragm got fatigued.

Section 4
BEHAVIOURAL CONTROL
OF
BREATHING AND DYSPNEA

Breathing Versatility

Jere Mead

Harvard School of Public Health, Boston, Massachusetts,
USA

ABSTRACT

The respiratory pump is highly versatile. It functions adequately
in a variety of circumstances. I will distinguish respiratory and
non-respiratory acts. The latter include transients (coughing,
sneezing, shouting, straining at stool, or during weight lifting),
prolonged static events (orientation relative to gravity, changes
in posture and in particular spinal attitude), and prolonged periodic events (talking, walking, running). I will distinguish and
give examples of three sorts of interactions: interruption, accommodation, and independence. Transient acts have little influence
on tissue oxygen because of the substantial buffering of gas reservoirs. Talking and singing are frequently prolonged. Here a rough
accommodation is achieved. The minute volume requirements for
phonation are approximately equal to those for gas exchange at
rest. But in exercise a mismatch develops. In other non-respiratory acts there is a high degree of respiratory homeostasis.
Mechanisms are both mechanical and neuromuscular, and incompletely
known. One example clearly involves control. The mid-positional
shifts accompanying postural changes, for example from recumbency
to the upright postures, produce very substantial changes in mechanical advantage of breathing muscles. The beautiful control of
ventilation in these circumstances requires substantial neural responses. Purely mechanical effects are important in other instances. Abdominal muscles are classified as expiratory: they increase
abdominal pressure, thereby displacing the diaphragm in the expiratory direction. But such increases in abdominal pressure push outward and upward on the lower rib-cage. During inspiration while
the diaphragm is contracting and thereby stiffened the inspiratory
influence of increasing abdominal pressure on the rib-cage wins.
As a result inspiration is not embarrassed by abdominal compres-
sion.
Changes in spinal attitude have very little influence on lung
volume. Spinal flexion compresses the trunk substantially in the
axial direction. But this influence is compensated by simultaneous
radial expansion of the rib-cage and abdomen.
These and further examples indicate a remarkable independence of
breathing from non-breathing acts. The relative importance of passive mechanical and active neuromuscular control in the homeostasis

is largely unknown.

The breathing pump occupies a body trunk which does much more than
simply breathe. We pull on it with our arms and legs. We confine
it with clothing. We twist it and bend it. We change its orientation with respect to gravity. We talk and sing and shout and cough
and sneeze. We lift heavy weights. And in health we do all of
these things without giving a thought to breathing.
Breathing is wonderfully versatile. I want to discuss the basis of
this versatility - specifically the interactions of breathing and
other acts. Amongst these other acts are short-acting ones: sneezing, coughing, breath-holding while straining - these are no problem because of the buffering capacity of our lung and tissue gas
reservoirs. In health we can stop breathing altogether for several
seconds without embarrassment to gas-exchange. To repeat, transient non-respiratory acts are no problem in health, thanks to gas
buffering.
What about more prolonged actions? Periodic motor acts such as
locomotion might be expected to induce rhythmic lung volume displacements, and it is easy to picture these as synchronized so as
to assist breathing. (Indeed, the synchronization of stepping and
breathing is a common experience.) To examine this possibility we
have recently isolated the specific contribution of locomotion to
lung volume change in running humans and have found it to be trivi-
al. From this point of view the advantages of synchronization
would appear to be vanishingly small.
This lack of effect is but one example of motor acts which might be
expected to influence lung volume - but which do not. Let me give
you some more examples.
We are taught that spinal flexing is an expiratory act and this
would seem to be borne out by the observation that unrestrained
subjects bend forward during an expired vital capacity effort.
Here is an easy experiment to test this: Compare vital capacity
measured during flexion with that measured during spinal extension
- i.e., ones begun bent over and completed fully erect. You will
find that they are trivially different. The substantial axial com-
pression and expansion associated with the spinal changes are compensated by equal and opposite radial displacements of the rib-cage
and belly wall. In fact, all spinal movements - flexion, extension
side-to-side bending and twisting - have little influence on lung
volume. They are essentially non-respiratory.
We are taught that contracting abdominal muscles - or pushing in
the belly wall - causes expiratory displacements. Indeed, abdominal wall muscles are classified simply as expiratory muscles. And
this is true during expiration! That is when the diaphragm is relaxed. But what about inspiration? Pushing in on the belly wall is
minimally embarrassing to inspiration because the associated outward displacement of the rib-cage in the zone of apposition of the
diaphragm to the rib-cage is in itself an inspiratory act. Inward
displacement of the belly wall tends to displace the diaphragm in
the expiratory direction and the rib-cage in the inspiratory direction. During expiration, with the diaphragm relaxed and under no
tension, the first influence wins. If the diaphragm contracts this
effect is decreased. The expiratory and inspiratory influences
then tend to balance out and any abdominal muscle contraction during inspiration becomes essentially non-respiratory!
Let me say more about the respiratory action of the rib-cage. The
rib-cage mainly pumps the abdomen, and its major influence on lung
volume is by way of its action on the abdomen. As it expands it
pulls out and upward on the abdomen and thereby lowers intra-

abdominal pressure. And this assists the diaphragm as follows:
The diaphragm causes inspiration by lowering pleural pressure.
But it simultaneously pushes down on the abdominal contents and increases intra-abdominal pressure. Thus the total pressure developed by the diaphragm - that is, transdiaphragmatic pressure - is
the sum of two components: a fall in pleural pressure, which acts
directly on the lungs, and a rise in abdominal pressure. To the
extent that active rib-cage expansion lowers abdominal pressure it
decreases the inspiratory increase in abdominal pressure, and
thereby allows the diaphragm to expend a larger fraction of its
total pressure on the lungs. In a very real sense this abdominal
pumping action of the rib-cage clears the path for the diaphragm.
It gets things out of the way.
And this action relates directly to the potential respiratory embarrassment of non-respiratory events. Pregnancy grossly encroach-
es on the abdomen but minimally embarrasses breathing. Ascites and
obesity, and even tight abdominal binders, are also abdominal en-
croachments which embarrass breathing surprisingly little. In
every instance the compensating influence of the rib-cage explains
the minimal respiratory embarrassment.
The only clear example of mutual dependence of breathing and non-
breathing that we are aware of is phonation. Singing and talking
are produced by relatively prolonged controlled outflow through the
phonating larynx, interspersed with quick, brief inspirations.
During ordinary speech the resulting minute ventilation is perfect-
ly adequate. But this accommodation of speech to breathing is relatively crude. It is impossible to carry out prolonged quiet
speech when the ventilation is driven, as during exercise. Speech
becomes "breathy" - with phonatory flows increased by intentional
laryngeal leaks - and the phrases are short. The ventilatory demands exceed and over-ride the speech demands.
Independence of breathing from other acts is the general rule.
Such independence may require neuromuscular coordination, or it may
be simply the result of passive mechanical features. The relative
importance of these meuromuscular and passive mechanical contributions to this independence is largely unknown as yet. The experimental tests are easy enough in most instances. They just haven't
been done! Perhaps some of you might be interested in doing them.
Again I will give examples.
First, one in which a neuromuscular mechanism clearly is involved.
Postural shifts are long-term non-respiratory acts which through
the action of gravity change lung volume and also the operating
lengths of respiratory muscles. In this circumstance simple mechanics cannot explain the independence of breathing from the postural effects. Neuromuscular adjustments are necessary and are clearly demonstrable. The remaining questions in this compensation are
the nature of the reflexes involved (if any) and the extent to
which this mechanism is influenced in disease. For example, does
the onset of dyspnea have any relationship to the failure of operational length compensation? Patients with emphysema and diminished
lung recoil breathe at progressively unfavorable operational
lengths. We make powerful adjustments to changes in operational
lengths without symptoms. Do such patients have the onset of dyspnea when this mechanism is exhausted?
I mentioned earlier the independence of lung volume and spinal
flexion. This requires compensating radial displacements of the
rib-cage and belly wall. As yet it is not known to what extent
this compensation requires neuromuscular activity. Preliminary
measurements of the influence of changes of spinal attitude produced and assumed passively during voluntary relaxation suggest
that passive mechanical events suffice. But the underlying

mechanisms are as yet unknown.

A viewpoint which encompasses most of what I have told you can be expressed as a hypothesis, namely that breathing and non-breathing are mainly organized for minimal respiratory embarrassment. I would like to close by expressing this hypothesis in terms of pressures.

Here is a simple observation you can make that demonstrates your capacity to isolate breathing and non-breathing. Milic-Emili made wonderful use of mouth pressure to measure respiratory drive and we will do the same. With a nose-clip in place and with lips sealed around a tube leading to a manometer (a simple water-filled tube will suffice) and with the glottis open, any mouth pressure changes reflect pleural pressure changes. Any voluntary or involuntary breathing efforts then produce obvious changes in mouth pressure. Next, hyperventilate off the mouthpiece sufficiently to minimize respiratory drive and then with the mouthpiece back in place perform a variety of non-breathing acts, making certain that you maintain an open glottis. You will find that you can easily bend, twist, alternately compress and expand your rib-cage and abdomen (the iso-volume maneuver), step in place - all while maintaining nearly constant mouth pressure. Little, if any, practice is required. To what extent does this result reflect simple mechanical features and to what extent motor control? The normal healthy lung transduces parenchymal and airway distension and rates of distension into neural outputs via the vagus nerve. Is it possible that the central nervous system reacts to these signals with positive feed-back with respect to respiratory demands and with negative feed-back with respect to other than respiratory demands? Whatever the answers to these questions may be, it is apparent that once again Nature is was ahead of us, preparing the way as it were. Physiologists have made most of their measurements of breathing in confining circumstances, thereby isolating breathing and allowing it to be measured with single variables. It appears that mechanisms exist which strongly support this isolation, even during free living.

Cellular Basis of Behavioral
Control of Breathing

J.M. Orem* and T.E. Dick[†]

*Department of Physiology, Texas Technical University
Health Sciences Center, Lubbock, TX 79430;
[†]Department of Medicine, Case Western Reserve
University, Cleveland, OH 44106, USA

ABSTRACT

Brainstem neurons that generate the rhythmic pattern of respiration have been
identified by relating their firing pattern to the breathing pattern. We have
applied a statistical test to evaluate the consistency and strength of the
respiratory modulation of their activity. In intact unanesthetized animals,
this test indicated that respiratory neurons varied greatly in their
relationship to respiration. For example, some neurons appeared highly
modulated by the respiratory pattern having an invariant relationship to
respiration whereas others appeared to be weakly modulated and highly variable.
Our recordings showed that weakly modulated respiratory cells were affected
greatly by sleep, decreasing their activity in NREM sleep. On the other hand,
invariant cells were affected slightly by sleep. Similarly, the activity of
these cell types differed greatly during the performance of a behavioral
respiratory task. In cats trained to stop inspiring at the sound of a tone,
invariant cells ceased firing during the task. In contrast, some highly
variable cells were activated intensely. These results suggested that the
highly variable, weakly modulated cells integrate inputs related to changes in
state of consciousness and to behavioral control of respiration.

KEYWORDS

Control of respiration; brainstem; respiratory neurons; sleep.

INTRODUCTION

Traditionally, respiratory neurons have been classified qualitatively on the
basis of the relationship between their firing pattern and the breathing
pattern. For example, a neuron that discharges with an increasing discharge
frequency during inspiration and that becomes inactive at the end of
inspiration would be described as an early-onset, augmenting inspiratory neuron
(Merrill, 1974). We found this system inadequate because it says nothing about
the degree to which a cell is respiratory. In intact, unanesthetized animals,
only some respiratory cells have highly correlated activity patterns. In other
cells, activity varies not only across a breath but also from breath to breath.
Accordingly, we developed a quantitative analysis to characterize the

consistency and strength of the respiratory activity of respiratory neurons
(Orem and Dick, 1983).

In this chapter we describe this quantitative, statistical method and show the
results of application of this method to characterize medullary neurons
recorded in cats during changes in the state of consciousness and during the
performance of a behavioral respiratory response. Finally, we propose an
hypothesis of the organization of the control of breathing during behavioral
and state changes.

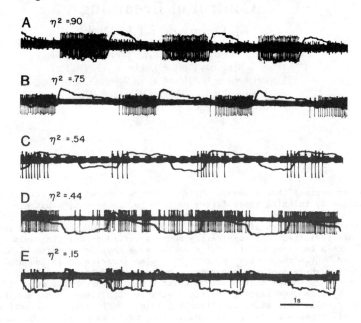

Fig. 1.   Variations in the consistency and signal strength
           of different respiratory neurons. Each trace (A-
           E) shows intratracheal pressure (inspiration is
           represented by a downward deflection) and the
           action potentials of a respiratory neuron. The
           consistency and signal strength of respiratory
           activity (quantified by the η^2 statistic) decrease
           from A to E. From Orem and Dick, 1983.

THE η^2 STATISTIC

The η^2 statistic is an effect-size statistic that can be calculated from the
results of the analysis of variance (ANOVA). We used the ANOVA to determine
whether the activity was significantly related to the respiratory cycle (Netick
and Orem, 1981). The ANOVA used was a subjects-by treatments design with 20-
iles of the respiratory cycle as the "treatment" variable and breaths
(typically, n = 50) as the "subjects" variable. The η^2 is the proportion of the
total variance (σ_t^2) of the neuronal activity over a series of breaths that is
comprised of the variance across fractions of the respiratory cycle (σ_m^2).

$$\eta^2 = \frac{\sigma_m^2}{\sigma_t^2} = \frac{\sigma_m^2}{\sigma_m^2 + \sigma^2} \qquad (1)$$

where σ^2 is the variance within fractions of the respiratory cycle, and σ_m^2 is the variance of means across fractions. σ_m^2 depends on the range of means across fractions of the cycle and also on how the means are dispersed over this range. σ_m^2 increases both as the range increases and as the values of the individual means tend to be distributed at the end points of the range. σ^2 is the variance across breaths within the individual fractions of the respiratory cycle. If the activity of a cell varies greatly from breath to breath, σ^2 will be large. Conversely, as the consistency of the discharge pattern across breaths increases, σ^2 will decrease, and η^2 will increase. Therefore, $1/\sigma^2$ is an index of the consistency of the respiratory activity of a cell. η^2 values can vary from 1.0 to 0.0 indicating, respectively, that all or none of the variability in the activity is accounted for by fractions (20-iles) of the respiratory cycle. In practice, η^2 was estimated as

$$\eta^2 = \frac{dfb(F)}{dfb(F) + dfw} \qquad (2)$$

where F is the F ratio, dfb is the degrees of freedom between groups, and dfw is the degrees of freedom within groups.

η^2 is a quantitative index of the strength of the respiratory modulation of a cell's activity. Presumably, high η^2-valued cells receive predominantly respiratory-modulated afferent input and have a highly modulated discharge pattern. In contrast, low η^2-valued cells must receive considerable nonrespiratory-modulated afferent input and are, therefore, poorly modulated.

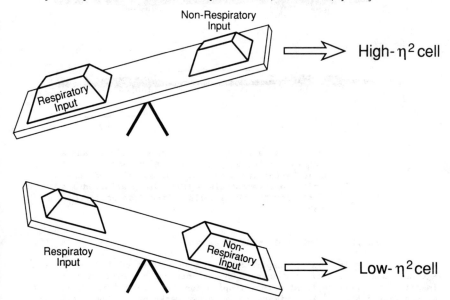

Fig. 2.   The hypothesized relationship between respiratory and nonrespiratory input and the η^2-value of respiratory activity.

THE WAKEFULNESS STIMULUS FOR BREATHING

In the early sixties, Fink (1961) reported that wakefulness was a stimulus to breathing. Many clinical reports support this idea (see, for example, Plum and Swanson, 1958; Severinghaus and Mitchell, 1962). The neural basis of the wakefulness stimulus is unknown. To obtain information about this, we recorded the activity of brainstem respiratory neurons during sleep and wakefulness (Orem et al., 1985). We found in a population of respiratory related cells (94 cells from eight cats) that the weakly modulated, low η^2-valued cells were preferentially affected by state changes. Indeed, many weak cells ceased firing during sleep. In contrast, high η^2-valued cells were affected little by state changes, and changes that occurred in their activity reflected changes in breathing pattern rather than state changes. In summary, changes in discharge rate from wakefulness to sleep are inversely related to the η^2 value of the cell's activity and, consequently, the effect of sleep on a respiratory neuron is proportional to the amount of nonrespiratory input contributing to its activity (Orem et al., 1985).

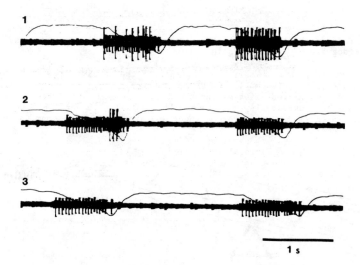

Fig. 3.   Activity of a low (large action potentials) and a high (small action potentials) η^2-valued cell during wakefulness (A), drowsiness (B), and nonrapid eye movement sleep (C). Sleep affected most of the low η^2-valued cells. From Orem et al., 1985.

BEHAVIORAL CONTROL OF BREATHING

We trained animals to stop inspiration using an operant conditioning technique. A tone and a small puff of dilute NH_4OH were presented at the onset of inspiration. Failure to stop that inspiration was punished by administration of additional NH_4OH. Approximately one to two weeks of one hour training sessions were required for the animals to learn this response.

During performance of this response, diaphragmatic activity was inhibited within 100ms (mean latency = 74ms). High η^2-valued inspiratory neurons in the dorsal and ventral groups were inhibited at latencies from ~40 to >200ms (mean latency = 81ms) (Orem, 1989). This inactivation of medullary inspiratory neurons during performance of the task indicates that behavioral control occurs in this case, at least in part, at the level of the brainstem. Interestingly, some low η^2-valued inspiratory neurons were activated during performance of the response. The relationship emerged that high η^2-valued cells were invariably inactivated during performance of this task, whereas some low η^2-valued cells were activated. This relationship held regardless of the phase-relationship of the cell, that is, high η^2-valued cells of all types, inspiratory, expiratory and phase-spanning, were inactivated during performance of the response. Similarly, low η^2-valued cells with various relations to the respiratory cycle (inspiratory, expiratory, and phase-spanning) were activated (Orem, 1987; 1989). The high η^2-valued cells that were inactivated included the expiratory cells of the Bötzinger group and late-onset inspiratory cells (Orem and Brooks, 1986; Orem, 1988) -- cell types with postulated inspiratory-inhibitory roles.

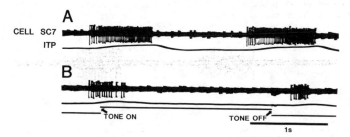

Fig. 4.   A high η^2-valued inspiratory cell during
          spontaneous breathing (A) and during the
          behavioral inhibition of inspiration (B). Note
          that this cell is inactivated during the
          behavioral inhibition of inspiration. From Orem
          and Brooks, 1986.

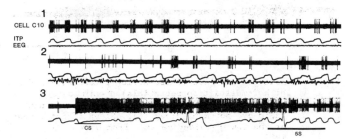

Fig. 5.   A low η^2-valued inspiratory cell that was
          activated when inspiration was stopped
          behaviorally. 1) Spontaneous activity of the cell
          during wakefulness: top trace, actional potentials
          of the cell; middle trace, intratracheal pressure;
          lower trace, electroencephalogram. 2) Spontaneous
          activity of the cell during drowsiness or non-REM
          sleep. Note that the activity of the cell
          decreased during sleep. 3) Intense activation of
          the cell during and after the behavioral
          inhibition of inspiration elicited by the
          conditioning stimulus (CS). From Orem, 1989.

A MODEL

We speculate that the high η^2-valued cells are rigidly controlled by respiratory related inhibitory and excitatory postsynaptic potentials and accordingly correspond to cells postulated to constitute the respiratory oscillator. The rigid sequences of excitatory and inhibitory postsynaptic potentials preclude the out-of-phase activation of those respiratory cells that may have inspiratory inhibitory roles during eupnea (e.g., late-onset inspiratory and augmenting expiratory). This, in turn, indicates a need for a type of respiratory cell that allows for the flexibility of behavioral control. We propose that the low η^2-valued cells provide this flexibility (Orem, 1987). Their low η^2-valued activity patterns indicate that they are not controlled rigidly by sequences of respiratory-related postsynaptic potentials and that they can be active at any time during the respiratory cycle. Furthermore, the intense activation of some of these cells is consistent with the possibility that they may mediate the behavioral inhibition of inspiration. As an abstraction, we propose that low η^2-valued cells integrate nonrespiratory afferents into the respiratory system. If this is the case, then an affect of non-REM sleep is a reduction in the amount of nonrespiratory afference to the respiratory system. This nonrespiratory afference appears related, in part, to mechanisms for behavior control.

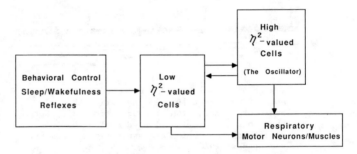

Fig. 6.   A schema showing the hypothesized relationship
           between high and low η^2-valued cells and their
           possible functional roles.

ACKNOWLEDGEMENT

The research of the authors described herein was supported by grant HL21257 from the National Heart, Lung, and Blood Institute.

REFERENCES

Fink, B.R. (1961). Influence of cerebral activity in wakefulness on regulation of breathing. J. Appl. Physiol. 16, 15-20.
Merrill, E.G. (1974). Finding a respiratory function for the medullary respiratory neurons. In: Essays on the Nervous System (R. Bellairs and E.G. Gray, eds.), pp. 451-468. Clarendon Press, Oxford.
Netick, A. and J. Orem. Erroneous classification of neuronal activity by the respiratory modulation index. Neurosci. Lett. 21, 301-306.
Orem, J. (1987). Inspiratory neurons that are activated when inspiration is inhibited behaviorally. Neurosci. Lett. 83, 282-286.
Orem, J. (1988). The activity of late inspiratory cells during the behavioral inhibition of inspiration. Brain Res. 458, 224-230.

Orem, J. (1989). Behavioral inspiratory inhibition: Inactivated and activated respiratory cells. *J. Neurophysiol.* 62, 1069-1078.

Orem, J. and E.G. Brooks (1986). The activity of retrofacial expiratory cells during behavioral respiratory responses and active expiration. *Brain Res.* 374, 409-412.

Orem, J. and T. Dick (1983). Consistency and signal strength of respiratory neuronal activity. *J. Neurophysiol.* 50, 1098-1107.

Orem, J., I. Osorio, E. Brooks and T. Dick (1985). Activity of respiratory neurons during NREM sleep. *J. Neurophysiol.* 54, 1144-1156.

Plum, F. and A.G. Swanson (1958). Abnormalities in central regulation of respiration in acute and convalescent poliomyelitis. *Arch. Neurol. Psychiatry* 80, 267-285.

Severinghaus, J.W. and R.A. Mitchell (1962). Ondine's curse -- Failure of respiratory automaticity while awake. *Clin. Res.* 10, 122.

Genetic Influences on Personality, Thresholds for Added Resistance and Dyspnea Sensation

Yoshikazu Kawakami,
Masaharu Nishimura, Shuichi Kobayashi
and Yasushi Akiyama

First Department of Medicine, School of Medicine,
Hokkaido University, Sapporo 060, Japan

ABSTRACT

Personality, threshold values for detecting added inspiratory resistance, and the visual analog scale (VAS) during chemical and mechanical stimuli were evaluated in adolescent and adult twins (49 pairs). Some personality elements (depression, nervousness, ascendance, social extroversion, hysteric trend, and anxiety) were influenced by genetic factors in adolescence. The threshold values correlated with nervousness, lack of objectivity, cooperativity, symptoms of easy fatigability, and anger in adolescent females but not in adolescent males. Personality elements were not influenced by genetic factors in adults. Correlations were seen between personality elements (depression and cyclic trend) and the threshold values in adult males but not in adult females. VAS scores during chemical and mechanical stimuli were little influenced by genetic factors. In adult males but not in females, anxiety scores correlated positively with the VAS-$\dot{V}_E$ relation and the VAS-PCO_2 relation during hypoxic, hypercapnic and mechanical interventions. The VAS-PCO_2, but not the VAS-$\dot{V}_E$, relation was augmented by hypoxia (endtidal PO_2 = 50 - 55 Torr). These results indicate genetic influence on some but not all personality elements in adolescence, the differential mode of influence of personality on threshold values and VAS between sexes in adolescence and adulthood, and little genetic influence on dyspnea sensation during chemical as well as mechanical stimuli in adults. Slight hypoxia has little dyspnogenic influence as analyzed by the VAS-$\dot{V}_E$ relation but it does as analyzed by the VAS-PCO_2 relation.

KEYWORDS

Behavioral control;twins;resistance detection;dyspnea;personality;
hypoxia;hypercapnia

Dyspnea is one of the important symptoms in cardiopulmonary disorders and may occur in healthy individuals as well. Although the cardiopulmonary function _per se_ is essential for producing this symptom, some studies indicate behavioral control of breathing and personality are involved in modifying dyspnea (Rosser and Guz, 1981; Dales et al.,1989). However, whether behavioral components in control of breathing and personality linked to dyspnea are genetically influenced or environmental (acquired) factors predominate during aging process is not known.

This study aimed to examine, by comparing monozygotic and dizygotic twins, genetic influence on behavioral control of breathing, sensation of dyspnea, and personality. The threshold was determined during room air breathing while the dyspnea sensation was quantitated during chemical and mechanical stimuli.

SUBJECTS AND METHODS

The subjects were 31 pairs of healthy adolescent twins (mean age, $16\pm SD$ 1 years, 20 pairs of monozygotic twins (MZ) and 11 pairs of dizygotic twins (DZ)) and 18 pairs of healthy adult twins (mean age, 49 ± 9.7 years for MZ and 43 ± 13.4 years for DZ). The male to female ratios were 13/7 for adolescent MZ, 7/4 for adolescent DZ, 4/5 for adult MZ, and 3/6 for adult DZ. Monozygosity in adolescent twins was defined as when all blood groups (ABO, Rh, MN, Kell, Lewis, Lutheran, P, and Xg), more than 7 finger prints, and physical appearances matched. In adult twins, HLA typing was used instead of blood groups.
The threshold values for detecting added inspiratory resistance were measured by randomly applying 17 kinds of flow resistances to the inspiratory side of the one-way valve and determining the mouth pressure (P) at which the subject detected the resistance 50% of occasion.

Personality was analyzed by questionnaires based on the Yatabe-Guilford test (YG), the Minnesota multiphasic personality inventory (MMPI), the Cornell medical index (CMI), and the manifest anxiety score (MAS). The analyses were performed independently by two specialists who had not known the zygosity of individual twin.

The adult twins were additionally analyzed for dyspnea grade during the following chemical and mechanical stimuli: 1)hyperoxic progressive hypercapnia, 2)hypoxic progressive hypercapnia, and 3)hyperoxic hypercapnia with an inspiratory resistive load (17 cmH_2O). During the progressive hypercapnia with hyperoxia, inspiratory PO_2 was kept at 150 Torr while inspiratory CO_2 concentration was gradually increased to an endtidal PCO_2 of approximately 50 Torr. During hypoxic progressive hypercapnia, endtidal PO_2 was maintained at 50 to 55 Torr while hypercapnia was progressively induced. A servocontrol system for regulating arterial blood gases was used throughout the chemical interventions (Kawakami et al.,1981). Minute ventilation ($\dot{V}_E$) was measured continuously with a hot-wire flowmeter and was standardized by predicted maximal voluntary ventilation (MVV).
Dyspnea was graded continuously by a method combining the visual analog scale with the Borg scale (called VAS in the following section). The subject adjusted the height of the red column with a knob every 30 sec to record how much dyspnea was felt compared to the limit of endurance.
Since the relations of VAS to $\dot{V}_E$ and VAS to endtidal PCO_2 were linear, dyspnea was graded by 1) VAS divided by $\dot{V}_E$ or endtidal PCO_2 and 2) VAS values at 40 (or 30) % of $\dot{V}_E$/predicted MVV and VAS values at endtidal PCO_2 of 55 (or 50) Torr.

When the variance in MZ pairs was significantly smaller than that in DZ pairs, genetic factors were thought to be predominant (analysis of covariance). The total variances (the sum of genetic and environmental forces) and the average values must be equal between MZ and DZ for this analysis. Unpaired t test was used for the comparison between the two groups (MZ vs. DZ and adolescence vs. adulthood). For the evaluation of changes in variables, paired t test was adopted. The significance level was assumed to be p=0.05.

RESULTS

Adolescent twins
The analysis of covariance in personality indicated genetic predominance in depression (F=4.08), nervousness (F=9.93), ascendance-dominance (F=4.35), social extroversion (F=8.91), hysteric trend (F=6.81), and anxiety (F=10.81) in adolescent twins. Other personality elements (cyclic trend, inferiority complex, lack of objectivity, cooperativity, aggressiveness, activity, rhathymia, thinking extroversion, manic trend, and psychosomatic symptoms other than anxiety in CMI) were not influenced by genetic factors.
Table 1 summarizes the correlation coefficients between personality elements and the threshold value P in adolescent twins. In males, only thinking extroversion and symptoms of the digestive tract correlated with P. In females, nervousness, lack of objectivity, cooperativity, symptoms of easy fatigability, and anger showed significant correlations with P.

Table 1. Correlation coefficients between personality elements and threshold values in adolescent twins.

YG Depression*	Cyclic trend	Inferiority complex	Nervousness*	Lack of objectivity
Male				
Female			-0.443	-0.556

Cooperativity	Aggressiveness	Activity	Rhathymia	Thinking extroversion
Male				0.427
Female 0.622				

Ascendance*	Social extroversion*	MMPI Hysteria*	Mania	CMI Digestive tract symptoms
Male				-0.304
Female				

Easy fatigability	Anger	Anxiety*		
Male				
Female -0.491	-0.406			

Only significant values are shown. Asterisks denote personality elements influenced by genetic factors. For abbreviations, see text.

<u>Adult twins</u>
No personality elements as analyzed by YG, MMPI, CMI, and MAS showed any genetic influence in adult twins. The only personality elements that correlated with P in males were depression (r=0.614) and cyclic trend (r=0.638). In females, P values did not correlate with any personality elements. There was no correlation between MAS-anxiety scores and ventilatory response to hypercapnia.

Variance values between MZ pairs for hypoxic hypercapnic ventilatory responses were significantly smaller than those in DZ pairs (F=5.16), indicating predominant genetic influence on hypoxic hypercapnic response. However, genetic traits were not seen in hyperoxic hypercapnic response and mechanically loaded hyperoxic hypercapnic response.

Dyspnea as analyzed by the VAS-$\dot{V}_E$ relation did not seem to be influenced by genetic factors during 3 interventions, since variances in neither VAS standardized by $\dot{V}_E$/predicted MVV nor VAS at 40% $\dot{V}_E$ of predicted MVV were different between MZ and DZ cotwins. The VAS-endtidal PCO_2 relation did not show any genetic influence either.
In adult males, the MAS-anxiety score correlated positively with every aspect of dyspnea as shown in Fig.1. However, no such correlation was seen in females.

Fig.1.Relation between VAS scores and personality.

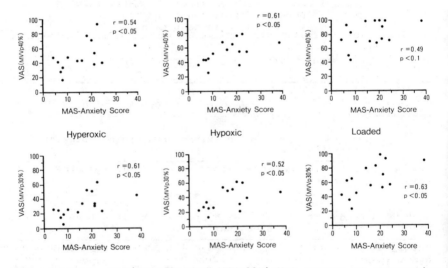

Abbreviations, VAS(MVVp40% and MVVp30%);VAS scores at respective 40 and 30% predicted maximal voluntary ventilation.

<u>Dyspnea during hyperoxic hypercapnia and hypoxic hypercapnia in adults</u>
Dyspnea grade as related to V_E was not different between hyperoxic and hypoxic hypercapnia except for VAS at 30% of predicted MVV, whereas the dyspnea grade as related to endtidal PCO_2 was significantly higher during hypoxic hypercapnia than during hyperoxic

hypercapnia (Fig.2).

Fig.2.Effect of hypoxia on VAS-ventilation
and VAS-PCO2 relations.

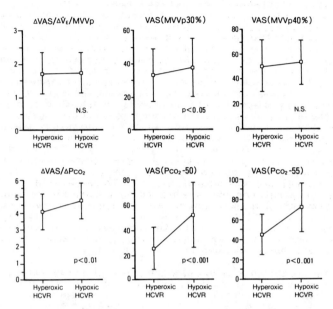

Vertical bars designate standard deviations. Abbreviations, Δ VAS/
ΔV̇E/MVVp;changes in VAS scores/changes in minute ventilation standardized by predicted maximal voluntary ventilation, VAS(MVVp30%
and MVVp40%);VAS scores at predicted MVV of 30% and 40%, respectively,ΔVAS/ΔPCO2 ;changes in VAS scores/changes in endtidal PCO2 ,
VAS/(PCO2 -50) and VAS(PCO2 -55);VAS scores standardized by endtidal
PCO2 at 50 and 55 Torr, respectively, HCVR;hypercapnic ventilatory
response. Other abbreviations are the same as in Fig.1.

DISCUSSION

The sensation of dyspnea originates from sensors in the
respiratory muscles and the lungs and its quality and quantity are
finally perceived in the cerebral cortex. Evidence suggests the
involvement of chemical and behavioral factors in modifying
dyspnea (Castele et al. 1985; Saunders et al. 1972). However, its
exact mechanisms are still not known.

Our previous studies indicate that the threshold for detecting
added inspiratory resistance is genetically determined in adolescence, not in adulthood (Kawakami et al., 1984). This suggests
that genetic factors controlling behavioral aspects of breathing
exist at least till adolescence. VAS scores during chemical, as
well as mechanical, stimuli were not influenced by genetic factors
in our adult twins, suggesting the absence of genetic influence on
behavioral control in adults.

Although the threshold seems to possibly relate to mechanisms of
dyspnea, the relation between the threshold and personality has

not been determined. This aspect must be important because a linkage between personality and dyspnea exists in the healthy population (Dales et al., 1989). Our present study disclosed that the threshold values in adolescent females correlate with some personality elements such as nervousness, lack of objectivity, cooperativity, symptoms of easy fatigability, and anger. Thus, a higher threshold value is associated with either lower nervousness, higher objectivity, higher cooperativity, lower easy fatigability, or lower anger. These correlations seem to be quite conceivable. It is of note that these personality elements are little influenced by genetic factors except for nervousness. Then, what factors determine the perception threshold for inspiratory resistance in adolescence from the genetic view point? Since personality elements are primarily cerebral cortical function and those elements not influenced by genetic components are related to the threshold, sensors in the respiratory muscles and the lungs and/or the afferent pathways must be the site of genetic action in adolescent females. However, sex is also an important factor determining the relation between personality and the threshold detection, since personality is little related to behavioral control in adolescent males. This difference between sexes in behavioral control of breathing is in line with a previous observation on the chemical control of normal subjects (Saunders et al., 1972): extroversion scores correlate with the ventilatory response to CO_2 only in females, not in males. Ventilatory response to hypercapnia is not pure reflex and is influenced by a behavioral component (Murphy et al., 1987).

Age possibly influences the relation between personality and behavioral control of breathing, since the threshold value for detecting added inspiratory resistance is a function of age in both sexes (Kawakami et al., 1984). Our present results indicate that the way of influence of personality on the threshold is quite different between adolescence and adulthood. An opposite relation of personality to hypercapnic ventilatory response is shown between young and old subjects (Tanaka et al., 1988). These results together with our present data, however, were obtained from cross sectional studies and longitudinal analyses are required for the firm conclusion as to the age effect.

Recent studies in healthy subjects (Dales et al., 1989) and patients with anxiety disorders (Tiller et al., 1987) indicate that dyspnea is associated with personality elements such as anxiety, anger, depression, and cognitive disturbance. However, our present study indicates that sex difference must be taken into account when analyzing the relation between personality and dyspnea.

It is interesting that the VAS-$\dot{V}_E$ relation is little influenced by hypoxia whereas the VAS-endtidal PCO_2 relation is augmented (Fig.2). This implies that dyspnea induced by hypoxic hypercapnia is practically comparable to that induced by hypercapnia alone at a given level of ventilation or at the same level of motor command. Therefore, we conclude from this analysis that either hypoxia of endtidal PO_2 down to 50-55 Torr has no dyspnogenic effect or hypoxia of this level has only a slight additional role as a dyspnogenic factor in hypercapnia.

Our results that added hypoxemia does not augment the dyspnea-ventilation relation during hypercapnia may not be extended to more intense hypoxemia. Hypoxic stimuli used in our study seem to be relatively weak in normal subjects, since ventilation does not usually increase till endtidal PO_2 is lowered to 60-50 Torr. However, our study has firmly established that superimposed hypoxia does not alter the dyspnea-ventilation relation during hypercapnic stimuli. Our study also supports a previous report that dyspnea during exercise is not altered after the correction of hypoxemia by oxygen inhalation in patients with chronic obstructive lung disease (Swinburn et al., 1984).

Hypercapnic responses under hypoxic condition were vigorously influenced by genetic factors in our adult twins. Our previous study conducted in other groups of twins indicated a stronger genetic influence on hypoxic response than on hypercapnic response, although both responses were governed by genetic components (Kawakami et al., 1985). Our present study seems to have confirmed this. Taking our present results of adults in the threshold and the VAS analyses into account, chemical control of breathing is more vigorously influenced by genetic factors than behavioral aspects of breathing. Thus, behavioral control seems to be a learned process in adulthood.

ACKNOWLEDGMENTS

The analyses of personality were kindly made by Dr. T. Sato, Department of Psychology, Sapporo Medical College and Dr. M. Hisamura, Director, Kohnan Hospital.

REFERENCES

Castele,R.J.,A.F.Connors and M.D.Altose.(1985). Effects of changes in CO_2 partial pressure on the sensation of respiratory drive. J.Appl.Physiol.,59,1747-1751.

Dales,R.E.,W.O.Spitzer,M.T.Schechter and S.Suissa.(1989). The influence of psychological status on respiratory symptom reporting. Am.Rev.Respir.Dis.,139,1459-1463.

Kawakami,Y.,T.Yoshikawa,Y.Asanuma and M.Murao.(1981). A control system for arterial blood gases. J.Appl.Physiol.,50,1362-1366.

Kawakami,Y.,A.Shida,T.Yoshikawa and H.Yamamoto.(1984). Genetic and environmental influence on inspiratory resistive load detection. Respir.45,100-110.

Kawakami,Y.,H.Yamamoto,T.Yoshikawa and A.Shida.(1985). Age-related variation of respiratory chemosensitivity in monozygotic twins. Am.Rev.Respir.Dis.,132,89-92.

Murphy,K.,A.Mier,L.Adams and A.Guz.(1990). Putative cerebral cortical involvement in the ventilatory response to inhaled CO_2 in conscious man. J.Physiol.,420,1-18.

Rosser,R.and A.Guz.(1981). Psychological approaches to breathlessness and its treatment. J.Psychosomat.Res.,25,439-447.

Saunders,N.A.,S.Heilpern and A.S.Rebuck.(1972). Relation between personality and ventilatory response to carbon dioxide in normal subjects:a role in asthma? Brit.Med.J.1,719-721.

Swinburn,C.R.,J.M.Wakefield and P.W.Jones.(1984). Relationship between ventilation and breathlessness during exercise in chronic obstructive airways disease is not altered by prevention of hypoxaemia. Cli.Sci.67,515-519.

Tanaka,Y.,Y.Nishibayashi,R.Maruyama,T.Morikawa,Y.Honda. (1988). Relationships among panic-fear personality, aging, and ventilatory activity. Tohoku J. Exp. Med.156,suppl.189-199.

Tiller,J.,M.Pain and N.Biddle.(1987). Anxiety disorder and perception of inspiratory resistive loads. Chest,91,547-551.

Optimization of Breathing Through Perceptual Mechanisms

N.S. Cherniack, Y. Oku, G.M. Saidel,
E.N. Bruce and M.D. Altose

Departments of Medicine and Biomedical Engineering,
Case Western Reserve University, Cleveland, OH 44106,
USA

ABSTRACT

The respiratory controller senses the forces and displacements it produces through signals from mechanoreceptors located in the respiratory passages, muscles, tendons and joints. It is possible that the controller takes the mechanics of the respiratory system into account in setting its activity and that this allows the controller to optimize the work or force it produces in breathing.

A number of different strategies have been proposed for how this optimization by the respiratory controller may operate. One concept is that chemoreceptors set the level of ventilation so that prescribed levels of arterial PCO_2 and PO_2 are obtained; and mechanoreceptor inputs determine the breathing patterns needed to produce that minute ventilation with minimum expenditure of energy or force. A modification of that idea is that a given level of chemical drive fixes the neural output of the controller and that neural output, in turn, determines ventilation according to the mechanical state of the thoracic bellows. Again, energy expenditure is minimized by adjusting breathing patterns using mechanoreceptor signals.

A more recent idea is that maintenance of arterial blood gas tensions and mechanical output are competing priorities for the respiratory controller and that the controller optimizes breathing so that both work output and deviations from desired blood gas tensions are minimized. Equations describing this possibility have been developed by Poon.

A difficulty with all these ideas is that it is unclear how the respiratory controller is able to sense its work or energy expenditure. Studies of respiratory sensation indicate that conscious humans can sense with considerable accuracy changes in ventilation, altered work, and altered force, though the anatomical basis for this perceptual ability remains to be clarified. It may be that these respiratory perceptions can be used by conscious humans to sense roughly energy expenditure by the respiratory muscles so as to achieve approximately minimum energy expenditures. Using psychophysical relations determined experimentally, it seems possible to modify the Poon equation so as to describe the perceptual contributions to optimization of breathing.

KEYWORDS

Dyspnea; respiratory sensations; optimization of breathing; energy cost of breathing; hypercapnia; exercise.

It is well established that higher brain centers, and in particular the cortex, can affect breathing (Fink, 1961; Orem, 1986, 1987, 1988; Plum, 1970; Plum and Leigh, 1981). Speaking, singing, and swallowing are obvious examples of voluntary acts which interrupt and modify ventilation. Noise, changes in light intensity, and even mental arithmetic can alter respiratory patterns and ventilation levels. The well-known effects of states of arousal and sleep are other examples of the respiratory actions of suprapontine regions of the brain (Orem et al., 1985; Phillipson and Bowes, 1986).

Respiratory movements and forces can be consciously perceived and evaluated quantitatively with reasonable accuracy (Killian and Jones, 1988; Zechman and Wiley, 1986). Stimulation of intercostal afferents and airway occlusion also produce evoked potentials that can be detected with external monitors (Davenport et al., 1986; Gandevia and Macefield, 1989). Respiratory sensations when sufficiently intense and unpleasant cause dyspnea and can be incapacitating (Killian and Jones, 1988).

Conscious effects on the respiratory response to external loads are well known (Altose et al., 1979; Zechman and Wiley, 1986). Anesthesia, opiates, and tranquilizers depress the immediate excitatory effects of loads on occlusion pressure. The diminished acute excitatory response of patients with chronic obstructive lung disease to loads may be an example of "learning" produced by continuous exposure to increased airway resistance (Altose et al., 1977). Sears has hypothesized that breathing patterns can be adjusted to new situations and eventually become automatic and subconscious, much as playing a musical instrument becomes "automatic" with learning (Sears, 1971). Separate monosynaptic and oligosynaptic pathways exist for the voluntary control of breathing and can be demonstrated by external transcranial magnetic stimulation (Gandevia and Plassman, 1988; Plum, 1970). It also has been demonstrated in conscious cats that breathing can be reflexly conditioned and that this involves stimulation of medullary neurons whose activity has only a loose or no correlation to the phases of breathing (Orem, 1986, 1987, 1988).

However, it remains much less certain whether respiratory sensations can produce any continuous voluntary effect on breathing patterns or breathing levels or whether such behavior would serve any useful purpose.

This paper examines the possibility that respiratory sensations can produce voluntary respiratory actions which then act continuously and subconsciously to modify the reflex control of breathing, particularly in circumstances where breathing is mechanically impaired and the work of breathing is excessive.

The idea that the respiratory controller takes into account the mechanics of the respiratory apparatus and the work of breathing is not new (Cherniack, 1985; Longobardo et al., 1980; Milic-Emili and Tyler, 1963; Otis et al., 1950; Poon, 1983). Observations on normal subjects breathing on loads (devices which impede the movement of air into and out of the lungs) and patients with chronic obstructive lung disease show that large increases in respiratory work lead to elevated levels of PCO_2. According to one idea, inspiratory work is relatively constant at any given level of PCO_2 (Milic-Emili and Tyler, 1963). If respiratory work becomes greater, ventilation must fall and PCO_2 must as a consequence rise. It has been reasoned that the increase in PCO_2 facilitated CO_2 elimination and allowed a steady state to be more easily maintained (Cherniack, 1985). Acid-base homeostasis could be maintained despite the rise in arterial PCO_2 by renal compensation. Clinically significant hypoxia would also result from the hypoventilation only if the increase in PCO_2 was quite severe (>60 mmHg).

Longobardo et al. (1980) suggested that the ventilatory response to CO_2 (Δventilation/ΔPCO_2) might be optimized so that the energy expended to remove the CO_2 accumulated by a period of inadequate breathing was minimized. This implies that the ventilatory responses to CO_2 which are usually considered to be reflexly determined were under some degree of higher brain center control. Recent experimental studies support the possibility of cortical modification of CO_2 response (Guz, this volume). Longobardo et al. (1980) reasoned because CO_2 delivery to the lungs was perfusion limited, excessive ventilatory responses to CO_2 might have little effect on the amount of CO_2 expired and as a consequence might waste energy. On the other hand, excessively low responses would prolong the time required to eliminate the excess CO_2 thereby increasing energy use. They showed that optimum CO_2 responses could be well defined, particularly when respiratory energy use was high as is the case in lung disease. Optimum ventilation-PCO_2 response slopes decreased as resting PCO_2 increased and became steeper with greater lung perfusion.

Other investigators have shown that at any given PCO_2 there are optimum levels of tidal volume, breathing frequency, air flow rate, and end-expiratory position which minimize energy costs, especially if they were already high (Otis *et al.*, 1950; Yamashiro *et al.*, 1975).

Recently Poon has suggested that ventilatory output is set by the respiratory controller so as to minimize a net operating cost made up of the conflicting requirements to maintain arterial PCO_2 and to decrease ventilation (and hence work) to a minimum (Poon, 1983). Poon's idea would mean that neither ventilation nor PCO_2 is fixed but the price of each is balanced against the other by the controller.

All of these ideas have foundered on the inability to demonstrate physiological mechanisms which would allow energy expenditure to be signaled to the brain. Studies of respiratory sensation suggest the possibility that sensory input arising from chemoreceptors and muscle proprioceptors modifies breathing patterns and ventilation levels so that the conscious sensory effects of breathing are minimized, in a sense to avoid the curse of being always consciously aware of breathing (Killian and Jones, 1988; Longobardo *et al.*, 1980). We will briefly examine the admittedly fragmentary evidence that supports this hypothesis. Then, using a mathematical model, we will show how the cortical control of breathing would allow the respiratory system to have the optimizing characteristics postulated by Poon (1983).

Several pieces of evidence suggest that breathing may be adjusted to minimize perceptual effects (Killian *et al.*, 1982; Oliven *et al.*, 1985; Sorli *et al.*, 1978; Tack *et al.*, 1983). Sensory effects produced by breathing are most directly related to the force used in producing respiratory movements (Killian *et al.*, 1982). Normal subjects asked to match tidal volumes while breathing through increasingly severe resistive or elastic loads behave as if they are to sense the product of pressure and volume (*i.e.* work), although pressure and volume do not have equal sensory effects (Tack *et al.*, 1983). When patients with obstructive lung disease are asked to breathe for long periods of time through loads, the degree of PCO_2 elevation that occurs is inversely related to the intensity with which they sense pressure. Patients, who experience greater sensory effects when producing pressure changes, breathe with smaller tidal volumes and hence use less force each breath (Oliven *et al.*, 1985). Hypercapnic patients with chronic obstructive lung disease differ from eucapnic patients primarily because they breathe more shallowly (Sorli *et al.*, 1978).

Studies in normal subjects indicate that the sense of dyspnea intensifies with isocapnic increases in ventilation whether they are produced voluntarily or by exercise (Chonan *et al.*, in press). However, if breathing is increased by hypercapnia, the sense of dyspnea is much greater than if it is produced voluntarily. This suggests that CO_2 and ventilation have independent effects on ventilation. This idea is supported by the dyspnogenic effects of CO_2 reported in paralyzed artificially ventilated patients (Patterson *et al.*, 1962).

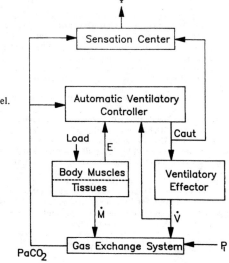

Fig. 1. Block diagram of the model.

shall consider a model which takes into account these experimental findings. The model udes a center of breathing sensation, an automatic CO_2 controller, mechanical effector, CO_2 respiratory plant as shown in fig. 1. The sensation center produces a discomfort x (Ψ) of breathing, which depends on C_{aut}, the automatic respiratory motor command, and '$_2$, the arterial CO_2 partial pressure.

discomfort index is measured as a psycho-physiological magnitude that grows as a power tion of the inputs ($\Psi = \Phi^n$) (Gottfried et al., 1978; Killian et al., 1981). The inputs ıde PCO_2 relative to a set point P_0 and mechanical loads related to command signals. er values of this relation have been reported from 1 up to nearly 4 (Chonan et al., 1987). ır model, we set all the exponents to 2 for simplicity:

$$\Psi = C^2_{aut} + K_1[PCO_2 - P_0]^2 \qquad (1)$$

e K_1 is a weighting constant. The rationale for these terms is as follows: An increase :entrally generated respiratory motor command signal causes dyspnea (Killian et al.,), as do afferent inputs from chemoreceptors (Chonan et al., 1987; Stark et al., 1981).

automatic (or non-willful) controller, which includes behavioral and non-behavioral ıonents, receives an inhibitory input of ventilation rate ($\dot{V}$) from the effector and an ıtory CO_2 signal from the plant ($PaCO_2$) to yield C_{aut}, which is enhanced by exercise. ostulate that the output dynamics of the command signal obeys:

$$\frac{dC_{aut}}{dt} = - W_0 C_{aut} - W_1 \dot{V} + W_2(E)[PCO_2 - P_0] \qquad (2)$$

ə C_{aut} is constrained to be positive. P_0 is the set point. The weighting factors W_0, and $W_2(E)$ are associated with neural activity related with CO_2 kinetics and self-decay, nhibition by ventilation feedback, and chemical stimulus. The weighting factor $W_2(E)$ ıds on the intensity of exercise. For simplicity, in this model, we consider the /-state metabolic rate $\dot{M}$ associated with exercise as a measure of the intensity of ise and let

$$W_2(E) = K_2 \dot{M} \qquad (3)$$

ə assume that there is no mechanical limitation, then the relationship between the command and total ventilation would be linear:

$$\dot{V} = K_3 C_{aut} \qquad (4)$$

K_3 is constant.

ompartment model (Chonan et al., 1988; ElHefnawy et al., 1988) adopted for the CO_2 plant ıics describes the PCO_2 dynamics of the lungs, muscle, and brain. This model assumes /eolar-arterial PCO_2 difference. Inputs of the plant are inspired CO_2 partial pressure metabolic rate, and alveolar ventilation ($\dot{V}_A$). We assume the relationship between $\dot{V}$ ı is

$$\dot{V}_A = \dot{V} - f V_D \qquad (5)$$

V_D is the dead space volume and f is the respiratory frequency.

e this mathematical model to simulate various physiological and psycho-physiological nents that have been reported in the literature. The purpose of these simulations is w that the same basic model can explain the behavior associated with exercise using ıd incremental inputs; and progressive hypercapnia by rebreathing.

ie

ıulate the effect of exercise at a fixed level of work, we assume that ıe time course beys first-order kinetics (fig. 2A) for a step increase of work rate:

$$\dot{M}(t) = \dot{M}_0[1 - \exp(-t/\tau)] \qquad (6)$$

τ is the time constant. $\dot{M}_0$ is the steady-state metabolic rate associated with the step stimulus caused by exercise. Furthermore, we assume that cardiac output increases linearly with metabolic rate:

$$\dot{Q} = K_4 \dot{M} + K_5 \tag{7}$$

This exercise stimulus leads to a biphasic increase in ventilation rate (fig. 2B), which after a short delay time rises to a plateau. The $PaCO_2$ decreases at the onset of exercise, shows damping oscillation, and comes back to a new baseline which is a little lower than at rest (fig. 2C). If the exercise stimulus $W_2(E)$ is significantly higher or lower (K_2 varied ± 25%), $\dot{V}$ changes by less than ± 0.5 L/min and $PaCO_2$ deviates only ± 1 torr from isocapnia in steady-state. The discomfort index also increases to a plateau with an inflection point caused by the $PaCO_2$ (fig. 2D).

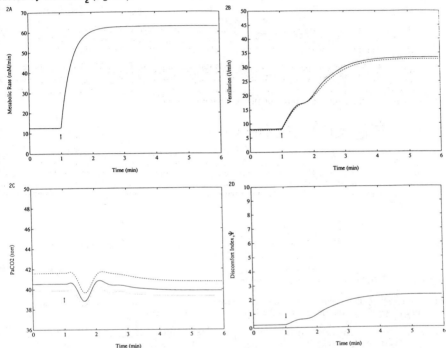

Fig. 2. The time course of (A) metabolic rate, (B) ventilation, (C) $PaCO_2$ and (D) discomfort index following a step change of work rate corresponding to the change in metabolic rate by 5 folds of the resting level. Dashed line: the response when the increase in metabolic rate is transmitted by 25% greater than the actual increase. Dotted line: the response when the increase in metabolic rate is transmitted by 25% less than the actual increase. The circulation time for this exercise is one-half the resting value. The scale factor of the discomfort index is altered to be able to compare with the experimental data measured by Visual Analog Scale for this and successive simulations. Arrow indicates the onset of the load.

<u>Rebreathing</u>

The hypercapnia induced by rebreathing requires an additional model equation for the PCO_2 dynamics of the rebreathing bag, as described by Chonan and co-workers (1988). The new variable (P_{BAG}) becomes the input P_I. During this simulation, the metabolic rate and cardiac output are assumed constant. Both PCO_2 and $\dot{V}$ increase rapidly during progressive hypercapnia (fig. 3A and 3B). Because both of these variables increase, the discomfort index (Ψ) is greater for this simulation than for the incremental exercise (fig. 4).

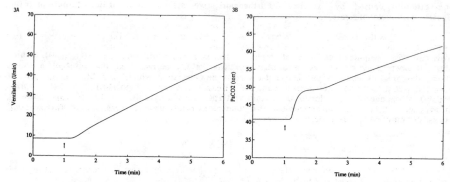

Fig. 3. The time course of (A) ventilation and (B) PaCO$_2$ following progressive hypercapnia. Arrow indicates the onset of the load.

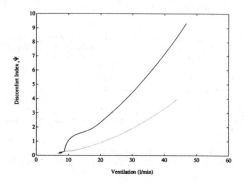

Fig. 4. Relationship between ventilation and discomfort index during progressive hypercapnia and incremental exercise.

The proposed model shows a possible controller structure which links the automatic regulatory process with the sensation and minimizes the operating cost.

The automatic ventilatory controller is assumed to receive (a) inhibitory feedback from lung or chest wall mechanoreceptors (perhaps tendon organs), which are stimulated by thoracic displacement, and (b) excitatory feedback from chemoreceptors. This assumption implies that feedback from mechanoreceptors attenuates dyspnea by reducing the activity of the automatic controller. This is consistent with the observations that static inspiratory efforts against a closed airway can extend breath-holding time (Rigg *et al.*, 1974) presumably by reducing the central motor command. Although such inhibitory and excitatory reflexes seem to be gated, we have not incorporated this feature in our model.

Our assumption that exercise augments the excitatory feedback from chemoreceptors corresponds to the concept that exercise and hypercapnia have synergistic effects on $\dot{V}$ (Poon and Green, 1985). We have assumed that this exercise stimulus reaches the ventilatory controller without any circulatory delay time. This does not imply that the exercise stimulus originates neurally, since Saunders (1980) has shown in his model that humoral signals may travel faster than the blood.

Optimal Controller Hypothesis

Our reflex control model can be related to optimal control models. The automatic controller tends to minimize the optimal control function suggested by Poon (1983):

$$J = \ln\dot{V}^2 + R(PCO_2 - P_0)^2$$

From our model, we calculate R ≈ 0.01, which is the value found by Poon. Furthermore, our model tends to minimize the discomfort index for perturbations about the operating point (V_0). In a simulated case, V_0 is about 20 L/min, which corresponds to the ventilation in moderate exercise. The basic behavior of C_{aut} is to minimize the discomfort associated with arterial chemical imbalance and respiratory mechanical effort. This concept is qualitatively the same as that of Poon. The spontaneously adopted ventilatory level is the minimum solution of the breathing sensation. This implies that the ventilation can be adequately controlled with behavioral and non-behavioral reflexes to minimize the respiratory discomfort in awake subjects (Longobardo et al., 1980). This possibility indicates the need for additional research in the interactions of mechanical and chemical inputs in both awake and asleep so that the mechanisms that are responsible for breathing patterns and breathing levels can be better understood.

REFERENCES

Altose, M.D., S.G. Kelsen and N.S. Cherniack (1979). Respiratory responses to changes in airflow resistance in conscious man. Respir. Physiol., 36, 249-260.

Altose, M.D., W.C. McCauley, S.G. Kelsen and N.S. Cherniack (1977). Effects of hypercapnia and inspiratory flow resistive loading on respiratory activity in chronic airways obstruction. J. Clin. Invest., 59, 500-507.

Cherniack, N.S. (1985). Potential role of optimization in alveolar hypoventilation and respiratory instability. In: Neurobiology of the Control of Breathing (C. von Euler and H. Lagercrantz, eds.), pp. 45-50. Raven Press, New York.

Chonan, T., A.M. Elhefnawy, O.P. Simonetti and N.S. Cherniack (1988). Rate of elimination of excess CO_2 in humans. Respir. Physiol., 73, 379-394.

Chonan, T., M.B. Mulholland, N.S. Cherniack and M.D. Altose (1987). Effects of constraining thoracic displacement and changes in chemical drive on the sensation of dyspnea. J. Appl. Physiol., 63, 1822-1828.

Chonan, T., M.B. Mulholland, J. Leitner, M.D. Altose and N.S. Cherniack (1990). Sensation of dyspnea during hypercapnia, exercise and voluntary hyperventilation. J. Appl. Physiol. (in press).

Davenport, P.W., W.A. Friedman, F.J. Thompson and O. Franzen (1986). Respiratory-related cortical potentials evoked by inspiratory occlusion in humans. J. Appl. Physiol., 60, 1843-1848.

ElHefnawy, A.M., G.M. Saidel and E.N. Bruce (1988). CO_2 control of the respiratory system: plant dynamics and stability analysis. Ann. Biomed. Eng., 16, 445-461.

Fink, B.R. (1961). Influence of cerebral activity in wakefulness on regulation of breathing. J. Appl. Physiol., 16, 15-20.

Gandevia, S.C. and G. Macefield (1989). Projection of low-threshold afferents from human intercostal muscles to the cerebral cortex. Respir. Physiol., 77, 203-214.

Gandevia, S.C. and B.L. Plassman (1988). Responses in human intercostal and truncal muscles to motor cortical and spinal stimulation. Respir. Physiol., 73, 325-338.

Gottfried, S.B., M.D. Altose, S.G. Kelsen, C.M. Fogarty and N.S. Cherniack (1978). The perception of changes in airflow resistance in normal subjects and patients with chronic airways obstruction. Chest, 73, 286-288.

Killian, K.J. and N.L. Jones (1988). Respiratory muscles and dyspnea. Clinics in Chest Med., 9, 237-244.

Killian, K.J., D.D. Bucens and E.J.M. Campbell (1982). Effect of breathing pattern on the perceived magnitude of added loads to breathing. J. Appl. Physiol., 52, 578-584.

Killian, K.J., S.C. Gandevia, E. Summers and E.J.M. Campbell (1984).   Effect of increased lung volume on perception of breathlessness, effort, and tension. *J. Appl. Physiol.*, 57, 686-691.

Killian, K.J., K. Mahutte and E.J.M. Campbell (1981).   Magnitude scaling of externally added loads to breathing. *Am. Rev. Respir. Dis.*, 123, 12-15.

Longobardo, G.S., N.S. Cherniack, and A. Damokosh-Giordano (1980).   Possible optimization of respiratory controller sensitivity. *Ann. Biomed. Eng.*, 8, 143-158.

Milic-Emili, J. and J.M. Tyler (1963).   Relationship between $PaCO_2$ and respiratory work during external resistance breathing in man. *Ann. N.Y. Acad. Sci.*, 109, 908-914.

Oliven, A., S.G. Kelsen, E.C. Deal, Jr., and N.S. Cherniack (1985).   Respiratory pressure sensation.   Relationship   to   changes   in   breathing   pattern   in   patients   with   chronic obstructive lung disease. *Am. Rev. Respir. Dis.*, 132, 1214-1218.

Orem, J. (1986). Behavioral control of breathing in the cat. *Brain Res.*, 366, 238-253.

Orem, J. (1987).   Inspiratory neurons that are activated when inspiration is inhibited behaviorally. *Neurosci. Lett.*, 83, 282-286.

Orem, J. (1988).   The activity of late inspiratory cells during the behavioral inhibition of inspiration. *Brain Res.*, 458, 224-230.

Orem, J., I. Osorio, E. Brooks and T. Dick (1985).   Activity of respiratory neurons during NREM sleep. *J. Neurophysiol.*, 54, 1144-1156.

Otis, A.B., W.O. Fenn, and H. Rahn (1950).   Mechanics of breathing in man. *J. Appl. Physiol.*, 2, 592-607.

Patterson, J.L., P.F. Mullinax, T. Gain, J.J. Krueger and D.W. Richardson (1962).   Carbon dioxide-induced dyspnea in a patient with respiratory muscle paralysis. *Am. J. Med.*, 32, 811-816.

Phillipson, E.A. and C. Bowes (1986).   Control of breathing during sleep. In: *Handbook of Physiology* (N.S. Cherniack and J.G. Widdicombe, eds.), Sect. 3, The Respiratory System, Vol. II, pp. 649-690. American Physiological Society, Bethesda MD.

Plum, F. (1970).   Neurological integration of behavioral and metabolic control of breathing. In: *Breathing: Hering-Breuer Centenary Symposium* (R. Porter, ed.), pp. 159-175. Churchill, London.

Plum F., and R.J. Leigh (1981).   Abnormalities of central mechanisms. In: *Regulation of Breathing* (T.F. Hornbein, ed.), Part II, pp. 989-1067. Marcel Dekker, New York.

Poon, C.S. (1983).   Optimal control of ventilation in hypoxia, hypercapnia and exercise. In: *Modelling and Control of Breathing* (B.J. Whipp and D.M. Wilberg, eds.), pp. 189-196. Elsevier, New York.

Poon, C.S. and J.G. Green (1985).   Control of exercise hyperpnea during hypercapnia in humans. *J. Appl. Physiol.*, 59, 792-797.

Rigg, J.R.A., A.S. Rebuck and D.J.C. Campbell (1974).   A study of factors influencing relief of discomfort in breath-holding in normal subjects. *Clin. Sci. Mol. Med.*, 47, 193-199.

Saunders, K.B. (1980).   Oscillations of arterial CO_2 tension in a respiratory model: some implications for the control of breathing in exercise. *J. Theor. Biol.*, 84, 163-179.

Sears, T.A. (1971).   Breathing: a sensori-motor act. In: *Sci. Basis Med. Annu. Rev.*, Chapter 7, pp. 129-147.

Sorli, J., A. Grassino, G. Lorange, and J. Milic-Emili (1978).   Control of breathing in patients with chronic obstructive lung disease. *Clin. Sci. Mol. Med.*, 54, 295-304.

Stark, R.D., S.A. Gambles and J.A. Lewis (1981). Methods to assess breathlessness in healthy subjects: a critical evaluation and application to analyze the acute effects of diazepam and promethazine on breathlessness induced by exercise or by exposure to raised levels of carbon dioxide. *Clin. Sci. Lond.*, 61, 429-439.

Tack, M., M.D. Altose and N.S. Cherniack (1983). The effects of aging on sensation of respiratory force and displacement. *J. Appl. Physiol.*, 55, 1433-1440.

Yamashiro, S.M., J.A. Daubenspeck, T.N. Lauretsen and F.S. Grodins (1975). Total work of breathing and optimization in CO_2 inhalation and exercise. *J. Appl. Physiol.*, 35, 522-525.

Zechman, F.W., Jr. and R.L. Wiley (1986). Afferent inputs to breathing respiratory sensation. *Handbook of Physiology* (N.S. Cherniack and J.G. Widdicombe, eds.), Sect. 3, The Respiratory System, Vol. II, pp. 449-474. American Physiological Society, Bethesda MD.

Ventilatory Response and Breathlessness in Deliberate Entrainment of Breathing and Pedaling Cycles During Cycle Exercise

Nariko Takano

Physiology Laboratory, Department of School Health,
Faculty of Education, Kanazawa University, Kanazawa
920, Japan

ABSTRACT

Ventilatory response and breathlessness during cycle exercise at aerobic work levels were examined under two breathing conditions: spontaneous breathing and deliberate entrainment of breathing rate (f) to pedal rate at a preferred coupling ratio. The pedal rate was 60 rpm for the 8 male subjects and 50 rpm for the 6 female subjects. During entrained cycling, 10 of the 14 subjects chose higher f, resulting in greater ventilatory response and less breathlessness, compared to those during non-entrained cycling. In the remaining 4 subjects, in whom entrained f was lower than spontaneous f, less ventilatory response and greater breathlessness were observed during the entrained cycling. These results suggest that the critical level of f at which breathlessness during cycling reaches its minimum does not always correspond to spontaneously adopted f, but can be shifted to a higher level when entrainment is made at a higher f than at a spontaneous f.

KEYWORDS

Entrainment of Breathing and Pedaling Rhythms; Ventilatory Response during Entrainment; Breathlessness during Exercise.

INTRODUCTION

During rhythmic exercise, respiratory rhythm occasionally entrains spontaneously to the exercise rhythm. In some sports, intentional entrainment (ENT) between the two rhythms is developed in order to accomplish favorable motor tasks and strength, and hence to improve total performance. The aim of the present study was to clarify the following points: (1) Is the ventilatory response at a given work rate identical when ENT is made and when breathing is driven reflexly ? (2) Does intentional ENT reduce the severity of dyspnea during rhythmic exercise ?

METHODS

Fourteen untrained subjects (8 males and 6 females) underwent a steady-state work test on a cycle ergometer with 4 different levels of aerobic work, equivalent to 0 (unloaded), 1/3, 2/3 and 1 times the work rate at the anaerobic threshold (AT), for 3 min at each work level. For the men, the pedal rate was 60 rpm and the mean work rate at AT was 165 W, while for the women they were 50 rpm and 100 W, respectively. The work test was performed under two different breathing conditions on separate days: (1) spontaneous breathing (Non-ENT) during pedaling, which was paced by a flashing light signal designed to prevent the development of intentional ENT, and (2) deliberate ENT at a preferred coupling ratio for each subject, in which the pedal rate was paced by a metronome designed to readily induce ENT. In the 3-min cycling period at each work rate, breathlessness during exercise was measured at the 1.5 th min by using a modified Borg rating scale, and averaged values of respiratory and metabolic variables during the last 1 min were obtained from the breath-by-breath measurements.

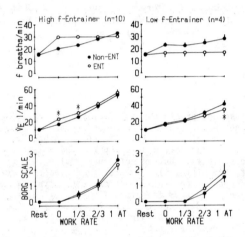

Fig. 1.   Respiratory responses and Borg scale for breathlessness during non-entrained and entrained
cycling. Values are means±SE. *: Significantly
different between the two cycling conditions.

RESULTS and DISCUSSION

The coupling ratio of pedaling to breathing rates chosen in ENT was 2:1 in 10 subjects, 4:1 in 3 subjects, and 3:2 in 1 subject. Change in the ventilatory response with ENT was not dependent on the coupling ratios but on the magnitude of breathing rate (f) in ENT relative to that in Non-ENT. As shown in Fig. 1, compared to spontaneous f, entrained f was higher in 10 of the 14 subjects, (high f-entrainers), except in the work at AT, while it was lower in the remaining subjects (low f-entrainers). Although the difference in f between the non-entrained and entrained cyclings was partly compensated by a reversed difference in tidal volume between the two cycling conditions, minute ventilation ($\dot{V}_E$) during entrained cycling was greater in the high f-entrainers and lower in the low-f entrainers, compared to that of non-entrained cycling. In both groups of entrainers, the difference in $\dot{V}_E$ between the two cycling conditions became more marked, as the disparity of f between the two conditions became greater. The difference between the two cycling conditions in ventilatory equivalents for metabolic variables ($\dot{V}_E/\dot{V}o_2$ and $\dot{V}_E/\dot{V}co_2$) showed a similar trend to that in $\dot{V}_E$ for both the high and low f-entrainers, and as a result, end-tidal Pco_2 during entrained cycling was lower in the high f-

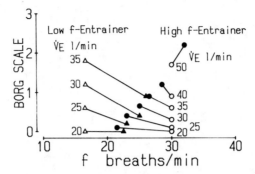

Fig. 2. Borg scale for breathlessness during cycling as
functions of f and $\dot{V}_E$. f was spontaneously driven
(closed symbol) and voluntarily entrained to
cycling rate (open symbol) in high f-entrainers
(circle) and low f-entrainers (triangle).

entrainers and higher in the low f-entrainers than that found during non-
entrained cycling. Yonge and Petersen (1983) have reported that
hyperventilation and hence hypocapnia during deliberately entrained cycling are
observed in untrained subjects, but not in highly trained subjects.

Figure 1 also shows that breathlessness during cycling against the work rate
tended to be less in ENT than in Non-ENT for the high f-entrainers, while the
tendency was reversed for the low f-entrainers, although the differences between
the two breathing conditions were not significant. Figure 2 shows the mean
value of breathlessness against f at 4 to 5 levels of $\dot{V}_E$ during non-entrained
and entrained cycling. Breathlessness during exercise was greater with
increasing $\dot{V}_E$, but for a given $\dot{V}_E$ it was less with increasing f, regardless of
breathing conditions, up to a certain level of f. Above this critical level of
f, breathlessness seemed to become greater with increasing f, as seen in the
case of $\dot{V}_E$ of 50 l/min. The critical f at which breathlessness reaches its
minimum has been reported to correspond to the spontaneously adopted f when
breathlessness is induced by hypercapnia (Cherniack et al., 1988). This would
not be the case in exercise, in which the critical f does not always correspond
to spontaneous f, but can be affected by the presence of ENT. If entrained f is
lower than spontaneous f during exercise, greater breathlessness may occur
during exercise with ENT than with Non-ENT, probably due to the secondarily
produced greater tidal volume which may act as a stronger dyspnogen (Cherniack
et al., 1988). On the other hand, if entrained f is higher than spontaneous f,
less breathlessness may occur during exercise with ENT, probably due to greater
respiratory efficiency as the result of the coordinated movement of the thorax
and abdomen (Garlando et al., 1985).

REFERENCES

Cherniack, N.S., T. Chonan and M.D. Altose (1988). Respiratory sensations
    and the voluntary control of breathing. In: Respiratory Psychophysiology
    (C. von Euler and M. Katz-Salamon, Ed.), MacMillan Press, London, pp. 35-45.
Garlando, F., J. Kohl, E.A. Koller and P. Pietsch (1985). Effect of coupling
    the breathing- and cycling rhythms on oxygen uptake during bicycle
    ergometry. Eur. J. Appl. Physiol., 54, 497-501.
Yonge, R.P. and S. Petersen (1983). Entrainment of breathing in rhythmic
    exercise. In: Modelling and Control of Breathing (B.J. Whipp and D.M.
    Wiberg, Ed.), Elsevier Sci. Pub., New York, pp. 197-204.

Effects of Hypoxia on Ventilatory Response at the Onset of Bicycle Exercise

M. Miyamura*, L. Xi*, K. Ishida[†],
F. Schena* and P. Cerretelli*

*Department of Physiology, Faculty of Medicine,
University of Geneve, Geneve, Switzerland
[†]Research Center of Health, Physical Fitness and Sports,
Nagoya University, Nagoya 464-01, Japan

In order to examine the effects of hypoxia on ventilatory response at the onset of dynamic exercise, the subject performed a bicycle exercise with rectangular load of 50 watts at 60rpm in both normoxic and hypoxic conditions. There are no statistical differences in the initial ventilatory response (d$\dot{V}$I and d$\dot{V}$E) between normoxia and hypoxia. our results suggest that neurogenic drive at onset of dynamic exercise is independent from PO2.

Ventilatory response;onset of exercise;hypoxia;hypocapnia

It is well known that the transition from rest to exercise is typically accompanied by an abrupt increase in pulmonary ventilation at the first exercise breath (phase I). According to Cunningham et al. (1966), neural stimuli do not immediately interact with any combination of chemical stimuli, either centrally or at the peripheral chemoreceptors. By contract, Asmussen (1973) noted that in the presence of existing chemical stimuli e.g. in hypercapnia, hypoxia, or combination of the two, the fast neurogenic component is very pronounced. Moreover, Springer et al. (1989) have recently found reduced phase I ventilatory responses as a result of hypoxia (15% O2) both in adults and children.

The present study, therefore, was undertaken to examine the effects of acute hypoxia on ventilatory response at the onset of dynamic exercise and possibly to settle with above contradictions.

Four healthy males participated in this study as subjects. All subjects familiar with the laboratory procedures required by the study. In order to ascertain the effects of hypoxia on ventilatory response at the onset of exercise, four tests were conducted for each subject on different days, i.e. 2 in normoxia (N) and 2 in hypoxia (H). In each test only the inspiratory ($\dot{V}$I) or the expiratory ($\dot{V}$E) responses were recorded at 30-45 min intervals. The subjects started breathing room air. After $\dot{V}$I (or, alternatively, $\dot{V}$E) was stabilized (3 min), subject asked to carry out a 50 watt exercise with 60 rpm (4 min) followed by a 3 min recovery period. Work onset and offset were marked by acoustic signals. During experiments the subjects sat on a saddle of a electrically braked bicycle ergometer (Bosch) with their feet on the pedal. The left pedal arm was kept in its frontal, horizontal position. The hypoxic trials were conducted while breathing 11% O2-N2 mixture from a series of Douglas bags.

M. Miyamura *et al.*

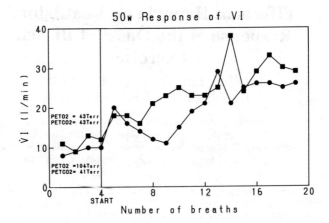

Fig. 1. An example of inspiratory response in transition from rest to exercise in normoxic and hypoxic conditions.

Pulmonary ventilation and gas exchange were determined breath-by-breath using a metabolic measurement apparatus (MMC 4400tc, Sensor medics); minute ventilation ($\dot{V}I$ or $\dot{V}E$), oxygen uptake ($\dot{V}O2$), carbon dioxide output ($\dot{V}CO2$), and end tidal pressure for O2 (PETO2) and for CO2 (PETCO2) were computed on-line. The rate of pedaling was also entered into the on-line breath-by-breath system.

Fig. 1 shows an example of inspiratory ventilatory response before and after submaximal ergometer exercise. $\dot{V}I$ increased immediately in response to the exercise stimulus. The ventilatory response was calculated as the difference (delta) between the mean of the first and second breath after the onset of exercise and the mean of 4 breaths preceding exercise. The average data of $\dot{V}I$ for the four investigated subjects are indicated in Fig. 2. The average values of resting $\dot{V}I$ were significantly (p< 0.05) higher in the hypoxia (13.4 $\pm$ 3.5 l/min) than that in the normoxia (10.3 $\pm$ 0.8 l/min). However, there are no statistical difference in the d$\dot{V}I$ between normoxia and hypoxia, despite a significant difference (p <0.05) between the absolute levels (H 31.2 $\pm$ 10.1 and 22.1 $\pm$ 2.9 l/min, respectively). Similar results were obtained in $\dot{V}E$.

The results of the present study indicate that the initial ventilatory response at the onset of exercise (both d$\dot{V}I$ and d$\dot{V}E$) is not affected by hypocapnic hypoxia. Our findings in agreement with those of Cunningham <u>et al</u>. (1966), but not with those of Asmussen (1973) and Springer <u>et al</u>. (1989). The discrepancy of the data in the phase I responses obtained by these authors could be explained by the difference in CO2 flow; Ward <u>et al</u>. (1983) reported that in man a decrease of pulmonary CO2 flow induced by a depletion of the body CO2 stores through volitional hyperventilation prior to exercise onset, diminishes the early phase of exercise hyperpnea. Although we unable to reproduce Ward's results, the alleged drop of phase I, attributed

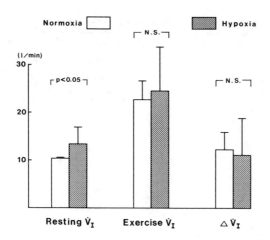

Fig. 2. Comparison of inspiratory volume in normoxia and hypoxia.

to reduced CO_2 flow, could have been hypothetically counterbalanced in the present experiments by hypoxia, either directly or indirectly. The first possibility seems to be ruled out by the cerebral vasopressor effect of hypoxia on the CNS. With regard to the indirect mechanism, whereby hypoxia could affect " per se " CO_2 flow to the lungs via an increase of the readjustment rate of cardiac output, this possibility is not supported by the results of Nakazono and Miyamoto (1987). They have reported that no remarkable difference in early transient (30 sec) response of cardiac output between hypoxia and hyperoxia.

From these results, it was suggested that the neurogenic component, besides being the primary factor controlling both $\dot{V}I$ and $\dot{V}E$, is not influenced by PO_2.

This study was supported by grant 3.088-0.87 from the Swiss National Foundation.

Asmussen,E. (1973) Ventilation at transition from rest to exercise. Acta Physiol. Scand.,89,68-78.
Cunningham,D.J.C., B.B.Lloyd and D.Spurr (1966) The relationship between the increase in breathing during the first respiration cycle in exercise and the prevailing background of chemical stimulation. J.Physiol.(Lond.),185,73-74P.
Nakazono,Y. and M.Miyamoto (1987) Effect of hypoxia and hyperoxia on cardiorespiratory responses during exercise in man. Jpn.J.Physiol.,37,447-457.
Springer,C., T.J.Barstow and D.M.Cooper (1989) Effect of hypoxia on ventilatory control during exercise in children and adults. Pediatr.Res.,25,285-290.
Ward,S.A., T.J.Whipp, S.Koyal and K.Wasserman (1983) Influence of body CO_2 stores on ventilatory dynamics during exercise. J.Appl.Physiol.,55,742-749.

PGE_2 Inhalation Increased Dyspnea During Exercise in Normal Subjects

O. Taguchi, Y. Kikuchi, W. Hida, N. Iwase,
M. Satoh, S. Okabe, T. Chonan and
T. Takishima

First Department of Internal Medicine, Tohoku
University School of Medicine, 1-1 Seiryo-machi,
Aoba-ku, Sendai 980, Japan

ABSTRACT

Whether vagal afferents from the lung affect the sensation of dyspnea has not
been determined. As inhaled PGE_2 has been shown to stimulate irritant receptors
and C-fibers in the lung, we examined the effects of aerosolized PGE_2 on the
sensation of exercise-induced dyspnea in eight normal male subjects. Exercise
tests were performed on a bicycle ergometer after either saline (0.9 vol%) or
PGE_2 (100 ug/ml) inhalation. The tests consisted of 3 min at rest followed by a
2 min 0 watt load after which the workload was increased by 50 watt at 2 min
intervals to 150 watt. We found that, although airway resistance and lung
volume did not change significantly between values after saline and those after
PGE_2 inhalation, inhaled PGE_2 significantly increased the magnitude of the
dyspneic sensation than did inhaled saline when compared at the same levels of
workload, ventilation and oxygen consumption during exercise. These results
suggest that afferent vagal activity from the lung contribute to the sensation
of dyspnea, probably through a direct effect on higher brain centers.

KEYWORDS

Control of breathing; prostaglandins; vagal afferents; Borg scale.

INTRODUCTION

Whether vagal afferents from the lung affect the sensation of dyspnea has not
been determined. However, we (Taguchi et al., 1989) have recently found that
airway anesthesia with 4 % lidocaine significantly decreased the intensity of
dyspneic sensation at the same levels of ventilation or occlusion pressure
during voluntary hyperpnea with histamine induced bronchoconstriction. In
contrast, airway anesthesia did not change the dyspneic sensation during
external resistive loading. Because histamine stimulates the vagal afferent
receptors, especially irritant receptors, and these receptors are blocked by
airway anesthesia, these results suggest that vagal afferents may increase the
intensity of the dyspneic sensation. To further confirm this hypothesis, we
examined the effects of prostaglandin E_2 (PGE_2) inhalation on the sensation of
exercise-induced dyspnea, because inhaled PGE_2 has been shown to stimulate
irritant receptors and C-fibers in the lung (Coleridge et al., 1976).

METHOD

Eight normal male subjects ranging in age from 30 to 41 yr were studied.   Four
of the subjects had had previous experience with respiratory and sensory
studies, and they knew the purpose of the study.   However, the other four
subjects were not aware of the general purpose of the study.

One hundred μg/ml of PGE_2 (Ono Pharmaceutical Co., Osaka, Japan) dissolved in
saline or saline (control, 0.9 vol%)was inhaled through a Bird nebulizer for 2
minutes.   This dose of PGE_2 is known to produce cough when inhaled by normal
subjects (Costello et al., 1985).

Airway resistance (Raw) and thoracic gas volume (Vtg) were measured with a body
plethysmograph (Gould 2800J, AUTOBOX) by the DuBois' panting method after saline
inhalation, and before and after exercise after PGE_2 inhalation.
Exercise tests were performed on a   bicycle ergometer after saline inhalation
and after PGE_2 inhalation on separate days.   The tests consisted of 3 min at
rest followed by a 2 min exercise with a 0 watt load after which the workload
was increased by 50 watt at 2 min intervals to 150 watts.   Minute ventilation
(V_E) and breathing frequency were monitored from an expiratory line through a
low resistance, non-rebreathing two-way mask (model 7900-M, Hans-Rudolph).
Samples of mixed expired gas were analyzed every 10 sec to calculate oxygen
consumption ($\dot{V}_{O2}$) and carbon dioxide production ($\dot{V}_{CO2}$) using a measurement cart
(Aerobic Processor, NEC-Sanei, Tokyo).   The sensation of dyspnea was measured on
a modified Borg scale at the end of each workload.

RESULTS

Raw tended to decrease after PGE_2 inhalation compared with that after saline,
however this difference did not reach statistical significance.   Mean values of
Vtg did not change significantly between those after saline and after PGE_2
inhalation.   Also exercise did not change Raw and Vtg significantly after PGE_2
inhalation.

There were basically no differences between results obtained from naive subjects
and those obtained from the subjects who were familiar with the apparatus and
were well informed about the general purpose of the study.   The mean values of
$\dot{V}_{O2}$, $\dot{V}_{CO2}$ and V_E did not change significantly at the same levels of workload
between those after saline and those after PGE_2 inhalation.   However, the
sensation of dyspnea significantly increased after PGE_2 inhalation than that
after saline inhalation, compared at the same levels of workload, oxygen
consumption and minute ventilation (Table 1).   These results suggest that vagal
afferents from the lung have an important role in the genesis of exercise-
induced dyspnea in normal subjects.

DISCUSSION

We have found that the sensation of dyspnea during exercise increased after PGE_2
inhalation at the same levels of workload, $\dot{V}_{O2}$, $\dot{V}_{CO2}$ and ventilation than after
saline inhalation.   Several possibilities must be consisted when seeking to
explain this observation.   First, mechanical changes in the lung produced by
inhaled PGE_2 seem to be unlikely, because airway resistance and Vtg did not
change significantly after saline and after PGE_2.   Second, as $F_{ET}CO2$ did not
increase, we think that possible changes in chemoreceptor activity may be
negligible.   Thus, the most possible explanation is that increases in vagal
afferent activity increase the sensation, because inhaled PGE_2 is known to
stimulate vagal irritant receptors and bronchial and pulmonary C-fibers in the
lung (Coleridge et al., 1976).   In fact, all our subjects produced coughs and

felt tightness of breathing and irritation in the chest after PGE$_2$ inhalation. We conclude that afferent vagal activity from the lung increases the sensation of dyspnea during exercise. Because the increase in dyspnea was not accompanied by an increase in ventilation, the sensation of dyspnea increased probably through a direct projection to the sensory cortex of the higher brain centers.

Table 1. Changes in $\dot{V}_{O2}$, $\dot{V}_{CO2}$, V_E and Borg scale during exercise after saline (S) and after PGE$_2$ (P) inhalation.

Workload		at rest	0watt	50watt	100watt	150watt
$\dot{V}_{O2}$	S	292±26	552±29	760±41	1214±36	1758±44
(ml/min)	P	258±24	505±47	721±38	1196±47	1643±72
$\dot{V}_{CO2}$	S	262±28	440±31	621±35	1096±34	1827±76
(ml/min)	P	239±29	422±35	587±40	1104±34	1824±74
V_E	S	9.7±0.9	16.0±1.6	21.7±1.4	33.7±1.5	55.1±3.3
(L/min)	P	9.7±1.3	15.8±1.6	20.7±1.9	35.4±1.9	58.2±3.4
Borg Scale	S	0.3±0.1	0.5±0.1	1.4±0.3	2.7±0.3	4.7±0.4
	P	0.7±0.1**	1.0±0.1**	2.2±0.2*	3.6±0.3*	6.1±0.4**

Values are means±SE in eight subjects. Symbols indicate significant difference from value after saline: *P<0.05, **P<0.01.

REFERENCES

Chonan, T., M.B. Mulholland, J. Leitner, M.D. Altose and N.S. Cherniack (1987). Comparisons of the sensation of dyspnea during hypercapnia, exercise and voluntary hyperventilation. Am. Rev. Respir. Dis., 135, A297.
Coleridge, H.M., J.C.G. Coleridge, K.H. Ginzel, D.G. Baker, R.B. Banzett and M.A. Morrison(1976). Stimulation of 'irritant' receptors and afferent C-fibers in the lungs by prostaglandins. Nature, 264, 451-453.
Costello, J.F., L.S. Dunlop and P.J. Gardner (1985). Characteristics of prostaglandin induced cough in man. Br. J. Clin. Pharmac., 20, 355-359.
El-Manshawi, A. K.J. Killian, E. Summers and N.J. Jones (1986). Breathlessness during exercise with and without resistive loading. J. Appl. Physiol., 51, 895-905.
Killian, K.J., S.C. Gandevia, E.Summers and E.J.M. Campbell (1984). Effect of increased lung volume on perception of breathlessness, effort, and tension. J. Appl. Physiol., 57, 686-691.
Taguchi, O., Y. Kikuchi, W. Hida, N. Iwase, S. Okabe, M. Satoh, T. Chonan, H. Inoue and T. Takishima (1989). The effects of airway anesthesia on the sensation of dyspnea in normal subjects. Am. Rev. Respir. Dis.,139, A322.

Effects of Vagal Afferent Stimulation on High-frequency Oscillation in Phrenic Nerve Activity of Rabbits

T. Hukuhara, Jr., W.-J. Yuan, K. Takano,
F. Kato and N. Kimura

Department of Pharmacology II, Jikei University School
of Medicine, Minato-ku, Tokyo 105, Japan

ABSTRACT

In aiming to elucidate the functional involvement of the phasic afferent inputs from pulmonary stretch receptors (PSR) in determination of the central respiratory rhythm and in modification of the high-frequency synchronization of the phrenic motoneuronal discharges, low-intensity afferent stimulation of the vagus nerve were performed in artificially ventilated rabbits. The effects of the electrical stimulation at various frequencies delivered during different phases within respiratory cycles were quantitatively analyzed.

KEYWORDS

Central respiratory mechanisms; respiratory rhythm; respiratory reflex; phrenic nerve; high-frequency oscillation; vagus afferent; power spectral analysis; Fourier analysis.

INTRODUCTION

It is commonly recognized that the afferent inputs from the PSRs to the central respiratory mechanisms modulate the final output from the central respiratory pattern generator and contribute to the adjustment of the rhythmic contractions of the respiratory muscles in mammals. Wyss (1939) has shown that the electrical sti⁻ula-tion of the fast-conducting afferent fibers in the vagus nerve in rabbits c⌐used reversed responses depending on the stimulus frequency and suggested the differential action of the PSR afferents on the respiratory center. It is also demonstrated that the respiratory unit discharges in the brain stem alter diversely by the vagal afferent stimulation depending on its frequency in rabbits, cats and dogs (Hukuhara et al., 1956) or in cats (Hukuhara, Jr. et al., 1966).

On the other hand, it is known that the central respiratory pattern generator produces other synchronized activity in a much higher frequency range (70-130 Hz) than the respiratory rhythm. This activity is designated as the high-frequency oscil-lation (HFO) and appears synchronously in the inspiratory discharges of the phrenic nerve and some of the cranial nerves involved in the phasic control of the upper airway resistance and subserve presumably the central coordination of the ven-tilatory movements (Dittler and Garten, 1912; Cohen, 1973; Kato et al., 1987).

The aim of this study is to determine whether the vagal afferents exert influences to the respiratory rhythm and phrenic HFO in a similar fashion or not and whether the effect is dependent on the timing and intensity of the afferent inputs.

METHODS

Experiments were performed on nine rabbits under ether-anesthesia. After bilateral vagotomy, the animals were paralyzed with gallamine and artificially ventilated under monitoring of the carbon dioxide level (end-tidal: 4.3 ± 0.5 %; mean$\pm$SD, n=9). Efferent discharges of the phrenic nerve were derived with bipolar platinum electrodes at the neck and recorded on magnetic tapes. The vagus nerve was stimulated at the central end of the section. Based on the evaluation of the conduction velocities for the fibers in the vagus nerve trunk, selective stimulation of A-alpha, beta and gamma afferent fiber groups was performed by adjusting the stimulus voltage (<0.5 V, 0.1 ms, 5-160 Hz). The following three modes of stimulation were applied for consecutive 30 s: i) stimulation during inspiratory phase (IS), ii) during expiratory phase (ES), and iii) continuous stimulation throughout both phases (CS).

After digitization of 20 s data of the phrenic nerve activity, total respiratory cycle duration (Tt), inspiratory time (Ti) and expiratory time (Te) were measured and the power spectral density function (0-256 Hz) was estimated. By means of the non-linear parameter estimation (Kato et al., 1987), the mean square values (MSV) of the HFO component representing the total amount of HFO-output were estimated.

RESULTS

Effect of Vagus Nerve Stimulation on Respiratory Cycle.

The CS, IS and ES consistently exerted an accelerative effect on the respiratory rhythm when stimulated at lower frequencies (5-80 Hz), that is, slight but significant shortening of Ti, Te and consequentially, Tt (Table 1). In contrast, stimulations at a higher frequency (160 Hz) prolonged Tt Te prominently when stimuli were delivered during expiratory phase or continuously (Table 1). No qualitative difference was observed between the effect of higher frequency IS and the lower frequency IS.

Table 1. Effect of vagus nerve stimulation on respiratory cycle and the mean square values of the phrenic HFO.

stimulation mode	freq. [Hz]	Tt[%]	Ti[%]	Te[%]	MSV of HFO[%]
CS	5	74.6±6.4*	86.6±11.5*	65.4±8.1*	32.3±14.9*
	80	53.5±15.7*	60.8±11.2*	49.4±24.9*	1.4±1.9*
	160	228.3±147.0*	88.4±18.7	346.3±304.2*	1.1±1.6*
IS	5	85.6±4.8*	93.2±12.6	82.4±11.7*	45.6±18.4*
	80	47.0±9.3*	61.5±17.5*	39.7±14.0*	2.9±4.2*
	160	46.3±18.9*	57.8±20.3*	40.1±19.3*	4.8±4.3*
ES	5	83.8±6.7*	84.7±12.7*	85.2±11.1*	57.3±16.9*
	80	59.3±11.1*	66.5±10.8*	56.4±19.7*	12.8±12.3*
	160	221.2±86.4*	117.0±24.9	303.9±148.0*	24.4±27.4*

Mean±standard deviation of the percentile to the control; n=8-9; *, P<0.05

Effect of Vagus Nerve Stimulation on HFO.

Independent of the timing and rate of the stimulus, the vagal afferent stimulation depressed the phrenic HFO. The MSV was decreased by each of the three modes of stimulation almost in a stimulus-frequency dependent fashion (Table 1). The CS was most potent, then IS, and ES was less effective, though the decrease in the MSV was significant (P<0.01) for each of these stimulation modes.

DISCUSSION

These results suggest that the vagal afferences, presumably from the pulmonary stretch receptors, could prominently modulate not only the respiratory rhythm, but also the oscillating state of the neural mechanism responsible for generation and formation of HFO in the phrenic activity. There was a pronounced difference, however, between the effects on them, that is, the influence of the vagal afferent inputs on the respiratory rhythm varied not only quantitatively but also qualitatively depending on the frequency and the timing within the respiratory cycle of the stimuli in contrast with the influence on the phrenic HFO which was consistently depressed regardless of the stimulus mode and frequency. The result of the lung inflation experiments presented by Richardson (1988) is in accordance with this diverse responses of the respiratory rhythm and phrenic HFO. Nevertheless, our observation that the phrenic HFO was prominently depressed by the vagus afferents is not consistent with the findings by Cohen et al. (1987) and Richardson (1988) who found that the HFO in the efferent discharges of the cranial nerves are eliminated but not that of the phrenic nerve by the lung-inflation during the inspiratory phase. This contradiction might be due to the differences in i) animal species, ii) anesthetic conditions, iii) spatiotemporal excitation pattern of the afferent fibers between lung-inflation and electrical stimulations, and in iv) sensitivity of the quantification of HFO. It is concluded that the activity of the neural networks controlling the respiratory rhythm and the respiratory motor outputs might consist of different neural organizations and are independently modified by the same afferent information from the PSR and react in a different manner to optimize respiratory movements in response to the extent of distinction of the lungs.

Partly supported by the Ministry of Education, Science and Culture, Japan, Grant-in-Aid for Developmental Scientific Research, No. 01870012 and by the Science Research Promotion Fund of Japan Private School Promotion Foundation (1988).

REFERENCES

Cohen, M.I. (1973). Synchronization of discharge, spontaneous and evoked, between inspiratory neurons. Acta Neurobiol. Exp., 33, 189-218.

Cohen. M.I., W.R. See, C.N. Christakos and A.L. Sica (1987). High-frequency and medium-frequency components of different inspiratory nerve discharges and their modification by various inputs. Brain Res., 417, 148-152.

Dittler, R. and S. Garten (1912). Die Zeitliche Folge der Aktionsstroeme in Phrenicus und Zwerchfell bei der natuerlichen Innervation. Z. Biol., 133, 420-450.

Hukuhara, T., H. Okada and S. Nakayama (1956). On the vagus-respiratory reflex. Jpn. J. Physiol., 6, 87-97.

Hukuhara, T. Jr., N. Kumadaki, H. Kojima, H. Tamaki, Y. Saji and F. Sakai (1966). Effects of electrical stimulation of n. vagus on the respiratory unit discharge in the brain stem of cats. Brain Res., 1, 310-311.

Kato, F., N. Kimura, K. Takano and T. Hukuhara, Jr. (1987). Quantitative spectral analysis of high frequency oscillation in efferent nerve activities with respiratory rhythm. In: Respiratory Muscles and Their Neuromotor Control (G.C. Sieck, S.C. Gandevia and W.E. Cameron, eds), pp. 263-267, Alan R. Liss, New York.

Richardson, C.A. (1988). Power spectra of inspiratory nerve activity with lung inflations in cats. J. Appl. Physiol., 64,, 1709-1720.

Wyss, O.A.M. (1939) Reizphysiologishe Analyse des afferenten Lungenvagus. Pfluegers Arch., 242, 215-233.

EMG Biofeedback Training of Painful Respiratory Muscles in Patients with Dyspnea

I. Saito*, Y. Saito[†] and K. Takaoka[‡]

*Sapporo Meiwa Hospital, Tsukisamu West 1-10,
Toyohira-Ku, Sapporo;
[†]Sapporo National Hospital;
[‡]Japan Steel Memorial Hospital, Japan

ABSTRACT

The subjects with functional dyspnea due to painful respiratory muscles were incorporated into the EMG biofeedback training program. Present relaxation training of respiratory muscles revealed an increase of %vital capacity, no definite change of Fev 1.0% and a decrease of EMG level in abdominal muscle. The physical activity showed better in the follow-up. It was suggested that biofeedback assisted training of respiratory muscle helps better respiration and available to rehabilitation.

KEYWORDS

Dyspnea, Painful respiratory muscle, EMG-biofeedback training, Biofeedback training

INTRODUCTION

Present study was performed to elucidate whether EMG biofeedback training (BFT) might have any influence on painful respiratory muscle group and respiratory function, especially %vital capacity(VC) and Fev 1.0%.

SUBJECTS

Among 25 subjects (12 male and 13 female) who suffered from functional dyspnea such as hyperventilation syndrome, and were painful in respiratory muscles, 18 subjects (5 male and 13 female) were incorporated into this program. 7 excluded subjects were all male and their %VC showed over 100%. These subjects were neglected from this program because %VC was an inappropriate parameter in these subjects.

APPARATUS

EMG-BFT: P-303(Cyborg Ltd.) and UT-201(Unique Medical Ltd.).
Spirometry: AS-300(Minato, Ltd.) & PM-50(portable spirometer, Hukuda Ltd.)

PROCEDURE

The target muscles were 1) abdominal rectal muscle & diaphragmaticmuscle, and 2) shoulder, neck and back muscle groups. The subjects were examined VC first instanding posture, then they were examined EMG level of the abdominal muscle and shoulder or neck in lying posture before and after EMG-BFT, and VC was examined again in standing posture. The numbers of relaxation training ranged 3-26(mean: 9) sessions. Each subject performed two of 7 minutes muscle relaxation training in one session. Spirometry was performed before and after BFT weekly or biweekly basis for clinical evaluation. Paired t-test was used for evaluation of VC and EMG-level, and Chi square test for clinical evaluation.

364   I. Saito *et al.*

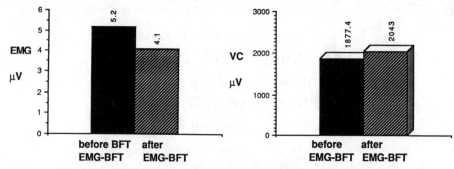

Fig.1.   EMG level showed a significant decrease
         (p<0.05) after EMG-biofeedback training.

Fig.2.   %vital Capacity showed a significant change
         (p<0.001) before and after EMG-biofeedback
         training of the abdominal rectus muscle.

RESULTS

I Physiological aspect:
1) EMG level was 5.2 ± 4.6μV before EMG-BFT, and 4.1 ± 3.2μV after EMG-BFT (p<0.05)(Fig. 1).
2) Vital capacity was 1877.4 ± 716ml after EMG-BFT (p<0.001)(Fig. 2).
3) There was no quantitative relationship between the mean decreased EMG level and the mean increase of %VC.

II Physical activity:
The physical activity of these patients was examined with Hugh-Jones criteria which was applied to evaluation of dyspnea. In Fig. 3, the left bars show the rate before BFT, and the right bars show those after BFT. Chi square test revealed that the distribution of the subjects changed through BFT(p<0.05).
The median shifted from Grade 3 to Grade 2 through BFT. In the 3 grade, the rate decreased from 42% to 17% and in the 2 grade, the rate increased from 42% to 65% significantly. It is concluded that EMG-BFT of abdominal muscle worked in increasing VC, and contributed to make the subjects' physical activity better.
As an example, A case of 37 years old housewife is introduced, who suffered from dyspnea and myalgia of shoulder, neck, chest and extremities with general lassitude. After 3 months' admission she was referred to the psychosomatic treatment. In the Fig. 4, two pieces of the chart(left side) show those taken during one month. The curve marked X indicates VC taken before BFT and the open circles indicate those after BFT. Open circles were over Xs indicating that subjects' %VC increased through relaxation training of respiratory muscles. The right figures indicate an increase of the %VC (x axis), a suggested increase of % inspiratory volume(y axis) and no definite change of Fev 1% after 3 months' training.

DISCUSSION

The mechanism of BFT is estimated to be central regulation of unnoticed physiological function such as heart rate, blood pressure, electromyogram etc.. This behavioral treatment has been applie widely.
Feldman (1976) and Kostes et al. (1977) applied this technique in the treatment of bronchial asthma of children. Holliday et al. (1983) and Tiep (1978) tried biofeedback approach in the treatmen of chronic lung diseases. Pepper and his group(1987a,b) has applied a diaphragmatic breathing to a field of health science.
The abdominal muscles have several roles, one is the maintenance and chang of posture, the co-operation of respiration with major respiratory muscles and the third is to protection from outside noxious interventions.
Although the reason why relaxation of abdominal muscle group works for better respiration is not clear, one of suggestions is that as the peripheral fringe of the diaphragmis supplied from the lower intercostal nerves (Anderson, 1978), present relaxation training of upper abdomen might induce a relaxation of the diaphragm through above-mentioned nerve supply and better diaphragmatic function. According to our experience, relaxation training of the abdominal muscle induces relaxation of the shoulder and neck muscle group in patients with chronic muscle contraction headache in EMG-level (Saito, 1988), this suggest a possibility of better thoracic respiration. Further study should be required to elucidate EMG relationship between the abdominal muscle relaxation and the diaphragm.

REFERENCES

Anderson, J. (1978). *Grant's Altas of Anatomy* (The William & Wilkins Company), 7th Asian Edition. Igaku Shoin Ltd./Tokyo, 2-120.

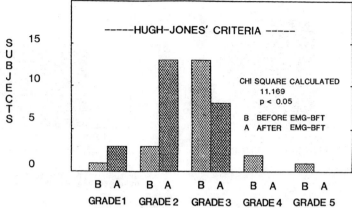

Fig. 3. The quality of life was evaluated with Hugh-Fohnes' criteria. The median shifted from Grade 3 to GRADE 2 and showed a significant modulation in the pattern (p<0.05) .

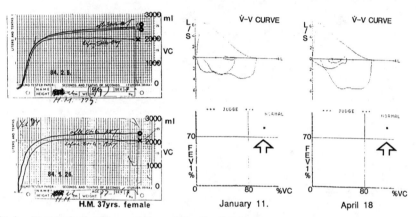

Fig. 4. An example of a 37 years old house wife. Her %vital capacity increased after EMG-biofeedback training within a session, and 3 months follow-up revealed her respiratory function was better.

Feldman, G.M. (1976). The effect of biofeedback training on respiratory resistance of the asthmatic children. *Psychosomatic Med.*, 38, 27-34.

Holliday, J.E., McDaniel, S. (1983). Comparison of biofeedback between emphysema patients and chronically anxious patients. *Biofeedback and Self-Regulation*, 8, 327-328.

Kostes, H., Glaus, K., Bricel, S. (1977). Muscle relaxation effects on speak expiratory flow rate in asthmatic children. *The Proceedings of The Biofeedback Research Society*, Orland, Fla..

Pepper, E., Smith, K., Waddel, D. (1987). Voluntary wheezing versus diaphrag breathing within inhalation (Voldyne) feedback. *Clinical Biofeedback and Health*, 10, 83-88.

Rolland, M. and Pepper, E. (1987). Inhalation volume change with inspirometer feedback and diaphragmatic breathing coaching. *Biofeedback and Self-Regulation*, 10, 89-97.

Saito, I., Yashiro, N., Okuse, S. (1988). Unpublished data.

Saito, I., Takaoka, K., Saito, Y. (1989). Self-regulation of abdominal muscle tension and respiratory function. Symposium, Modulated by Naifeh, K.: Breathing for Health; An overview of breathing techniques used to enhance self-regulation. 20th Annual Meeting of Association for Applied Psychophysiology and Biofeedback. San Diego, *Biofeedback-Audio Tape*, BSA89-12(II).

Tiep, B. et al. (1978). Respiratory feedback: two non-invasive approaches in the treatment of patients with chronic obstructive lung diseases. *Proceedings of The San Diego Biochemical Symposium*. Academic Press, Inc., New York.

The Effect of Abdominal Rectal Massage in Subjects with Functional Dyspnea and Chronic Obstructive and Restrictive Lung Diseases

I. Saito*, Y. Saito† and K. Takaoka‡

*Sapporo Meiwa Hospital, Tsukisamu West 1-10,
Sapporo; and Hokkaido University, School of Medicine;
†Sapporo National Hospital;
‡Japan Steel Works Memorial Hospital, Japan

ABSTRACT

The massage assisted relaxation of the abdominal muscle was performed in the functional dyspnea group (A group) and the dyspnea group with organic respiratory diseases. In A group, the vital capacity(VC) and the forced ventilatory capacity(FVC) increased and EMG-level decreased after the massage with no definite change in the %forced expiratory volume in one second(Fev1.0%). In B group, although VC increased significantly after the massage, no relevant change was observed in FVC, Fev1.0% and EMG-level. It is suggested that stroking massage is one of the candidates in the self-aid rehabilitative techniques for better respiration in subjects with dyspnea, specially in the case of functional dyspnea.

KEYWORS

Abdominal massage, Vital capacity, Forced vital capacity, Dyspnea.

Dyspneic subjects suffers from vicious cycle of physical disorders and psychological trouble, then meet social difficulties. Prevous report revealed that the soft abdominal massage was helpful in reducing the chronic pain of the abdominal rectus muscle of contraction type(Saito,1988), and we happened to observe this simple maneuvers worked as good as EMG biofeedback relaxation technique(1990) when applied to these subjects. We notice too that abdominal massage produces relaxation in shoulder and neck muscle groups concomitantly(1989). Present study was performed to elucidate whether the massage assisted abdominal muscle relaxation might have any influence on respiratory function.

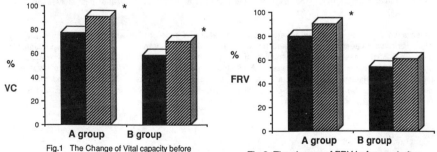

Fig.1 The Change of Vital capacity before and after the abdominal massage. * p<0.05

Fig.2 The change of FRV before and after the abdominal massage. * p<0.05

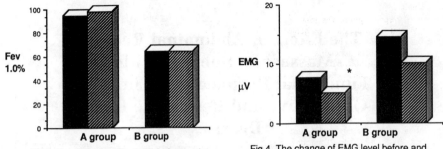

Fig.3 The change of Fev1.0% before and
after the abdominal massage.

Fig.4 The change of EMG level before and
after the abdominal massage. * p<0.05

SUBJECTS

The subjects are divided into 2 groups, A group is consisted of 14 subjects(5 male & 9 female) who range
in age from 16 to 60(mean; 39.6). They were suffered from functional dyspnea such as hyperventilation
syndrome and so on. B group is 15 subjects (5 male & 10 female) who range in age 53 to 75(mean;64.8).
These subjects suffered from organic dyspnea of chronic obstructive and/or restrictive lung diseases as
emphysema and old tuberculosis.

APPARATUS

Electromyograph: P-303(Cyborg Ltd.).   Spirometer: AS-300(Minato,Ltd.) & Discom-14(Chest Co.).

PROCEDURE

The subjects were examined respiratory function with a spirometer first, then lay down on the bed, and
practised stroking the surface of their abdomen with both palms 100 times or for 5 minutes.
They were examined again respiratory function. The results were evaluated with paired t-test.

RESULTS

A group:
  1) VC was 77.4 ± 21.9% before the massage and 90.8 ± 19.6% after the massage (p<0.05) (Fig.1).
  2) FVC showed 80.2 ± 21.6% before the massage and 90.0 ± 18.4% after the massage (p<0.05) (Fig.2).
  3) Fev1.0% was 95.1 ± 27.8% before the massage and 97.8 ± 27.9% after the massage (NS) (Fig.3).
  4) EMG level showed 7.8 ± 8.8 µV before the massage and 5.2 ± 5.5 µV after this intervention (p<0.05)
     (Fig.4).
B group:
  1) VC showed 58.9 ± 26.4% before the massage and 70.1 ± 29.1% after this intervention (p<0.05) (Fig.1).
  2) FRV showed 54.0 ± 19.1% before the massage and 61.5 ± 21.8% after the massage (NS) (Fig.2).
  3) Fev1.0% was 64.4 ± 19.9% before the massage and 64.5 ± 13.9% after the massage (NS) (Fig.3).
  4) EMG level showed 14.6 ± 15.5 µV before the massage and 10.2 ± 8.7 µV after this intervention (NS)
     (Fig.4).

As an example of the massabge assisted relaxation training, a case of 47 years old male is shown in Fig.5.
After this patient caused a car accident, he was seized with a panic and was admitted as hyperventilation
syndrome. After massage relaxation training of the abdominal muscle, his VC increased and V-V curve
showed faster from 6.5 l/sec to 7.7 l/sec. As stated in the preface, the abdominal massage mtigate
myalgia in many cases. Fig.6 shows a case of 28 years old lady who was admitted due to abdominal pain
and deppresion. Her subjective unit of tentative pain shifted from 70 to 40 in the epigatrium and from 60
to 30 in both sides of ileocecal parts.

Discussion

Stroking massage of the abdominal muscle showed significant increase of VC in both groups of functional and
organic respiratory diseases. However, FVC and EMG-level showed a discrepancy between both groups

with siginicant better results in the functional dyspnea group. The result indicates that the dyspnea of oraganic respiratory diseases is more refractory than those of the functional diseases. The mechanis by which the stroking massage produced about 10% increaseof VC is speculated as follows; 1) relaxation of the abdominal muscle faccilitated expiratory respiration as shown in this study that EMG-level of the abdominal muscle decreased after the stroking massage, and 2) as our previous study revealed(Saito,1987) revealed, the stroking massage of the abdomen turned less painful and tentative in the abdominal muscle and such mitigation of myalgia might cause sufficient muscle movement. As for forerunning application of massage technique to muscle relaxation training, Mdders (1980) succeeded in the conjunctive use of massage in a group therapy of patients with chronic muscle contraction headache. McKenie (1983) reported that the massage worked on better effect on autonomic nervous function. As the fatigue of respiratory muscle groups has been the major issues in therecent respirology, the stroking massageis one of the possibilities for such intervention.

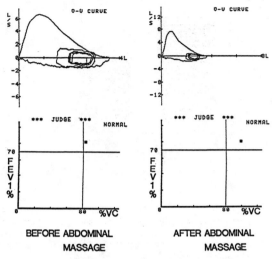

Fig. 5 An example of the spirometry in 47 years old male.

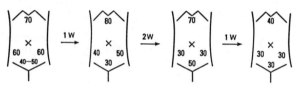

Fig. 6 Subjective score of abdominal pain(the muximum is 100). 28 years old female.

REFERENCES

Conner,W.H.(1974). Effect of brief relaxation training on autonomic response to anxiety-evoking stimuli. *Psychophysiology,* 11: 591-9.

Madders,J.(1980). Group relaxation: In: *Stress and Tension Control,* Mc Guigan, F.J., Sime, W.E. & Wallace,J.M.(ed.), Plenum Press, NY and London, p.141-145.

McKennie,A.A.,Wilson,F.,Watson,N.,Scott,D.(1983). Anxiety states: A preliminary report on the value of connective tissue massage. *Journal of Psychosomatic research,* 27: 125-129.

Saito,I.,Saito,Y.Nishino,T.,Ishikawa,M.,Yasiro,N.,Okuse,S.(1987). The use of biofeedback in the treatment of chronic abdominal pain characterized by muscle contraction. Presented at *The 1st International Conference on Biobehavioral Self-Regulation and Health.* Honolulu, Proceedings: No.36.

Saito,I.,Saito,Y.,Takaoka,K.(1990).EMG biofeedback training of painful respiratory muscles in patients with dyspnea. In: *Control of Breathing and Dyspnea* (T.Takishima & N.S Chernick, ed.), In press. Pergamon Press plc., Oxford.

Takaoka,K.,Saito,I.(1988). Effect of soft abdominal massage on vital capacity in subjects with dyspnea. *Japanese Journal of Biofeedback Research.* 16. 47.

Is a New Demand Valve Oxygen Regulator Useful for Patients with Home Oxygen Therapy?

Kazuo Machida*, Naohiro Nagayama*,
Yoshiko Kawabe*, Yoshihiro Otsuka*,
Toshihiko Haga* and Yoshiyuki Honda†

*Tokyo National Chest Hospital, 3-1-1 Takeoka, Kiyose,
Tokyo 204;
†Department of Physiology, School of Medicine, Chiba
University, 1-8-1 Gaibi, Chiba 280, Japan

ABSTRACT

A new demand valve oxygen regulator (TER-20) was tested for patients with
chronic respiratory failure during rest and exercise, and considered useful in
oxygenation, operability, perceived sensation and sparing effect of oxygen.

KEYWORDS

demand oxygen delivery; chronic respiratory failure; exercise; home oxygen
therapy

OBJECT

The long-lasting usage of portable oxygen supply is an urgent need for
patients with home oxygen therapy. Such instrument with demand valve oxygen
regulator, which permits oxygen flow only during inspiratory period, has been
reported useful (Cotes et al., 1956; MaDonnel et al., 1986; Bower et al.,
1988; Tiep et al., 1985, 1987). The purpose of this study is to clarify
whether a new demand valve oxygen regulator apparatus (TER-20) is useful for
patients with chronic respiratory failure (CRF).

APPARATUS AND ITS OPERATION

The portable oxygen system consists of oxygen cylinder with flow meter, demand
oxygen delivery system (TER-20) and nasal cannula. Fig. 1 shows overview and
schematic illustration of the system. TER-20 supplies oxygen during the
inspiratory period, by incorporating a microcomputer system which detects the
two preceding respiratory cycles and determines the timing and period oxygen
delivery. This apparatus, 400g in weight, can adjust the rate of oxgen flow
in variable degrees, and have the sensitivity to open the value for oxyten
inflow in two steps. It can also alter the pulsatile oxygen flow to the
continuous one.

Apparatus and its operation

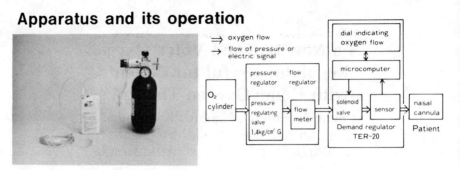

Fig. 1. Overview and schematic illustration of the portable oxygen system

SUBJECTS AND METHOD

The subjects were 14 patients with CRF(8 males and 6 females). The underlying diseases were 10 tuberculosis sequalae, 3 chronic bonchitis and 1 chronic pulmonary emphysema. Lung function in terms of %VC, FEV1, FEV1% were 37.0+ 12.8%, 581+125 ml and 63.0+20.0% respectively. Arterial blood during with room air breathing exhibited Pa_{O2} 59.0+6.2 torr, Pa_{CO2} 61.3+11.2 torr and pH 7.37+0.03.

Three experimental runs (room air breathing, breathing with pulse oxygen flow and that with continuous oxygen flow) were conducted by a crossover method, during both sitting (lasting for each 5 or 20 minutes) and walking on a treadmill with a slow speed (lasting for each 5 minutes). During the tests, Sa_{O2} (measured by Biox-3740 and Pulsox-7 pulse oximeter), pulse rate, signal of opening the valve, nasal pressure, breathing pattern (by Respigraph), the amounts of oxygen consumed (by weight) and arterial blood gas at rest were monitored.

Table 1. Comparison among room air breathing, breathing with pulse oxygen flow and continuous O_2 flow during rest and exercise (N=12)

			SaO₂ %	Pulse rate min	Respiratory frequency min	Sensitivity
Rest	O. 0.83±0. 55 l min	RA	92.9±1.9	87.9±10.0	21.9±6.9	
		C	96.3±1.3⁺	85.3±10.9*	21.8±5.8	
		P	96.4±1.6⁺	85.6± 9.5*	21.5±6.2	High 8 Low 4
Exercise	1.54±0. 35 km hr O. 2.08±1. 10 l min	RA	91.1±3.1	101.8±12.1	28.4±7.5	
		C	95.7±1.8**	97.3± 9.2**	26.4±6.1	
		P	95.7±2.1**	97 ± 9.2**	25.7±7.2	High 1 Low 11

*P<0.05. **P<0.01. † P<0.001   compared with room air breathing

Comparison of consumed O₂ between P and C

P/C ⟨ Rest   34.3±6.9(21~47) %
     Exercise 27.6±5.7(18~40) %

Table 2. Comparison among room air breathing, breathing with
pulse oxygen flow and continuous O_2 flow at rest

	Room air	Continous O_2 (C)	Pulse O_2 (P)
		Mean ± SD　(N=13)	
PaO_2 torr	63.4 ± 7.6	87.1 ± 9.7[†]	86.3 ± 8.1[†]
$PaCO_2$ torr	58.5 ± 7.7	61.0 ± 11.4[*]	59.6 ± 9.0
PH	7.37 ± 0.03	7.36 ± 0.03	7.37 ± 0.03
Pulse Rate min	87.2 ± 10.1	84.0 ± 11.0[*]	83.4 ± 10.4[**]
SaO_2%	90.8 ± 2.3	96.0 ± 1.7[**]	96.1 ± 1.9[**]
Respiratory frequency min	21.3 ± 5.7	21.9 ± 5.6	23.4 ± 6.8
O_2 flow l min		0.88 ± 0.56	0.88 ± 0.56

[*] $P < 0.05$, [**] $P < 0.01$, [†] $P < 0.001$,
compared with room air breathing
Comparison of consumed O_2 between P and C
$P/C = 31.3 \pm 5.1 (24.7 \sim 41.7)$ %

RESULTS

SaO_2 and PaO_2 during rest and exercise, were improved by oxygen breathing
compared to room air breathing, with no significant difference between two
types of oxygen flow breathing (Table 1 and Table 2). Comsumed oxygen volume
by pulse oxygen flow method was 31.3 or 34.3% (rest) and 27.6% (exercise) of
that by continuous one. The valve operated almost satisfactorily and nasal
discomfort by pulse oxygen flow was not noticed.

DISCUSSION

Demand oxyten delivery system (DODS) conserves oxygen by a bolus of
pressurized oxygen in early inspiration. DODS has been generally shown to
reduce consumed oxygen volume to 1/3 to 1/2 levels of that by steady oxygen
flow. Sensitive operation of the demand valve, attenuating click sound on
oxygen delivery so as to avoid annoying the patients with noise and taking a
safe measure for machine failure are required for successful use. TER-20,
satisfying these conditions, decreased consumed oxygen volume by pusatile one
to about 1/3 of that by continuous one.

REFERENCES

Cotes JE, Gilson JC (1956). Effect of oxygen on exercise ability in chronic
oxygen respiratory insufficiency-use of portable apparatus. Lancet, 1,
872-876.
Tiep BL, Nicotra MD, Carter R, Phillips R, Otsap B (1985). Low concentration
oxygen therapy via a demand oxygen delivery system.
Chest, 87, 636-638.
McDonnell TJ, Wanger JS, Senn S, Cherniack RM (1986). Efficacy of pulsed
oxygen delivery during exercise. Respiratory Care, 31, 883-888.
Bower JS, Brook CJ, Zimmer K, Davis D (1988) Performance of a demand oxygen
saver system during rest, exercise and sleep in hypoxemic patients. Chest,
94, 77-80.
Tiep BL, Carter R, Nicotra B, Berry J, Phillips RE, Otsap B (1987). Demand
oxygen delivery during exercise. Chest, 91, 15-20.

Subject Index

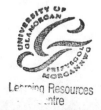